HUMAN IMMUNOLOGY

PATIENT-BASED RESEARCH

ANNALS OF THE NEW YORK ACADEMY OF SCIENCES
Volume 1062

HUMAN IMMUNOLOGY
PATIENT-BASED RESEARCH

Edited by Ralph M. Steinman

The New York Academy of Sciences
New York, New York
2005

♾ *The paper used in this publication meets the minimum requirements of the American National Standard for Information Sciences—Permanence of Paper for Printed Library Materials, ANSI Z39.48-1984.*

Library of Congress Cataloging-in-Publication Data

Human immunology : patient-based research / edited by Ralph M. Steinman.
p. ; cm. —(Annals of the New York Academy of Sciences ; v. 1062)
Includes bibliographical references and index.
ISBN 1-57331-606-7 (cloth : alk. paper) — ISBN 1-57331-607-5 (pbk. : alk. paper)
1. Immunology—Congresses. 2. Immune system—Pathophysiology—Congresses. 3. Infection—Immunological aspects—Congresses. 4. Allergy—Immunological aspects—Congresses. 5. Cancer—Immunological aspects—Congresses. I. Steinman, Ralph M. II. New York Academy of Sciences. III. Series.
[DNLM: 1. Immune System—physiopathology—Congresses. 2. Autoimmunity—physiology—Congresses. 3. Hypersensitivity—immunology—Congresses. 4. Infection—immunology—Congresses. 5. Neoplasms—immunology—Congresses. W1 AN626YL v.1062 2005 / QW 504 H918 2005]
Q11.N5 vol. 1062
[QR180.3]
500 s—dc22
[616.07'9]

2005033672

GYAT / PCP

ISBN 1-57331-606-7 (cloth)
ISBN 1-57331-607-5 (paper)
ISSN 0077-8923

ANNALS OF THE NEW YORK ACADEMY OF SCIENCES

Volume 1062
December 2005

HUMAN IMMUNOLOGY

PATIENT-BASED RESEARCH

Editors
RALPH M. STEINMAN

This volume is the result of a conference entitled **Human Immunology: Patient-Based Research** presented by the New York Academy of Sciences and The Dana Foundation, and held May 16–18, 2005, in New York, NY.

CONTENTS

Part II. Infection

Part III. Autoimmunity

Part IV. Allergy and Inflammation

Cosponsor

- THE DANA FOUNDATION

The New York Academy of Sciences believes it has a responsibility to provide an open forum for discussion of scientific questions. The positions taken by the participants in the reported conferences are their own and not necessarily those of the Academy. The Academy has no intent to influence legislation by providing such forums.

Foreword

RALPH M. STEINMAN

The Rockefeller University, New York, New York 10021, USA

Three years ago, the Dana Foundation began a program to support researchers who were asking fundamental immunological questions of patients. This new Dana program extended the interest of the Foundation in immunology, as manifest by support for research in neuroimmunology and immune imaging. To bring together the grantees who are studying immunology in patients, Dana partnered with the New York Academy of Sciences to hold a meeting at the Academy. Many of the contributions are represented in this volume.

The potential for immunology to understand and treat disease is real, but the underlying science is intricate and challenging, requiring research on patients as well as on simpler model systems. There are several illustrations of the potential of immune-based interventions. For example, the rejection of transplants can be blocked by immune suppressive drugs. The many symptoms of rheumatoid arthritis can be blocked by interfering with a product called tumor necrosis factor (TNF). The majority of newly approved drugs against cancer are actually immune antibodies that react with the cancers and then mobilize other immune cells against the tumor. Clearly, research on immune-based clinical conditions holds promise.

Scientists make their discoveries by studying problems and unknowns directly; this sets the stage for new therapies and vaccines. For example, the TNF that was just mentioned as a critical mediator in arthritis and other inflammatory diseases, was discovered independently by two groups of scientists working in New York on animal models for disease. Lloyd Old and his colleagues at the Sloan-Kettering Institute wanted to understand how components from bacteria could sometimes induce death or necrosis of tumors, while Tony Cerami and his group at the Rockefeller University wanted to understand why animals lost so much weight during infection and became emaciated or cachetic. TNF was pinpointed as the culprit in both instances. However, while Old and Cerami figured out the problems that they were addressing —tumor necrosis and cachexia—they did not study inflammatory diseases or patients. Instead, it was Marc Feldmann and Ravinder Maino in London, who turned to patients and figured out that TNF was the culprit in other disease settings, initially arthritis, but now inflammatory bowel disease, psoriasis, and more. The scientific enterprise, and the public that supports it, would do well to grow its efforts in patient-based research.

This volume illustrates ongoing progress from immunology research in patients that is being supported by the Dana Foundation. The findings in most cases could not have been anticipated from research on simpler experimental systems such as mice. For example, were you aware of the following?

Ann. N.Y. Acad. Sci. 1062: ix–xi (2005).
doi: 10.1196/annals.1358.001

(1) The most common form of leukemia in adults, chronic lymphocytic leukemia, is actually two diseases that differ in the types of antigen receptors as well as prognosis.
(2) Cancers like multiple myeloma and breast cancer have premalignant stages that are recognized by the immune system, and a patient's immune response—not just the tumor itself—changes when premaligancy develops into frank cancer.
(3) According to new gene-array criteria, the immune system of patients with advanced melanoma appears to be suppressed, as if the patient was a transplant recipient receiving immunosuppressive drugs.
(4) In autoimmune diseases like rheumatoid arthritis and systemic lupus erythematosus, the "bad" autoantibody–producing immune cells actually are made in higher numbers early on during their development.
(5) In addition to autoantibodies, the autoimmune disease lupus is characterized by a marked increase in interferon production, which very likely aggravates the disease. A source of this interferon is now evident; complexes of autoantibodies with self-antigens are recognized by a combination of receptors on dendritic cells, which then pour out the interferon.
(6) Self-constituents that are attacked in autoimmune diseases share a chemical identity, being subject to digestion by a specific enzyme found in immune cells.

Enormous progress continues to be made in immunology from simpler systems, particularly studies of mice. Each year sees major breakthroughs and hundreds of less earth-shattering but significant, hard-earned, and clever advances. Yet research on patients is also essential. The causes of diseases in humans, for example, the cancers and the infections, are different from those that cause disease in mice. The standards of human research are different, not simply because of the demands of testing something new in humans, but because the criteria are more long term and the test systems more intricate. Human research requires not only that one *dissect* what is going on, as is typically the goal of research in mice, but also that onr takes this information and *directs* the immune system to benefit the patient. Again, scientists need to study unknowns directly to figure them out. Research on patients with an immune component to their disease, and research evaluating new interventions and therapy, are really another kind of scientific research, the careful systematic study of a problem that leads to discovery.

Yet there is an imbalance in our research enterprise in that research on patients is so underrepresented relative to research on simpler systems. The latter are essential, but our culture needs to *grow* or *add* a new capacity to study patients. The science and the safeguards are in place, but they require "patient" support. This is what the Dana Foundation is aiming to do. Have a look at <www.dana.org>, where you will see: the new programs in human immunology; the joint fellowships with the Irvington Institute to support postdoctoral training in patient-based immunology research; an annual award through the American Association of Immunologists to recognize outstanding researchers in this field given for the first time this year to Dr. Fred Rosen at the Center for Blood Research in Boston; a newspaper called *Immunology in the News* (subscriptions are free); and new books, including the illuminating volume called *Fatal Sequence* by Dr. Kevin Tracey, one of the pioneers in the aforementioned TNF research.

As in its other programs in neuroscience and arts in education, the trustees and employees of the Dana Foundation seek to stimulate and inform. The meeting represented here is an example, one that required a delightful partnership with another organization devoted to the advancement of science worldwide, the New York Academy of Sciences. On behalf of the participants, I wish to thank several people. From the Dana Foundation, I thank Andrea Nadosy, Rebecca Husmann, Abby Slovonic and Carolyn Asbury, and from the New York Academy of Sciences, I am grateful to Reneé Wilkerson Brown, Rashid Shaikh, and Ellis Rubinstein. We are also grateful to the editorial department of the *Annals,* and particularly Trumbull Rogers, for seeing these proceedings through the press. We all recognize the support and spirit of the leadership of the Dana Foundation and the New York Academy of Sciences.

B-Cell Chronic Lymphocytic Leukemia, a Clonal Disease of B Lymphocytes with Receptors that Vary in Specificity for (Auto)antigens

NICHOLAS CHIORAZZI,[a,b,c] KATERINA HATZI,[a] AND EMILIA ALBESIANO[a]

[a]*Feinstein Institute for Medical Research, North Shore—LIJ Health System, 350 Community Drive, Manhasset, New York 11030, USA*

[b]*Department of Medicine, North Shore University Hospital, 300 Community Drive, Manhasset, New York 11030, USA*

[c]*Departments of Medicine and of Cell Biology, Albert Einstein School of Medicine, Bronx, New York, USA*

ABSTRACT: B-Cell chronic lymphocytic leukemia (B-CLL) is an incurable disease that is relatively common among aging Caucasians. Patients with this leukemia can be divided into prognostic categories using clinical staging parameters, as well as molecular features [presence or absence of IgV_H mutations in rearranged V_HDJ_H segments that code for the leukemic B cell's receptor for antigen (BCR)]. In addition, the deduced amino acid structure of the BCRs from patients that fall into different prognostic categories is shared, to varying degrees, within these groups. In this paper, the molecular features of the genes that code for the BCRs of B-CLL patients are reviewed, and these are comapred to antibodies of known specificity. These comparisons suggest that the BCRs of many cases resemble autoantibodies, and in some cases, antibodies to microbial antigens. Antigen-binding analyses confirm these impressions, and also indicate that polyreactivity appears to distinguish cases with worse clinical outcomes differ from those with better outcomes. The persistence of autoreactivity and polyreactivity is somewhat surprising, because *IgV* DNA sequence analyses suggest that many of the B cells that become leukemic have undergone one form or another of receptor editing. Thus, B-CLL appears to be a disease of B-cell clones that have undergone various types of receptor reconfiguration and yet retain inappropriate antigen-binding properties.

KEYWORDS: B-cell; lymphocytic leukemia; B lymphocytes; autoanigens

Address for correspondence: Nicholas Chiorazzi, M.D., Feinstein Institute for Medical Research, North Shore—LIJ Health System, 350 Community Drive, Manhasset, NY 11030. Voice: 516-562-1085; fax: 516-552-1022.
nchizzi@nshs.edu

Ann. N.Y. Acad. Sci. 1062: 1–12 (2005). © 2005 New York Academy of Sciences.
doi: 10.1196/annals.1358.002

INTRODUCTION

B-Cell chronic lymphocytic leukemia (B-CLL) is the most prevalent leukemia affecting the aging Caucasian population.[1] The disease starts later in life; its incidence is rare before the fourth decade, but increases with each decade thereafter.[2] As the post–World War II "baby boomer" population ages, the disease will likely become even more common.

Patients suffering from B-CLL often follow divergent clinical courses, with some patients living decades after diagnosis and dying with the disease, not from it, whereas others decline and die relatively rapidly, despite chemotherapy. The median survival of patients with the indolent form of the disease is >25 years, and with the more aggressive form of the disease is <8 years.

At this point, B-CLL remains an incurable disease and none of the currently employed therapies prolong life span.[3] Many patients develop an associated immune deficiency as the leukemia progresses and ~15% of all patients experience an episode of autoimmune hemolytic anemia or thrombocytopenia during the course of the illness,[1] although the precise mechanisms responsible for these complications are not defined.

The disease presents a dilemma for both patients and physicians. Because of the dichotomy in clinical outcome and the ineffectiveness of available treatment modalities, it is difficult to justify an aggressive treatment regimen early in the disease. Furthermore, treating patients early in the disease has not led to an extension of life span. Therefore, most patients diagnosed in the initial phases of the disease are not treated, but rather are followed closely until evidence for disease progression arises.

In an attempt to deal with this dilemma, Rai *et al.*,[4] and subsequently Binet *et al.*,[5] devised clinical staging systems that are invaluable guides to clinicians for determining the phase of a patient's illness and the need for therapy. These staging systems were aided recently by the recognition that the clinical course that a patient might follow (indolent vs. aggressive) could be predicted[6, 7] based on the presence or absence of somatic mutations in the genes coding for the variable (V) region of the immunoglobulin molecule (Ig) produced by the leukemic B lymphocyte.[8] The precise reasons for this association remain unclear, but current opinions are that the association relates to the ability of the leukemic B cell to bind specific antigens, before and after leukemic transformation,[9] since surface membrane Ig serves as the B-cell antigen receptor (BCR). Studies are currently underway to determine if this *IgV* marker is of sufficient reliability to warrant its use in the initial phases of the disease as an indicator for early and aggressive treatment.

The observation that patients with B-CLL can be divided into subgroups based on the presence or absence of somatic mutation,[8] and that this categorization has prognostic relevance,[6,7] has proved to be an important jumping off point for the study of the disease. It has spurred clinical investigators to look for other markers to define these subgroups, and several have been identified.[6,10–16] It has also engendered considerable interest on the part of basic and clinical investigators into understanding how somatic mutations in IgV genes affect the biology of the B lymphocytes that become malignant.[17,18]

In this chapter we address the possibility that the ability of the B-CLL cell's BCR to bind antigen is an integral determinant of the cell biology of the leukemic cell and its influence on clinical outcome. In particular, we will develop the hypothesis that

B cells with a polyreactive, autoantigen-binding BCR are at the highest risk for evolving into a B-CLL cell associated with poor outcome, V_H unmutated type, thereby implying that B-CLL is a disease of autoreactive B cells and that disease severity is determined by the extent to which these B cells have "successfully" or "unsuccessfully" eliminated polyreactivity by changing the structure of their BCRs.

ANTIGEN DRIVE AND SELECTION IN THE DEVELOPMENT OF B-CLL

In order to address the question whether B-CLL cells derive in a random fashion or are selected from a pool of B cells having specific antigen-binding characteristics, several laboratories analyzed the rearranged V_HDJ_H/V_LJ_L segments that encode the receptor's antigen-binding site (reviewed in Refs. 17 and 18). Finding evidence for restricted use of specific IgV segments, and especially the association of specific V, (D), and J, in the leukemic B cells of unrelated patients would indicate that the disease evolved in a nonstochastic fashion, and that this evolution was either caused by specific antigen selection of BCRs of restricted structure or that the evolution from a normal B cell to a B-CLL cell could have occurred within a B-cell subset that was preselected for BCRs of a restricted structure (or both). Indeed, studies of rearranged IgV segments in B-CLL suggest those B cells destined to become B-CLL cells are selected nonrandomly for discrete BCR structural characteristics that can be slightly, moderately, or remarkably discriminating, based on the deduced primary structure of the BCR. Whether this selection process acts on any B cell or B cells from specific anatomic compartments is still an open question.

In brief, these analyses revealed evidence for biased use, compared with the normal B-cell repertoire, of certain V_H (but not V_L) genes; the selective association of specific V_H, D, and J_H segments to yield characteristic and relatively unique IgV_H rearrangements with HCDR3s that differ in length, charge, and composition; the selective pairing of certain V_HDJ_H with specific V_LJ_L segments; and the conservation of FR structure and/or the alteration of CDR structure by limiting replacement mutations to CDRs.[17,18]

WHAT TYPES OF ANTIBODIES DO THE BCRS OF B-CLL CELLS RESEMBLE?

Antibodies that react specifically with autoantigens as well as "polyspecific" antibodies that react with multiple antigens, including autoantigens, can exhibit distinct features. These features are listed here:

- Biased use of individual V_H and/or V_L genese;
- Preferential association of V_H, D, J_H or V_L, J_L segments;
- Relatively unique H and L CDR3s as regards to length, charge, and composition;
- Selective pairing of individual V_H and V_L genes;
- Accumulation of more replacement mutations than predicted by statistical alogorithms in the CDR and/or accumulation of less replacement mutations than predicted in the FR.

Many of these characteristics are found in the H- and L-chain V gene rearrangements found in B-CLL patients, and interestingly, they may differ among those patients who have a worse or better clinical course.

IgV$_H$ and V$_L$ Use

Among the patients who experience a dismal outcome and have the unmutated V_H genotype, the genes that are clearly overexpressed in relation to the normal B-cell repertoire are *V_H1-69* and *V_H4-34*.[8] Both of these genes are commonly expressed in monoclonal gammopathies with known autoreactivity and in autoimmune conditions. For example, *V_H1-69* is found often among patients with mixed cryoglobulinemia and Waldenstrom's macroglobulinemia, clonal diseases of B cells reactive with human IgG (rheumatoid factors).[19–21] This finding was first made with the use of anti-idiotypic antibodies, and one of these antibodies was used to demonstrate expression of this V_H gene on the surface of B-CLL cells.[19] In addition, *V_H4-34* is expressed in every case of cold agglutinin disease, another monoclonal abnormality involving B cells that bind the i/I antigen on human red blood cells.[22–24] Anti-DNA antibodies from patients with systemic lupus erythematosus also can utilize *V_H 4-34*.[25] This gene may be so inherently autoreactive that it is prevented from maturing to Ig-secreting plasma cells.[26]

Other genes commonly used by B-CLL cells, that may or may not be more utilized than by normal B cells, are *V_H3-07*, *V_H3-23*, and *V_H3-21*.[8,27,28] These genes are not known to associate with monoclonal autoreactive neoplasms or with systemic autoimmunity. As expected, these genes are most often identified among B-CLL patients with the mutated genotype and the better clinical course. *V_H3-21*, however, is especially interesting because it can also be associated with aggressive disease, even when it is expressed in a mutated form.[27,28]

Unlike the H-chain V gene repertoire, V_L use in B-CLL is not different from that of normal human B lymphocytes.[29] However, among those gene segments found often rearranged in B-CLL cells are some of those used by autoreactive B lymphocytes. For example, *IGKV3-20* is often found associated with *V_H1-69* in rheumatoid factor-producing monoclonal B cells in the gammopathies mentioned earlier.[30]

Association of Specific V, (D), and J

In transgenic mice, autoreactive B cells frequently home to the marginal zones of the spleen,[31] an area highly enriched in B lymphocytes that respond to T-cell–independent antigens and provide a first line of defense against blood-borne microbial antigens.[32] One might, therefore, postulate a relationship between antibodies to TI-2 microbial determinants and autoantibodies, and indeed autoantibodies can protect against bacterial infection,[33] and antibodies to bacteria can convert to autoantibodies after minimal structural alteration.[34,35]

As mentioned earlier, the mAb/BCRs of B-CLL cells can be composed of H- and L-chain rearrangements that are restricted to specific V_H, D, J_H, and/or V_L, J_L gene segments, as are antibodies to carbohydrate and other nonprotein epitopes.[36–39]

Unique H and L CDR3s

B-CLL cells of unmutated, poor-outcome patients differ considerably from those of mutated, better-outcome patients not only in the respective absence or presence

```
CLL122

VH3-07               D1-14                        D3-3              N2          JH4b
----------         ---a---->         -------------------------->          ---------------
tgtgcgagag     ttagggacccacgctggg  ttacgattttggagtggttatta         ct   tactttgactactgg

CLL263

VH1-69      P          D1-14                        D2-2               N2          JH5b
-----------          -------a->          ------------------------->           ---------------
tgtgcgagaga t   tctctcggaaccgctagc    attgtagtagtaccagctgctatg    ggt    tggttcgacccctgg

CLL394

VH1-69                   N1                         D3-16                            D1-20           P          JH4b
--------                                ------------------------------t-->       -a--------a->        -----------------
tgtgcgag            tacccaacgggtccc  tattatgattacgtttggggggagttatcgtgat   gggtaatctaactggaccga agt actactttgactactgg

CLL156

VH1-45         N1                   D2-2                D5-18                              JH5b
------                       --------------------->    <-------                       ------------t-----
tgtgca       ttggccgaa       agtagtaccagctgcataaac agtgtctgtatcaccccagaaacaggt   agctggttcgacccctgg
```

FIGURE 1. Four examples of likely D segment to D segment fusions in B-CLL cells.

of V gene mutations but also in CDR3 characteristics. For example, unmutated B-CLL cases have HCDR3 lengths significantly longer than those of mutated B-CLL cases as well as normal human B cells.[8,40,41] These longer HCDR3s result from the use of certain D and J_H segments (e.g., J_H6), and also from the occurrence of D segment to D segment fusions (D–D) that can occur in the course of IgV recombination (FIG. 1). In our experience, HCDR3 DNA sequences consistent with D–D fusions are found in 6% of B-CLL cases. Although D–D fusions are rare in the adult human B-cell repertoire,[42] they are common in certain inbred strains of mice that spontaneously develop systemic lupus erythematosus-like disease.[43] Whatever the reason, long HCDR3 segments are frequently found among polyreactive autoantibodies in both man and mouse.

Furthermore, HCDR3s of unmutated B-CLL cells can be formed from discrete V_H, D, and J_H segments (e.g., $V_H1\text{-}69 + D3\text{-}3 + J_H6$,[40,41] and $V_H4\text{-}39 + D6\text{-}13 + J_H5$[44]) differing from those in mutated B-CLL cases (e.g., $V_H3\text{-}07 + J_H6$,[8] and $V_H3\text{-}21 + J_H6$[27,28]). Similar associations can be found in LCDR3s (e.g., *IGKV1-39* + $J\kappa2$ and *IGLV3-21* + $J\lambda3$).[29] These associations frequently yield H and L CDR3s of similar amino acid composition with unique, often charged residues at the V_H/D, D/J_H, and V_L/J_L junctions, features that are also common among autoantibodie,[45,46] and antibodies to carbohydrates and other nonprotein determinants.[36,47–49]

Selective Pairing of V_H and V_L Genes and V_HDJ_H and V_LJ_L Rearrangements

Some B-CLL cases exhibit remarkably similar BCRs comprising identical V_H, D, and J_H, and V_L and J_L segments.[50–52] These cases also show considerable similarity in H and L CDR3 structure, despite the inconsistencies inherent in V, (D), J rearrangement. For example, among unmutated cases, the $V_H4\text{-}39/D6\text{-}13/J_H5$ rearrangement can pair with the $V\kappa1\text{-}39/J\kappa1$ rearrangement leading to highly similar HCDR3 (xxGYSSSWYG/Sx(x)NWFDP) and LCDR3 (an invariant arginine at the V_L–J_L

junction) motifs.[44] It is also striking that all of these patients express a BCR of the IgG isotype, which is unusual for B-CLL cases (<8%). Similar stereotypic rearrangements involving other IgV segments can be found among other members of the unmutated group.[50–52] This phenomenon, however, is not restricted to unmutated cases, since similar associations can be found in mutated B-CLL,for example, *V_H3-21/?/J_H6* paired with *Vλ2-14*,[51] and *V_H4-34/D5-5/J_H6* paired with *Vκ2-30/Jκ1/2*.[50]

The necessity of selective pairing of V gene segments in autoantibodies has been elegantly demonstrated in animals that are transgenic for autoreactive BCRs.[53,54] The finding that autoreactive rearrangements underwent *in vivo* change in V_H/V_L pairing has led to the recognition of an essential salvage mechanism operating in autoreactive B cells, namely, receptor editing.[53,54]

Type and Location of Ig V_H Gene Mutations

BCRs of mutated B-CLL cases exhibit evidence for antigen selection and drive, as defined by the accumulation of less replacement mutations than predicted in the FR and more replacement mutations than predicted in CDR.[55,56] These findings are similar to those described for antibodies to defined exogenous antigens as well as to autoantigens.[57] It is important to remember that although IgV somatic mutations can refine antigen-binding specificity, such changes can also lead to autoreactivity and polyreactivity. Presumably BCR specificity is triaged against high-affinity autoreactivity, but may not eliminate lower threshold autoreactivity or polyreactivity.

ANTIGEN REACTIVITY OF THE BCR/MAB OF B-CLL CELLS

Thus the DNA and deduced amino acid sequence data are suggestive that at least some of the cases, primarily unmutated B-CLL, are autoreactive and/or polyreactive. In fact, this is consistent with early studies of B-CLL mAb collected from either *in vitro* differentiation experiments[58,59] or somatic cell hybridization experiments.[60] These studies showed a large fraction of B-CLL-derived mAb were reactive with classic autoantigens (e.g., DNA, IgG, thyroglobulin, actin, myosin) in solid-phase immunoassays and in immunofluorescent analyses of fixed and permeabilized human cells. Another characteristic of B-CLL mAb was polyreactivity, which occurred in many of the samples. In these studies, however, polyreactivity and autoreactivity were not correlated with IgV mutation status.

Recently, Herve *et al.*[61] expressed B-CLL mAb as recombinant IgG1 molecules and demonstrated that the majority reacted with a similar battery of autoantigens and with foreign antigens (e.g., LPS), and that this reactivity was often multispecific. Furthermore, they correlated the capacity to bind specific autoantigens and multiple antigens with the level of somatic mutation detected in the rearranged V_HDJ_H segments of the various cases. These data were striking and significant in that the majority of unmutated mAb were polyreactive/multispecific, whereas a minority of the mutated mAb possessed this feature. The discrimination was made between cases with selective autoreactivity and multispecific autoreactivity, which correlated with the presence or absence of IgV somatic mutations. This conclusion was corroborated when some of the mAb were converted back to the germline sequence and polyreactivity returned in several instances.[61]

HAVE PRECURSORS OF B-CLL CELLS UNDERGONE RECEPTOR EDITING DURING DEVELOPMENT?

The specificity of BCRs in developing B cells is closely monitored. In particular, B cells with BCRs of high and moderate affinities for autoantigen are usually either deleted or forced to undergo secondary rearrangements at the L-chain and H-chain loci. B cells with BCRs that are reconfigured to an acceptable structure are then permitted to progress further down the differentiation pathway. These processes occur primarily centrally in the bone marrow, but may take place in the periphery on occasion.

However, it is possible for such secondary rearrangements to permit allelic inclusion, allowing the original rearrangement to remain functional with a diminished frequency of pairing with the existing V_HDJ_H segment, or in conjunction with deletion events involving V genes up- and downstream of the existing V segment, so that the original rearrangement is excluded. Secondary rearrangements involving the H chain (V_H replacement) retain the structure of the existing D/J_H and swap the originally rearranged V_H for another upstream V_H gene.[62,63] In contrast, refinements involving the L-chain locus occur in several ways. For example, a completely new V_L/J_L rearrangement can be made on the same allele using a V_L segment upstream of the existing V_L and a J_L segment downstream of the existing V_L.[53,54]

Since most B-CLL cells appear to be monoclonal expansions of autoreactive and or polyreactive B cells, it is likely that the precursors of the leukemic clone have undergone one or several secondary attempts at receptor reconfiguration. However, given their retained "inappropriate" reactivity, these cells may have "failed" the process, and continued to survive by other means. Although the available DNA sequences do not support a single mechanism for receptor reconfiguration among B-CLL cells, many leukemic clones exhibit at least one feature reminiscent of these processes.

Although it is difficult to confidently assign receptor editing in an individual clone without prior knowledge of the structure of its B-cell receptor, nevertheless certain features of normal (and B-CLL) cells suggest that editing may have occurred. For example, cells expressing 5′ V_L genes with 3′ J_L genes are more likely to have undergone this process than cells expressing 3′ V_L genes with 5′ J_L. Therefore, we examined the 111 B-CLL cases in our series that express a κ chain (n = 155)[29] and focused on those VκJκ rearrangements involving a 3′ Jκ segments (defined as Jκ 3, 4, or 5) and determined how many were associated with 5′ Vκ (defined as genes 5′ of IGKV1-17). Of the 111 VκJκ rearrangements, 33 use 3′ Jκ segments and 24 (~73%) were linked with 5′ Vκ genes. Furthermore, within those 24 cases expressing 5′ Vκ/3′ Jκ rearrangements, 19 (~80%) were unmutated. Analogous data leading to similar conclusions were reported recently by Stamatopoulos *et al.*[64]

With regard to V_L mutations, 73.9% of the Vκ genes 5′ of *IGVK1-17* (regardless of the associated Jκ) were unmutated, whereas 46.5% of the Vκ genes located 3′ (within the interval from *IGKV4-1* to *KV1-17*) were mutated. In contrast, unmutated and mutated Vλ genes were distributed uniformly along the λ locus.[29]

V_H replacement is analogous to V_L editing, with the exception that the original D/J_H rearrangement can remain intact. This replacement event requires the presence of cryptic heptamer-like sequences embedded in the coding regions of V_H genes. V_H replacement was originally identified in B-cell lines[62,65–67] and transgenic mice expressing autoreactive BCRs,[68–70] and has recently been extensively studied *in vitro* using a human pro–B-cell line that spontaneously matures and undergoes this process.[71] These latter studies emphasized "footprints" in the new V_HDJ_H representing residual sequences from the replaced V_H. Since these extra nucleotides are 3′ of the new V_H gene, they yield longer HCDR3s, often with charged amino acids.[71] This phenomenon is especially intriguing in B-CLL, since long HCDR3s containing charged residues are frequently seen and an example of V_H replacement in B-CLL has been reported.[72] Our preliminary analyses suggest that at least 5% of B-CLL V_HDJ_H rearrangements contain footprints consistent with V_H replacement.

Finally, as mentioned previously, allelic inclusion can be interpreted to be another form of receptor editing. B-CLL cells can exhibit allelic inclusion at the V_H locus.[73] In our cases, we have detected the expression of two V_HDJ_H rearrangements in 5% of cases by reverse transcription polymerase chain reaction. We have also found evidence for allelic inclusion at the L-chain locus in ~7% of our cases. To ascertain that allelic inclusion is, in fact, occurring at the single-cell level requires confirmation, such as from single-cell DNA sequencing.

CONCLUSIONS AND QUANDARIES

The data reviewed here collectively suggest that B-CLL is a disease of antigen-selected B lymphocytes, in which the antigen selection has culled out B cells with varying degrees of autospecificity, ranging from narrow to broad and multispecific. Examples of various types of receptor editing can be found in B-CLL, and it is not evident that these processes are more frequent than in the normal B-cell repertoire, where at least 33% of B cells have reconfigured their BCRs.[74,75] Nevertheless, another "type" of receptor reconfiguration, somatic mutation of Ig V genes, has altered the breadth of autoreactivity by diminishing or eliminating polyreactivity, and this type of receptor change may relate to the clinical course and outcome for patients with this disease.

Several inconsistencies and questions remain, however. For example, what degree of cross-reactivity do B-CLL mAb/BCRs have with foreign molecules, such as microbes? Could there be a dynamic, intermittent interplay between autoreactivity and exoreactivity that nurtures the B-CLL population and permits it to survive, expand, and eventually transform to a leukemic cell? Similarly, if leukemic precursors have undergone typical attempts at receptor reconfiguration, why have they remained auto and polyreactive? Have these processes traded one autoreactive receptor for another, albeit possibly more tolerable to the immune system and thereby failed to abrogate the survival or growth advantage that antigen-binding might provide to the leukemic cell? Examples of such "maladaptive" editing for both the H- and L-chain loci have been found in mice expressing autoreactive receptors,[76,77] and in human *in vitro* rearrangements.[71]

These types of questions will be more difficult to address and answer in humans where the original genetic structure of the antigen-binding site is not known and where genetic manipulation is not possible. Nevertheless, as more information becomes available about the structures of normal, autoreactive, and leukemic BCRs, the answers to these questions will emerge. In addition, identifying the cause of those "experiments of nature" that have been so revealing for inherited human immunodeficiency diseases may also provide clues and insights into these dilemmas.

ACKNOWLEDGMENTS

These studies were supported in part by RO1 grants CA 81554 and CA 87956 from the National Cancer Institute and a M01 General Clinical Research Center Grant (RR018535) from the National Center for Research Resources. The Peter J. Sharp Foundation, The Marks Family Foundation, the Jean Walton Fund for Lymphoma & Myeloma Research, and the Joseph Eletto Leukemia Research Fund also provided support for these studies.

We thank the present and past members of the Laboratory of Experimental Immunology, Feinstein Institute for Medical Research, North Shore—LIJ Health System, and Dr. Manlio Ferrarini and his colleagues in the Division of Medical Oncology C, Istituto Nazionale per la Ricerca sul Cancro, Genoa, Italy, for the work that we have discussed in this manuscript.

[*Competing interests*: The authors declare that they have no competing financial interests.]

REFERENCES

1. Cheson, B.D. 2001. The chronic lymphocytic leukemias. *In* Cancer: Principles and Practice of Oncology. V.T. Devita, Jr., S. Hellman & S.A. Rosenberg, Ed.: 2447–2465. Lippincott Williams & Wilkins. Philadelphia.
2. Rai, K.R. 1997. Chronic lymphocytic leukemia in the elderly population. Clin. Geriatr. Med. **13:** 245–249.
3. Rai, K.R. *et al.* 2000. Fludarabine compared with chlorambucil as primary therapy for chronic lymphocytic leukemia. N. Engl. J. Med. **343:** 1750–1757.
4. Rai, K.R. *et al.* 1975. Clinical staging of chronic lymphocytic leukemia. Blood **46:** 219–234.
5. Binet, J.L. *et al.* 1981. A new prognostic classification of chronic lymphocytic leukemia derived from a multivariate survival analysis. Cancer **48:** 198–206.
6. Damle, R.N. *et al.* 1999. Ig V gene mutation status and CD38 expression as novel prognostic indicators in chronic lymphocytic leukemia. Blood **94:** 1840–1847.
7. Hamblin, T.J. *et al.* 1999. Unmutated Ig VH genes are associated with a more aggressive form of chronic lymphocytic leukemia. Blood **94:** 1848–1854.
8. Fais, F. *et al.* 1998. Chronic lymphocytic leukemia B cells express restricted sets of mutated and unmutated antigen receptors. J. Clin. Invest. **102:** 1515–1525.
9. Chiorazzi, N., K.R. Rai & M. Ferrarini. 2005. Chronic lymphocytic leukemia. N. Engl. J. Med. **352:** 804–815.
10. Hamblin, T.J. *et al.* 2002. CD38 expression and immunoglobulin variable region mutations are independent prognostic variables in chronic lymphocytic leukemia, but CD38 expression may vary during the course of the disease. Blood **99:** 1023–1029.
11. Jelinek, D.F. *et al.* 2001. Analysis of clonal B-cell CD38 and immunoglobulin variable region sequence status in relation to clinical outcome for B-chronic lymphocytic leukaemia. Br. J. Haematol. **115:** 854–861.
12. Krober, A. *et al.* 2002. V(H) mutation status, CD38 expression level, genomic aberrations, and survival in chronic lymphocytic leukemia. Blood **100:** 1410–1416.
13. Rosenwald, A. *et al.* 2001. Relation of gene expression phenotype to immunoglobulin mutation genotype in B cell chronic lymphocytic leukemia. J. Exp. Med. **194:** 1639–1647.

14. WIESTNER, A. *et al.* 2003. ZAP-70 expression identifies a chronic lymphocytic leukemia subtype with unmutated immunoglobulin genes, inferior clinical outcome, and distinct gene expression profile. Blood **101:** 4944–4951.
15. CRESPO, M. *et al.* 2003. ZAP-70 expression as a surrogate for immunoglobulin-variable-region mutations in chronic lymphocytic leukemia. N. Engl. J. Med. **348:** 1764–1775.
16. RASSENTI, L.Z. *et al.* 2004. ZAP-70 compared with immunoglobulin heavy-chain gene-mutation status as a predictor of disease progression in chronic lymphocytic leukemia. N. Engl. J. Med. **351:** 893–901.
17. CHIORAZZI, N. & M. FERRARINI. 2003. B cell chronic lymphocytic leukemia: lessons learned from studies of the B cell antigen receptor. Annu. Rev. Immunol. **21:** 841–894.
18. STEVENSON, F. & F. CALIGARIS-CAPPIO. 2004. Chronic lymphocytic leukemia: revelations from the B-cell receptor. Blood. **103:** 4389-95.
19. KIPPS, T. J., *et al.* 1989. Developmentally restricted immunoglobulin heavy chain variable region gene expressed at high frequency in chronic lymphocytic leukemia. Proc Natl Acad Sci U S A. **86:** 5913-7.
20. SILVERMAN, G.J. & D.A. CARSON. 1990. Structural characterization of human monoclonal cold agglutinins: evidence for a distinct primary sequence-defined VH4 idiotype. Eur. J. Immunol. **20:** 351–356.
21. SILVERMAN, G.J. *et al.* 1988. Idiotypic and subgroup analysis of human monoclonal rheumatoid factors. Implications for structural and genetic basis of autoantibodies in humans. J. Clin. Invest. **82**: 469–475.
22. SILBERSTEIN, L.E. *et al.* 1991. Variable region gene analysis of pathologic human autoantibodies to the related i and I red blood cell antigens. Blood **78:** 2372–2386
23. THOMPSON, K.M. *et al.* 1991. Human monoclonal antibodies against blood group antigens preferentially express a VH4-21 variable region gene-associated epitope. Scand. J. Immunol. **34:** 509–518.
24. PASCUAL, V. *et al.* 1992. VH restriction among human cold agglutinins. The VH4-21 gene segment is required to encode anti-I and anti-i specificities. J. Immunol. **149:** 2337–2344.
25. STEVENSON, F.K. *et al.* 1993. Utilization of the VH4-21 gene segment by anti-DNA antibodies from patients with systemic lupus erythematosus. J. Autoimmun. **6:** 809–825.
26. PUGH-BERNARD, A. *et al.* 2001. Regulation of inherently autoreactive VH4-34 B cells in the maintenance of human B cell tolerance. J. Clin. Invest. **108:** 1061–1070.
27. TOBIN, G. *et al.* 2002. Somatically mutated Ig V(H)3-21 genes characterize a new subset of chronic lymphocytic leukemia. Blood **99:** 2262–2264.
28. TOBIN, G. *et al.* 2003. Chronic lymphocytic leukemias utilizing the VH3-21 gene display highly restricted V{lambda}2-14 gene use and homologous CDR3s: implicating recognition of a common antigen epitope. Blood **101:** 4952–4957.
29. GHIOTTO, F. *et al.* 2006. Immunoglobulin light chain variable region gene sequence analyses of B-CLL cells reveal similarities and differences to the heavy chain variable region gene repertoire. Mol. Med. In press.
30. KIPPS, T.J. *et al.* 1988. Autoantibody-associated kappa light chain variable region gene expressed in chronic lymphocytic leukemia with little or no somatic mutation. Implications for etiology and immunotherapy. J. Exp. Med. **167:** 840–852.
31. LI, Y., H. LI & M. WEIGERT. 2002. Autoreactive B cells in the marginal zone that express dual receptors. J, Exp, Med. **195:** 181–188.
32. MARTIN, F. & J. KEARNEY. 2002. Marginal-zone B cells. Nat. Rev. Immunol. **2:** 323–335.
33. BRILES, D. E. *et al.* 1981. Antiphosphocholine antibodies found in normal mouse serum are protective against intravenous infection with type 3 streptococcus pneumoniae. J. Exp. Med. **153:** 694–705.
34. RUDIKOFF, S. *et al.* 1982. Single amino acid substitution altering antigen-binding specificity. Proc. Natl. Acad. Sci. USA **79:** 1979–1983.
35. DIAMOND, B. & M. D. SCHARFF. 1984. Somatic mutation of the T15 heavy chain gives rise to an antibody with autoantibody specificity. Proc. Natl. Acad. Sci. USA **81:** 5841–5844.
36. INSEL, R.A., E.E. ADDERSON & W.L. CARROLL. 1992. The repertoire of human antibody to the Haemophilus influenzae type b capsular polysaccharide. Int. Rev. Immunol. **9:** 25–43.

37. ADDERSON, E.E. *et al.* 1992. Immunoglobulin light chain variable region gene sequences for human antibodies to Haemophilus influenzae type b capsular polysaccharide are dominated by a limited number of V kappa and V lambda segments and VJ combinations. J. Clin. Invest. **89:** 729–738.
38. ADDERSON, E.E. *et al.* 1991. Restricted Ig H chain V gene usage in the human antibody response to Haemophilus influenzae type b capsular polysaccharide. J. Immunol. **147:** 1667–1674.
39. ADDERSON, E.E. *et al.* 1993. Restricted immunoglobulin VH usage and VDJ combinations in the human response to Haemophilus influenzae type b capsular polysaccharide. Nucleotide sequences of monospecific anti-Haemophilus antibodies and polyspecific antibodies cross-reacting with self antigens. J. Clin. Invest. **91:** 2734–2743.
40. JOHNSON, T.A., L.Z. RASSENTI & T.J. KIPPS. 1997. Ig VH1 genes expressed in B cell chronic lymphocytic leukemia exhibit distinctive molecular features. J. Immunol. **158:** 235–246.
41. WIDHOPF, G.F., II & T.J. KIPPS. 2001. Normal B cells express 51p1-encoded Ig heavy chains that are distinct from those expressed by chronic lymphocytic leukemia B cells. J. Immunol. **166:** 95–102.
42. CORBETT, S.J. *et al.* 1997. Sequence of the human immunoglobulin diversity (D) segment locus: a systematic analysis provides no evidence for the use of DIR segments, inverted D segments, "minor" D segments or D-D recombination. J. Mol. Biol. **270:** 587–597.
43. KLONOWSKI, K.D. & M. MONESTIER. 2000. Heavy chain revision in MRL mice: a potential mechanism for the development of autoreactive B cell precursors. J. Immunol. **165:** 4487–4493.
44. GHIOTTO, F. *et al.* 2004. Remarkably similar antigen receptors among a subset of patients with chronic lymphocytic leukemia. J. Clin. Invest. **113:** 1008–1016.
45. RADIC, M.Z. *et al.* 1993. Residues that mediate DNA binding of autoimmune antibodies. J. Immunol. **150:** 4966–4977.
46. COCCA, B.A. *et al.* 2001. Structural basis for autoantibody recognition of phosphatidylserine-beta 2 glycoprotein I and apoptotic cells. Proc. Natl. Acad. Sci. USA **98:** 13826–13831.
47. MILNER, E.C. & J.D. CAPRA. 1982. VH families in the antibody response to p-azophenylarsonate: correlation between serology and amino acid sequence. J. Immunol. **129:** 193–199.
48. JESKE, D.J. *et al.* 1984. Junctional diversity is essential to antibody activity. J. Immunol. **133:** 1090–1092.
49. SANZ, I. & J. CAPRA. 1987. VK and JK gene segments of A/J Ars-A antibodies: somatic recombination generates the essential arginine at the junction of the variable and joining regions. Proc. Natl. Acad. Sci. USA **84:** 1085–1089.
50. MESSMER, B.T. *et al.* 2004. Multiple distinct sets of stereotyped antigen receptors indicate a key role for antigen in promoting chronic lymphocytic leukemia. J. Exp. Med. **200:** 519–525.
51. TOBIN, G. *et al.* 2004. Subsets with restricted immunoglobulin gene rearrangement features indicate a role for antigen selection in the development of chronic lymphocytic leukemia. Blood **104:** 2879–2885.
52. WIDHOPF, G.F., II *et al.* 2004. Chronic lymphocytic leukemia B cells of more than 1% of patients express virtually identical immunoglobulins. Blood **104:** 2499–2504.
53. GAY, D. *et al.* 1993. Receptor editing: an approach by autoreactive B cells to escape tolerance. J. Exp. Med. **177:** 999–1008.
54. TIEGS, S.L., D.M. RUSSELL & D. NEMAZEE. 1993. Receptor editing in self-reactive bone marrow B cells. J, Exp, Med. **177:** 1009–1020.
55. JUKES, T.H. & J.L. KING. 1979. Evolutionary nucleotide replacements in DNA. Nature **281:** 605–606.
56. KLEIN, U., K. RAJEWSKY & R. KUPPERS. 1998. Human immunoglobulin (Ig)M+IgD+ peripheral blood B cells expressing the CD27 cell surface antigen carry somatically mutated variable region genes: CD27 as a general marker for somatically mutated (memory) B cells. J. Exp. Med. **188:** 1679–1689.

57. SHLOMCHIK, M.J. *et al.* 1987. The role of clonal selection and somatic mutation in autoimmunity. Nature **328:** 805–811.
58. BROKER, B.M. *et al.* 1988. Chronic lymphocytic leukemic cells secrete multispecific autoantibodies. J. Autoimmun. **1:** 469–481.
59. STHOEGER, Z.M. *et al.* 1989. Production of autoantibodies by CD5-expressing B lymphocytes from patients with chronic lymphocytic leukemia. J. Exp. Med. **169:** 255–268.
60. BORCHE, L. *et al.* 1990. Evidence that chronic lymphocytic leukemia B lymphocytes are frequently committed to production of natural autoantibodies. Blood **76:** 562–569.
61. HERVE, M. *et al.* 2005. Unmutated and mutated chronic lymphocytic leukemia derive from common self-reactive B cell precursors despite expressing different antibody reactivity. J. Clin. Invest. **115:** 1636–1643.
62. KLEINFIELD, R.W. & M.G. WEIGERT. 1989. Analysis of VH gene replacement events in a B cell lymphoma. J. Immunol. **142:** 4475–4482.
63. ZHANG, Z., P.D. BURROWS & M.D. COOPER. 2004. The molecular basis and biological significance of VH replacement. Immunol. Rev. **197:** 231–242.
64. STAMATOPOULOS, K. *et al.* 2005. Immunoglobulin light chain repertoire in chronic lymphocytic leukemia. Blood **106:** 3575–3583.
65. KLEINFIELD, R. *et al.* 1986. Recombination between an expressed immunoglobulin heavy-chain gene and a germline variable gene segment in a Ly 1+ B-cell lymphoma. Nature **322:** 843–846.
66. RETH, M. *et al.* 1986. A novel VH to VHDJH joining mechanism in heavy-chain-negative (null) pre-B cells results in heavy-chain production. Nature **322:** 840–842.
67. BROKAW, J.L., S.M. WETZEL & B.A. POLLOK. 1992. Conserved patterns of somatic mutation and secondary VH gene rearrangement create aberrant Ig-encoding genes in Epstein-Barr virus-transformed and normal human B lymphocytes. Int. Immunol. **4:** 197–206.
68. CHEN, C. *et al.* 1995. Immunoglobulin heavy chain gene replacement: a mechanism of receptor editing. Immunity **3:** 747–755.
69. CASCALHO, M., J. WONG & M. WABL. 1997. VH gene replacement in hyperselected B cells of the quasimonoclonal mouse. J. Immunol. **159:** 5795–5801.
70. BERTRAND, F.E., R. GOLUB & G.E. WU. 1998. V(H) gene replacement occurs in the spleen and bone marrow of non-autoimmune quasi-monoclonal mice. Eur. J. Immunol. **28:** 3362–3370.
71. ZHANG, Z. *et al.* 2003. Contribution of Vh gene replacement to the primary B cell repertoire. Immunity **19:** 21–31.
72. STAMATOPOULOS, K. *et al.* 1996. Evidence for immunoglobulin heavy chain variable region gene replacement in a patient with B cell chronic lymphocytic leukemia. Leukemia **10:** 1551–1556.
73. RASSENTI, L.Z. & T.J. KIPPS. 1997. Lack of allelic exclusion in B cell chronic lymphocytic leukemia. J. Exp. Med. **185:** 1435–1445.
74. LOUZOUN, Y. *et al.* 2002. Analysis of B cell receptor production and rearrangement. Part I. Light chain rearrangement. Semin. Immunol. **14:** 169–190; Discussion, 221–22.
75. WARDEMANN, H. *et al.* 2003. Predominant autoantibody production by early human B cell precursors. Science **301:** 1374–1377.
76. BRARD, F. *et al.* 1999. Somatic mutation and light chain rearrangement generate autoimmunity in anti-single-stranded DNA transgenic MRL/lpr mice. J. Exp. Med. **190:** 691–704.
77. SEKIGUCHI, D.R., R.A. EISENBERG & M. WEIGERT. 2003. Secondary heavy chain rearrangement: a mechanism for generating anti-double-stranded DNA B cells. J. Exp. Med. **197:** 27–39.

Harnessing the Immune System Against Human Glioma

KAVITA M. DHODAPKAR, DEVI BANERJEE, AND RALPH M. STEINMAN

Laboratory of Cellular Physiology and Immunology, The Rockefeller University, New York, New York 10021, USA

ABSTRACT: Our studies are directed toward immune resistance to glial tumors, particularly in children. Initial experiments indicate that it is possible to boost both innate natural killer T lymphocytes and adaptive CD4+ and CD8+ T cells by targeting the appropriate antigens to dendritic cells. Our hypothesis is that optimal vaccination approaches against cancer will need to recruit both innate and adaptive defense mechanisms.

KEYWORDS: vaccine; tumor immunity; dendritic cells; Fcγ receptor; glioma

BRAIN TUMORS AS A THERAPEUTIC CHALLENGE IN PEDIATRIC ONCOLOGY

Childhood cancers represent the success story of modern oncology, with high cure rates for many tumors. Brain tumors, however, remain a glaring exception and now represent the leading cause of cancer-related mortality in children. The most common subtype are glial tumors. Despite recent advances in surgical techniques, radiation therapy as well as chemotherapy, the prognosis of patients with high-grade glioma remains dismal.[1,2] The median survival of patients with glioblastoma multiforme, a high-grade glial tumor, is only 52 weeks after current therapy. The location of tumor, and the procedures of surgical resection, as well as radiation therapy, all result in neurologic deficits and toxicities, including learning disabilities. There also is an increased risk for second malignancy in survivors. Systemic chemotherapy is often attempted in these patients, either as an adjunct to surgery and radiation, or at the time of relapse. However, the clinical benefit is modest, at best, and again associated with considerable morbidity. Therefore, brain tumors represent the most dominant therapeutic challenge in pediatric oncology today.

Address for corresppondence: Kavita Dhodapkar. M.D., The Rockefeller University, Laboratory of Cellular Physiology & Immunology, 1230 York Ave., New York, NY 10021. Voice: 212-327-8191; fax: 212-327-8875.

dhodapk@mail.rockefeller.edu

Ann. N.Y. Acad. Sci. 1062: 13–21 (2005).
doi: 10.1196/annals.1358.003

THE CHALLENGE OF IMMUNOTHERAPY FOR GLIOMA

The limitations of current therapies point to the urgent need for novel approaches to glioma.[3] One approach is to harness the immune system against these tumors. An advantage of immune targeting is the exquisite specificity of the immune system, which should allow for tumor-specific therapies. Brain tumors, like other tumors, express several alterations that have the potential to serve as antigenic targets for immune recognition. However, the brain parenchyma resists the generation of immunity to even foreign antigens placed *in situ*. In contrast, there are examples in mice where immunity to antigens within the brain can be initiated, very often by presenting antigens outside the brain, in the periphery. This suggests that one obstacle to spontaneous immunity to brain tumors is at the level of optimal generation of immune responses *in situ*. Studies in mice suggest that if an adequate antitumor immune response can be generated in the periphery, it is able to mediate protection against glioma.[4,5] Our research looks for mechanisms that will enhance immune-based resistance to tumors.

Harnessing the immune system against brain tumors presents two distinct considerations.[3] First, the brain parenchyma is unique in that it lacks resident dendritic cells (DCs), and resists priming of T-cell immunity *in situ*. Second, access of T cells to this tissue may also be restricted by the blood–brain barrier. Naïve T cells cross this barrier poorly,[6] whereas activated T cells readily do so, as seen in neuroinflammatory disorders like multiple sclerosis, in animal models of allergic encephalitis, and in paraneoplastic cerebellar degeneration.[6,7] However, these very considerations may also restrict the ability of brain tumors to tolerize the immune system, including the induction of regulatory or suppressive T cells. Therefore, one could reason that brain tumors may pose less of an obstacle than other tumors in terms of immune silencing. Direct study of patients and manipulation of their immune system *in vivo* is needed to understand and overcome the lack of spontaneous immunity to brain tumors.

HYPOTHESIS: PARTICIPATION OF BOTH INNATE AND ADAPTIVE IMMUNITY IN PROTECTIVE IMMUNITY TO BRAIN TUMORS

Recent studies have shown that both innate and adaptive immune mechanisms can be recruited to resist cancer. Most of the attention in tumor immunology has been on adaptive CD4+ and CD8+ T cells. T cells recognize peptide antigens presented on MHC class I and II products. T cells are capable of extensive clonal expansion, acquisition of helper and killer functions, and development of immunologic memory. Innate lymphocytes recognize additional targets in tumors and can mediate helper and killer functions, but they are not thought to undergo extensive clonal expansion or to acquire memory. One type of innate lymphocyte is the NK-T cells, which express a T cell type of antigen receptor, but recognize glycolipid ligands in the context of the CD1 family of antigen-presenting molecules. Our research is directed to the recruitment of both innate and adaptive immunity, because these systems may recognize distinct targets and can cooperate to improve resistance. A critical cell that links both of these arms together is the DC. Therefore we feel that optimal targeting of tumor antigens to DCs, as well their activation will be key to eliciting glioma immunity *in vivo*.

DENDRITIC CELLS AS A TOOL TO BOOST ANTITUMOR IMMUNITY

DCs are efficient antigen-presenting cells that reside in the peripheral tissue in an immature state, designed to capture antigens and dying cells, but needing to differentiate further to induce immunity.[8,9] Upon exposure to defined stimuli, sometimes termed "danger" signals, DCs differentiate or mature and become capable of stimulating different types of innate and adaptive immunity. Recent direct studies of DCs in mouse lymphoid tissues have shown that the uptake of antigens by DCs under noninflammatory conditions can lead to the induction of tolerance *in vivo*.[10,53,54] Addition of activating stimuli, such as CD40 ligation or signals derived from innate lymphocytes differentiates the DCs and leads to immunity. Thus DCs have the capacity to mediate both immunity and tolerance, and the nature of T-cell responses generated to tumor or viral antigens may depend on the context in which DC–T cell interactions occur *in vivo*. Importantly, DCs process and present antigens on many different types of presenting molecules, such as MHCI, MHCII, and CD1. DCs also travel to the lymph nodes to identify and stimulate specific T cells and innate lymphocytes. We are therefore studying mechanisms to allow DCs to expand NK-T and T cells that can attack glioma.

STUDIES ON INVARIANT NK-T CELLS IN GLIOMA PATIENTS

Invariant NKT (iNKT) cells are innate lymphocytes that show restricted T-cell receptor usage, particularly a receptor that comprises Vα24 and Vβ11 segments in humans, as well as certain natural killer-cell or NK markers, like CD161. NKT cells recognize glycolipid antigens presented on CD1d molecules.[11] Naturally occurring ligands are just beginning to be identified in self-tissues and in some microbes.[12–14] A synthetic ligand α-galactosyl ceramide (α-GalCer) initially isolated from a marine sponge, was identified as a potent stimulator of these cells.[15] Upon activation, NK-T cells secrete large amounts of cytokines and are able to mediate antitumor effects, both directly and indirectly by recruiting other innate NK cells and by maturing DCs to initiate adaptive T-cell immunity. iNKT cells have been postulated to play a role in immunesurveillance in carcinogen-induced tumors in mice.[16]

A number of studies have shown a defect in both the number and function of circulating NKT cells in patients with systemic cancers.[17–20] However, glioma is different in that the growth of tumors is restricted to the brain, and therefore the relevant glycolipids may not gain access to peripheral NKT cells. We have studied the iNKT cells from the blood of glioma patients, first from adults,[21] and more recently from children (unpublished). Surprisingly, the number of circulating iNKT cells in these patients are comparable to those seen in healthy controls. Furthermore, in contrast to studies in other cancers, these NKT cells can rapidly secrete IFN-γ and proliferate in response to mature DCs loaded with α-GalCer. The expanded iNKT cells also are functional, being able to secrete IFN-γ and to kill glioma cells upon challenge. Importantly, glioma cells express CD1d and can be recognized by DC-activated NKT cells in a CD1d-dependent manner. Together these data point to NKT cells as logical targets to improve immunotherapy of glioma.

TARGETING TUMOR ANTIGENS TO DENDRITIC CELLS FOR ADAPTIVE T-CELL IMMUNITY

Because tumors by themselves are poor inducers of immunity, it has been proposed that the generation of effective antitumor immunity *in vivo* depends on the presentation of tumor antigens by professional antigen presenting cells.[22] Indeed, bone marrow–derived cells are critical for generating antitumor immunity in mice.[22] Subsequent studies have shown that DCs are the principal cells that capture tumor antigens and efficiently activate naive T lymphocytes,[23,53] and in particular that DCs cross present antigens from many different sources for presentation by MHC class I molecules to CD8+ T cells.[24] Efficient cross presentation of antigens by DCs likely requires specific receptors and distinct processing pathways, though these remain to be defined *in vivo*. Furthermore, effective CD8+ T-cell immunity to cross presented antigens likely requires the participation of CD4+ helper T cells, which can be mobilized simultaneously by DCs capturing dying cells *in vivo*.[23] Whole tumor cells, as opposed to defined tumor antigens, are therefore being used to load DCs for purposes of immune analysis and therapy. This approach is of particular interest for cancers like glioma, where dominant tumor antigens remain unknown. The ability to load whole tumor cells to DCs provides the opportunity to simultaneously elicit CD4 and CD8+ T-cell responses to multiple tumor-derived antigens.[25] Several studies have shown that human DCs can acquire antigen from dying (both apoptotic and necrotic) tumor cells and elicit tumor specific killer T cells.[8] Our current approach, as discussed below, is to target tumor antigens via antitumor antibodies and the Fcγ receptor on DCs.

DENDRITIC CELL–MEDIATED IMMUNIZATION IN GLIOMA

The recognition that it is feasible to elicit an immune response to glial tumor by immunization in the periphery, has prompted several studies of active immunization in glioma.[26] In animal models of brain tumors, DCs pulsed *ex vivo* with either dying tumor cells, peptides eluted from the tumor cells, or tumor RNA have been shown to mediate antitumor effects. Immunization with these antigen loaded DCs led to prolonged survival compared to control animals.[4,27,55] Increased intra and peri-tumoral CD4+ and CD8+ T cells have been seen in animals that receive DCs as compared to control animals. Also, tumor-specific cytotoxic T-lymphocyte response can be demonstrated in some studies. A number of recent phase I/II studies in humans also have demonstrated the feasibility and safety of using autologous DCs pulsed with either tumor peptides,[28] tumor lysate pulsed DCs,[29–31] DC loaded with tumor-derived RNA,[32] and DCs fused with glioma cells.[33]

FcγR AND ANTITUMOR MONOCLONAL ANTIBODIES

Antitumor antibodies have emerged as effective therapeutic agents for several human cancers, most notably anti-CD20 antibodies for therapy of lymphoma. Several mechanisms of action have been proposed to help explain the clinical efficacy of antitumor antibodies, including a direct effect on tumor cells, the recruitment of innate effector mechanisms, such as antibody-dependent cytotoxicity (ADCC) and complement dependent cytotoxicity (CDC).[34] In a mouse model, the efficacy of antitumor antibodies was clearly dependent on FcγR and not just direct antibody-based recognition of the tumor.[35] The dominant mechanism of the antitumor effect studied in these experiments was ADCC. However, these results do not exclude other mechanisms, including recruitment of adaptive immune effectors via DCs. It was indeed shown that CD8+ T-cell depletion *in vivo* prevents treatment of established solid tumors with antitumor antibodies.[36] A role for adaptive immunity is, however, suggested by the clinical observations of more durable clinical responses in some patients in spite of persistence of small amounts of tumor cells.

ENHANCING ANTITUMOR IMMUNITY BY TARGETING TUMOR ANTIGENS TO Fcγ ON DCS

Targeting model antigens to FcγR on murine DCs led to enhanced MHC I restricted antigen presentation.[37] In addition, a striking enhancement in both MHC I and II presentation of ovalbumin was demonstrated upon targeting the antigen to FcγR on murine DCs using liposomes.[38] Two models for antigen processing in FcR-mediated cross presentation have been proposed: one involving antigen entry into the cytosol, and another involving proteolysis in phagolysosomes and their fusion with vesicles containing newly synthesized MHC I. Recently, Akiyama *et al.* showed that mouse DCs present apoptotic tumor cells, tagged with a hapten antigen and coated with antihapten antibody, and this leads to improved protection as compared to DCs loaded with apoptotic cells alone.[39]

We reasoned that antitumor monoclonal antibodies (MoAb) may be effective tools to target tumor antigens from whole human tumor cells to Fcγ receptor on DCs. To test this, we first opsonized myeloma tumor cells with antisyndecan-1 monoclonal antibody and fed these opsonized tumors to DCs. Surprisingly, uptake of opsonized tumors by DCs was comparable to that of nonopsonized cells. However, DCs loaded with opsonized tumors were much more effective at eliciting tumor-specific killer T cells *in vitro* compared to DCs loaded with apoptotic or necrotic tumors.[40] This process was dependent on uptake of tumors via Fcγ receptors and was inhibited after blockade with anti-FcγR antibodies.[41] Therefore, uptake of antibody-coated tumor cells by DCs leads to enhanced presentation of tumor antigens expressed by these tumor cells. Similar findings have been reported for other human tumors and tumor antigens.[42,56] Together, these data provide an approach to exploit antitumor monoclonal antibodies to target tumor antigens to DCs to boost adaptive immunity. Recruitment of adaptive immunity may be critical for durable effects seen with monoclonal antibody therapy in the clinic.

MANIPULATING THE BALANCE OF Fcγ RECEPTORS TOWARD ENHANCED ANTIGEN PRESENTATION

The Fcγ receptor system comprises both activating and inhibitory receptors. The inhibitory receptors have an immune tyrosine inhibitory motif (ITIM) in their cytoplasmic domain, while the activating Fc receptors instead mobilize an activating motif (ITAM), for example, through an associated signaling γ chain. The biologic outcome of signaling via the Fcγ receptor is determined by the balance between activating and inhibitory receptors, both of which are generally coexpressed and coengaged.[43,57] For example, in the case of human monocyte-derived DCs, the dominant Fcγ receptor is CD32, which is expressed as activating CD32A and inhibitory CD32B receptors.

It has been demonstrated that targeting of antigen to Fcγ receptors on DCs leads to Th1 CD4+ and CD8+ effector responses *in vivo*.[45] Tumor immunity specific for the ovalbumin-expressing tumors was provided by immunization with wild-type, but not FcγR-deficient DCs loaded with ovalbumin-containing immune complexes. Interference with the inhibitory signal delivered by FcγRIIB on DCs (using FcγRIIB KO mice) converted immune complexes into effective DC maturation agents and resulted in effective T-cell activation. Applying this approach to immunization with DCs, pulsed *ex vivo* with immune complexes, antigen-specific CD8+ T cells were generated *in vivo*, achieving efficient protective immunity in a murine melanoma model, in which the immune response is directed to ovalbumin transduced into the melanoma.[46]

We hypothesized that selective blockade of inhibitory Fcγ receptors in the presence of an activating signal provided by Ig/immune complexes would enhance both maturation and antigen presentation by human DCs. To test this, we utilized pure populations of monocyte-derived DCs, which express both activating and inhibitory FcγRII receptors. Blockade of inhibitory Fcγ receptors using an FcγRIIb-specific antibody led to upregulation of DC maturation markers, such as CD80, CD86, CD83, and HLA-DR, as well as secretion of IL-12p70. These effects were only seen in the presence of an activating stimulus provided by Ig/immune complexes in the normal serum. When these DCs were fed with tumor cells, they were also efficient at stimulating antitumor T-cell immunity in culture, without the need for additional exogenous maturation stimulus.[47] Taken together, these data imply that immune complexes in the serum normally serve to maintain tolerance through their binding to inhibitory FcRs on DCs, but they can be converted to potent immunogenic stimuli by selective engagement of activating FcγRs. The inhibitory Fcγ receptors are therefore part of the regulatory control system aimed at preventing inadvertent DC maturation and autoimmunity. Exploiting this aspect of FcR biology has the potential to enhance the clinical efficacy of antitumor monoclonal antibodies as well as DC vaccination against cancer and infections.

IMPROVING ANTIBODY MEDIATED TARGETING OF GLIOMA

To extend our observations to human glioma, our ongoing research is emphasizing the epidermal growth-factor receptor (EGF-R). Binding of ligand activates the intrinsic tyrosine kinase activity of the EGF-R, resulting in cellular proliferation.[48]

EGF-R is commonly over expressed in glial tumors including glioblastoma multiforme (GBM).[49] In a recent study, EGF-R expression correlated with poorer prognosis, especially in younger patients with this tumor.[50] Monoclonal antibodies directed against this receptor can inhibit the growth of malignant tumor cells and are undergoing clinical trials.[51,52,58] In our experiments, we will primarily utilize antibodies against EGF-R as a strategy to opsonize tumor cells *in vitro* prior to feeding tumors to DCs. Other potential targets on the surface of glioma cells includc an aberrant IL-13 receptor, as well as a variant of EGF receptor. Ongoing studies in our lab are trying to optimize the conditions for loading antigens from these cells onto DCs and to elicit glioma-specific T-cell immunity. These studies will then serve as the basis for clinical studies in order to boost glioma-specific immunity in patients *in vivo* by DC vaccination. As discussed earlier, we intend to mobilize both innate and adaptive cells to harness the potential of the immune system against cancer.

[*Competing interests:* The authors declare that they have no competing financial interests.]

REFERENCES

1. Broniscer, A. & A. Gajjar. 2004. Supratentorial high-grade astrocytoma and diffuse brainstem glioma: two challenges for the pediatric oncologist. Oncologist **9:** 197–206.
2. Reddy, A.T. & J.C. Wellons III. 2003. Pediatric high-grade gliomas. Cancer J. **9:** 107–112.
3. Pollack, I.F., H. Okada & W.H. Chambers. 2000. Exploitation of immune mechanisms in the treatment of central nervous system cancer [In Process Citation]. Semin. Pediatr. Neurol. **7:** 131–143.
4. Liau, L.M. *et al.* 1999. Treatment of intracranial gliomas with bone marrow-derived dendritic cells pulsed with tumor antigens. J. Neurosurg. **90:** 1115–1124.
5. Heimberger, A.B. *et al.* 2000. Bone marrow-derived dendritic cells pulsed with tumor homogenate induce immunity against syngeneic intracerebral glioma. J. Neuroimmunol. **103:** 16–25.
6. Hickey, W.F., B.L. Hsu & H. Kimura. 1991. T-lymphocyte entry into the central nervous system. J. Neurosci. Res. **28:** 254–260.
7. Albert, M.L. *et al.* 1998. Tumor-specific killer cells in paraneoplastic cerebellar degeneration. Nat. Med. **4:** 1321–1324.
8. Banchareau, J. & R.M. Steinman. 1998. Dendritic cells and the control of immunity. Nature **392:** 245–252.
9. Mellman, D. *et al.* 2001. Dendritic cells: specialized and regulated antigen processing machines. Cell **106:** 255–258.
10. Hawiger, D. *et al.* 2001. Dendritic cells induce peripheral T cell unresponsiveness under steady state conditions i*n vivo*. J. Exp. Med. **194:** 769–779.
11. Bendelac, A. *et al.* 1995. CD1 recognition by mouse NK1+ T lymphocytes. Science **268:** 863–865.
12. Kinjo, Y. *et al.* 2005. Recognition of bacterial glycosphingolipids by natural killer T cells. Nature **434:** 520–525.
13. Mattner, J. et al. 2005. 2005. Exogenous and endogenous glycolipid antigens activate NKT cells during microbial infections. Nature **434:** 525–529.
14. Zhou, D. *et al.* 2004. Lysosomal glycosphingolipid recognition by NKT cells. Science **306:** 1786–1789.
15. Cui, J. *et al.* 1997. Requirement for Va 14 NKT cells by glycosylceramides. Science **278:** 1623–1626.
16. Crowe, N.Y., M.J. Smyth & D.I. Godfrey 2002. A critical role for natural killer T cells in immunosurveillance of methylcholanthrene-induced sarcomas. J. Exp. Med. **196:** 119–127.

17. MOLLING, J.W. et al. 2005. Peripheral blood IFN-gamma-secreting Valpha24+Vbeta11+NKT cell numbers are decreased in cancer patients independent of tumor type or tumor load. Int. J. Cancer **116:** 87–93.
18. YONEDA, K. *et al.* 2005. The peripheral blood Valpha24+ NKT cell numbers decrease in patients with haematopoietic malignancy. Leuk. Res. **29:** 147–152.
19. YANAGISAWA, K. *et al.* 2002. Impaired proliferative response of V alpha 24 NKT cells from cancer patients against alpha-galactosylceramide. J. Immunol. **168:** 6494–6499.
20. DHODAPKAR, M.V. *et al.* 2003. A reversible defect in natural killer T cell function characterizes the progression of premalignant to malignant multiple myeloma. J. Exp. Med. **197:** 1667–1676.
21. DHODAPKAR, K.M. *et al.* 2004. Invariant natural killer T cells are preserved in patients with glioma and exhibit antitumor lytic activity following dendritic cell-mediated expansion. Int. J. Cancer **109:** 893–899.
22. HUANG, A.Y.C. *et al.* 1994. Role of bone marrow-derived cells in presenting MHC class I-restricted tumor antigens. Science **264:** 961–965.
23. IYODA, T. *et al.* 2002.The CD8+ dendritic cell subset selectively endocytoses dying cells in culture and *in vivo*. J. Exp. Med. **195:** 1289–1302.
24. JUNG, S. *et al.* 2002. *In vivo* depletion of CD11c(+) dendritic cells abrogates priming of CD8(+) T cells by exogenous cell-associated antigens. Immunity **17:** 211–220.
25. BERARD, F. *et al.* 2000. Cross-priming of naive CD8 T cells against melanoma antigens using dendritic cells loaded with killed allogeneic melanoma cells. J. Exp. Med. **192:** 1535–1544.
26. FECCI, P.E. *et al.* 2003. The history, evolution, and clinical use of dendritic cell-based immunization strategies in the therapy of brain tumors. J. Neurooncol. **64:** 161–176.
27. OKADA, H. *et al.* 1998. Bone marrow-derived dendritic cells pulsed with a tumor-specific peptide elicit effective anti-tumor immunity against intracranial neoplasms. Int. J. Cancer **78:** 196–201.
28. YU, J.S. *et al.* 2001. Vaccination of malignant glioma patients with peptide-pulsed dendritic cells elicits systemic cytotoxicity and intracranial T-cell infiltration. Cancer Res. **61:** 842–847.
29. YU, J.S. *et al.* 2004. Vaccination with tumor lysate-pulsed dendritic cells elicits antigen-specific, cytotoxic T-cells in patients with malignant glioma. Cancer Res. **64:** 4973–4979.
30. YAMANAKA, R. *et al.* 2003. Vaccination of recurrent glioma patients with tumour lysate-pulsed dendritic cells elicits immune responses: results of a clinical phase I/II trial. Br. J. Cancer **89:** 1172–1179.
31. STEINER, H.H. *et al.* 2004. Antitumor vaccination of patients with glioblastoma multiforme: a pilot study to assess feasibility, safety, and clinical benefit. J. Clin. Oncol. **22:** 4272–4281.
32. KOBAYASHI, T. *et al.* 2003. Tumor mRNA-loaded dendritic cells elicit tumor-specific CD8(+) cytotoxic T cells in patients with malignant glioma. Cancer Immunol' Immunother. **52:** 632–637.
33. KIKUCHI, T. *et al.* 2004. Vaccination of glioma patients with fusions of dendritic and glioma cells and recombinant human interleukin 12. J. Immunother. **27:** 452–459.
34. LEVY, R. 2000. A perspective on monoclonal antibody therapy: where we have been and where we are going. Semin. Hematol. **37**(Suppl. 7): 43–46.
35. CLYNES, R.A. *et al.* 2000. Inhibitory Fc receptors modulate *in vivo* cytoxicity against tumor targets. Nat. Med. **6:** 443–446.
36. DYALL, R. *et al.* 1999. Cellular requirements for the monoclonal antibody-mediated eradication of an established solid tumor. Eur. J. Immunol. **29:** 30–37.
37. REGNAULT, A. *et al.* 1999. Fcgamma receptor-mediated induction of dendritic cell maturation and major histocompatibility complex class I-restricted antigen presentation after immune complex internalization. J. Ex. Med. **189:** 371–380.
38. MACHY, P., K. SERRE & L. LESERMAN. 2000.Class I-restricted presentation of exogenous antigen acquired by Fcgamma receptor-mediated endocytosis is regulated in dendritic cells. Eur. J. Immunol. **30:** 848–857.

39. Akiyama, K. *et al.* 2003. Targeting apoptotic tumor cells to Fc gamma R provides efficient and versatile vaccination against tumors by dendritic cells. J. Immunol. **170:** 1641–1648.
40. Dhodapkar, K. *et al.* 2002. Anti-tumor monoclonal antibodies enhance cross presentation of cellular antigens and the generation of tumor specific killer T cells by dendritic cells. J. Exp. Med. **195:** 125–133.
41. Dhodapkar, K.M. *et al.* 2002. Antitumor monoclonal antibodies enhance cross-presentation of cellular antigens and the generation of myeloma-specific killer T cells by dendritic cells. J. Exp. Med. **195:** 125–133.
42. Groh, V. *et al.* 2005. Efficient cross-priming of tumor antigen-specific T cells by dendritic cells sensitized with diverse anti-MICA opsonized tumor cells. Proc. Natl. Acad. Sci. USA **102:** 6461–6466.
43. Ravetch, J.V. & S. Bolland. 2001. IgG Fc receptors. Annu. Rev. Immunol. **19:** 275–290.
44. Geissmann, F. *et al.* 2001. A subset of human dendritic cells expresses IgA Fc receptor (CD89), which mediates internalization and activation upon cross-linking by IgA complexes. J I.mmunol. **166:** 346–352.
45. Rafiq, K., A. Bergtold & R. Clynes. 2002. Immune complex-mediated antigen presentation induces tumor immunity. J. Clin. Invest. **110:** 71–79.
46. Kalergis, A.M. & J.V. Ravetch. 2002. Inducing tumor immunity through the selective engagement of activating Fc receptors on dendritic cells. J. Exp. Med. **195:** 1653–1659.
47. Dhodapkar, K.M. *et al.* 2005. Selective blockade of inhibitory Fc{gamma} receptor enables human dendritic cell maturation with IL-12p70 production and immunity to antibody-coated tumor cells. Proc. Natl. Acad. Sci. USA **102:** 2910–2915.
48. Carpenter, C.D. *et al.* 1991. Structural analysis of the transmembrane domain of the epidermal growth factor receptor. J. Biol. Chem. **266:** 5750–5755.
49. Bredel, M. *et al.* 1999. Epidermal growth factor receptor expression and gene amplification in high-grade non-brainstem gliomas of childhood. Clin. Cancer Res. **5:** 1786–1792.
50. Simmons, M.L. *et al.* 2001. Analysis of complex relationships between age, p53, epidermal growth factor receptor, and survival in glioblastoma patients. Cancer Res. **61:** 1122–1128.
51. Bianco, R. *et al.* 2005. Monoclonal antibodies targeting the epidermal growth factor receptor. Curr. Drug Targets **6:** 275–287.
52. Shin, D.M. *et al.* 2001. Epidermal growth factor receptor-targeted therapy with C225 and cisplatin in patients with head and neck cancer. Clin. Cancer Res. **7:** 1204–1213.
53. Liu, K. *et al.* 2002. Immune tolerance after delivery of dying cells to dendritic cells in situ. J. Exp. Med. **196:** 1091–1097.
54. Bonifaz, L. *et al.* 2002. Efficient targeting of protein antigen to the dendritic cell receptor DEC-205 in the steady state leads to antigen presentation on major histocompatibility complex I and peripheral CD8+ T cell tolerance. J. Exp. Med. **196:** 1627–1638.
55. Ashley, D.M. *et al.* 1997. A genetically modified allogenic cellular vaccine generates MHC class I restricted cytotoxic responses against tumor associated antigens and protects against CNS tumor in vivo. J. Neuroimmunol. **78:** 34–46.
56. Selenko, N. *et al.* 2001. CD20 antibody (C2B8) -induced apoptosis of lymphoma cells promotes phagocytosis by dendritic cells and cross-priming of CD8+ cytotoxic T cells. Leukemia **15:** 1619–1626.
57. Toshiyuki, T. 2002. Roles of Fc receptors in autoimmunity. Nat. Rev. Immunol. **2:** 580–592.
58. Mendelsohn, J. & J. Baselga. 2003. Status of epidermal growth factor receptor antagonists in the biology and treatment of cancer. J. Clin. Oncol. **21:** 2787–2799.

Immune Response to Premalignancy

Insights from Patients with Monoclonal Gammopathy

MADHAV V. DHODAPKAR

Laboratory of Tumor Immunology and Immunotherapy, The Rockefeller University, and Hematology Service, Memorial Sloan Kettering Cancer Center, New York, New York 10021, USA

ABSTRACT: Many patients with preneoplastic gammopathy remain clinically stable, in spite of the presence of multiple genomic abnormalities in tumor cells. Our hypothesis is that the development of clinical cancer depends not just on the genomic changes in tumor cells, but also their interactions with the host-tumor microenvironment. Recent studies have shown that the host immune system is capable of responding to preneoplastic cells. Improved understanding of this response may provide novel opportunities for early detection and immune prevention of cancer.

KEYWORDS: myeloma; dendritic cells; inflammation; cancer; prevention

INTRODUCTION

Multiple myeloma (MM) is a common B-cell malignancy characterized by clonal expansion of transformed plasma cells in the bone marrow.[1] Natural history of MM is characterized by disease progression, and the development of anemia, lytic bone disease, and infections. However although clonal expansion of transformed plasma cells is an essential prerequisite for the development of MM, the most common clinical presentation of such expansions *in vivo* is not MM, but the development of monoclonal gammopathy of undetermined significance (MGUS). MGUS has been estimated to occur in up to 1–3% of the elderly population, and represents a preneoplastic state. However, most patients with MGUS will generally remain stable throughout their life, and only a small proportion (estimated at about 1% per year) will develop MM.[2]

Recent application of interphase cytogenetics and genomic technologies has yielded the surprising finding that many of the cytogenetic and genomic changes in tumor cells initially identified in myeloma can now also be detected in the tumor cells in MGUS.[3, 4] These findings therefore suggest the possibility that clinical outcome in myeloma depends not only on the properties of the tumor cells themselves, but also changes in the host tumor microenvironment and their interactions with the

Address for correspondence: Madhav V. Dhodapkar, M.D., Laboratory of Tumor Immunology and Immunotherapy, The Rockefeller University, 1230 York Avenue, New York, NY 10021. Voice: 212-327-7118; fax: 212-327-7119.

dhodapm@rockefeller.edu

Ann. N.Y. Acad. Sci. 1062: 22–28 (2005). © 2005 New York Academy of Sciences.
doi: 10.1196/annals.1358.004

tumor cells. An important component of this microenvironment are the cells of the immune system. Therefore improved understanding of the immune microenvironment in myeloma might provide newer approaches for therapy and prevention of this cancer. Understanding the status of the host immune response is an essential first step for optimal development of therapeutic approaches targeting the immune system in MM.

MECHANISMS OF IMMUNE CONTROL AND SURVEILLANCE OF TUMORS

The fact that nearly all tumors (and their "preneoplastic" counterparts) express antigenic determinants that can be potentially recognized by the immune system is now well established.[5–7] Molecular basis of this has come in part from the understanding that genetic instability of tumors leads to a tremendous array of genetic and cellular alterations in each tumor cell.[7] Surprisingly, in some instances (such as melanoma), when the specificity of T cells infiltrating tumors was determined, the immune response was found to be directed against nonmutated tissue differentiation antigens also expressed by normal tissue counterparts.[8] Nonetheless, although tumors are derived from "self" tissues, they appear to be sufficiently "foreign" or "altered" to allow their potential recognition by the immune system.[9] The inability of the immune system to protect against tumors thus seems largely not due to the lack of antigenic targets on tumor cells, but due to the inability of the host to mount a protective immune response.

The immune system has several components that can theoretically be recruited to protect from tumors.[10] CD4+ and CD8+ T cells are the adaptive arms of cell-mediated immunity, able to differentiate upon antigen encounter to produce cytokines and lytic products, to clonally expand, and to establish memory. Natural killer (NK) and NKT cells have innate functions, already prepared to kill and produce cytokines upon tumor recognition.[11,12] NK and NKT cells do grow upon exposure to cytokines like IL-2, but they are not known to establish memory with either expanded cell numbers or improved function. Finally, antibodies or humoral immune system may kill tumor cells either directly or by recruiting innate effector mechanisms such as complement or antibody dependent cytotoxicity. Recent studies in mice have demonstrated the role of interferon-γ and lymphocytes in protection against spontaneous and carcinogen-induced tumors in mice.[13] Interactions of the immune system with the developing tumors might lead to "editing" of these tumors *in vivo*. Evidence has now emerged for the role of both adaptive and innate lymphocytes (NK or NKT) cells in immune surveillance.[13]

MYELOMA/MGUS AS A MODEL FOR TUMOR IMMUNOLOGY AND IMMUNOTHERAPY

Myeloma provides several unique features to study the capacity of the human immune system to resist tumors. In this tumor, there is ready access to both autologous tumors and immune effector and antigen-presenting cells from the tumor bed, and these can be purified without the need for *in vitro* culture. Tumor cells express several well-defined antigens, such as tumor-derived monoclonal Ig, or cancer-testis antigens.[14] The secreted monoclonal Ig may not only be a potentially useful tumor-specific antigen (particularly for CD4+ T-cell responses), but also provides a unique tumor-specific serum marker for easy detection of "minimal residual disease." Perhaps the most important aspect of this tumor model is the availability of a defined preneoplastic state in the form of MGUS.

DETECTING ANTITUMOR T CELLS IN THE MYELOMA TUMOR BED

For our initial studies on anti-tumor immunity in myeloma, we first focused on T cells from the tumor bed of patients with newly diagnosed myeloma. These patients by definition have failed to control their tumors *in vivo*. When T cells from the blood or marrow of these patients were tested for the recognition of freshly isolated autologous tumors, there was no detectable reactivity.[15] These T cells were, however, capable of reacting to viral antigens and to polyclonal mitogens, indicating the lack of global T-cell dysfunction. Prior studies in our lab had shown that targeting tumor antigens to Fcγ receptors on DCs using anti-tumor monoclonal antibodies was an efficient approach to elicit an anti-tumor T-cell response in culture.[16,17] Thus DCs loaded with opsonized tumor cells were more efficient at generating anti-tumor T-cell immunity compared to DCs loaded with apoptotic or necrotic tumors. To extend this approach to primary tumors, we first coated tumor cells with anti-syndecan-1 antibody, and used autologous DCs loaded with these tumors to stimulate T cells. Importantly, T cells from the myeloma marrow could be reliably activated *ex vivo* to kill autologous tumors, even though these patients had progressive myeloma.[15] These expanded T cells were specific for autologous tumors and did not recognize DCs loaded with allogeneic tumor cells, or nontumor cells from the marrow. Interestingly, the T cells also did not recognize DCs loaded with tumor derived Ig. In other words, clinical progression in myeloma was not due to the deletion of anti-tumor T cells from the tumor bed, and these T cells can be reliably activated to kill autologous tumors, if properly activated by targeting tumor antigens to DCs. The presence of myeloma specific T cells in the marrow has now been confirmed by other labs as well.[18] Taken together these data support approaches to boost myeloma-specific T-cell immunity *in vivo* in patients using antigen-loaded DCs.

TUMOR IMMUNITY IN PRENEOPLASTIC GAMMOPATHY

As noted earlier, many of the genomic changes found in myeloma tumor cells have now also been observed in the tumor cells in MGUS. Therefore, we decided to test whether T cells in MGUS patients could directly recognize autologous preneoplastic cells. To ths end, we first purified autologous preneoplastic cells from MGUS patients and loaded them onto autologous monocyte-derived DCs. T cells from the bone marrow of MGUS or myeloma patients were then tested for the recognition of these APCs. Freshly isolated T cells from the myeloma marrow failed to recognize these DCs. In contrast, fresh T cells from bone marrow of MGUS patients readily secreted interferon-γ in short-term effector assays.[19] This response consisted of both

CD4+ and CD8+ T cells, and was specific for antigens expressed by autologous tumors, as DCs loaded with allogeneic tumors were not recognized. Interestingly, these T cells also did not recognize DCs loaded with tumor-derived Ig. The presence of T cells specific for tumor-derived Ig has been previously demonstrated in both myeloma and MGUS. However, these T cells do not appear to be major components of the immune response that we measured. MGUS-specific T cells in the tumor bed also recognized autologous MGUS cells, but not nontumor cells from the same marrow. Taken together, these data suggest that the human immune system is capable of immune recognition of preneoplastic cells, and that the nature of T-cell response against preneoplasia may differ from that against clinical cancer.

STUDYING IMMUNE RESPONSE AGAINST PRENEOPLASIA: THE NEXT STEPS

The finding that the immune system has the capacity to recognize and specifically respond to preneoplastic cells in MGUS leads to several new questions about its significance. One of the first steps is improved understanding of the specific antigenic targets of this response. Evaluation of antitumor immunity in other human preneoplastic states is also warranted. To this end, we have recently begun a collaborative effort with Dr. Finn at the University of Pittsburgh, which is supported in part by the Dana Foundation. The goals of this consortium are to characterize the nature of the host immune response in MGUS, as well as in smokers and patients with dysplastic epithelial lesions. Particular attention will be paid to two known targets of host response in other preneoplastic states, namely, muc-1 and cyclin B1. Immunity to these antigens has been extensively studied in the Finn laboratory.[20,21] Furthermore, data from mouse models suggests that harnessing immunity against these antigens may be of value for immune prevention of cancer. We have also begun to screen sera from MGUS patients for the presence of antibody responses against a panel of tumor-associated antigens, in collaboration with Drs. Scanlan and Gure at the Ludwig Institute (New York). Preliminary data from these studies confirm the presence of antibody responses against some of these antigens in MGUS. These data therefore provide additional support to the hypothesis that the immune system of these patients is capable of responding to antigens expressed on preneoplastic cells. Ongoing studies are trying to further characterize the nature of immune response to antigenic targets identified in these studies.

IMMUNE SURVEILLANCE VERSUS IMMUNE STIMULATION

The new studies of immune recognition of preneoplastic cells in humans raise important, but yet unanswered questions about the biologic and clinical impact of immune recognition of preneoplasia on the natural history and biology of human tumors. The immune surveillance hypothesis postulated by MacFarlane and Burnet, including its critics and supporters, has occupied a central place in tumor immunology for the last four decades.[13, 22] Recent elegant studies in immune-deficient mice have provided support for the role of both interferon-γ and innate as well as adaptive lymphocyte-dependent mechanisms in immune control of cancers.[13]

On the other hand, evidence has also accumulated that under some circumstances, chronic immune activation or inflammation may promote the persistence of tumor cells *in vivo*.[23–25] It is important to point out that both of these possibilities are not mutually exclusive. For example, a low-level immune response may help suppress tumor growth but fail to eradicate it, depending on the proliferative rate and clonogenic potential of the targeted subpopulation, and the nature of tumor antigen being targeted. At the same time, growth factors/chemokines in the inflammatory microenvironment may promote genomic instability, for example, by downregulating p53 function, and eventually promoting tumor-immune escape.[25] Immune recognition of preneoplasia may therefore be a two-edged sword, and contribute to sculpting of tumors with reduced immune responsiveness and a greater potential to grow independent of its microenvironment over time.[13] The dependence of early tumor growth on their microenvironment is now being increasingly appreciated.[26] The balance of positive and negative effects of the microenvironment on tumor growth may modulate the evolution of tumors.

IMPLICATIONS FOR THE CLINIC: EARLY DETECTION AND IMMUNE PREVENTION

Taken together, our preliminary data suggest that the host immune response in the bone marrow of MGUS patients is distinct from that in myeloma. The immune recognition of preneoplastic states has several important clinical implications. First, the detection of immune responses against defined tumor antigens may serve as a tool for early detection of cancer. Most of the current efforts on early detection of tumors are based on identifying molecules expressed by tumor cells.[27] An alternative, however, may be to instead detect the specific response of the host to this clonal growth. Detection of antitumor antibodies is an attractive platform, because it is less sensitive to artifacts associated with sample processing, as has been a challenge with current proteomic approaches.

These data also have important implications for harnessing the immune system for prevention of cancer.[28] Patients with premalignancy are at an increased risk for the development of cancer, although only a proportion will develop cancer in their lifetime. This coupled with the long natural history of these lesions provides an opportunity to target these lesions for the prevention of cancer. One distinct advantage for targeting preneoplasia is that the clonal tumor itself can be a surrogate for efficacy. However, these patients exhibit considerable heterogeneity and therefore an important first step is to understand the clinical heterogeneity of these tumors. Those at higher risk for malignant transformation may then be suitable candidates for targeted prevention. The nature of host response to preneoplasia (e.g., identifying those with a blunted response) may itself allow the identification of such target populations.

The field of tumor immunotherapy has provided the basis for several approaches to boost immunity, including peptides, DNA vaccines, viral vectors, cytokines, and dendritic cell (DC) vaccines.[29] In principle, these same approaches can now also be tested for boosting immunity for prevention of cancer. Our emphasis has been on the use of DCs as potent antigen-presenting cells for boosting immunity.[30,31] An important aspect of DCs is their ability to acquire and cross-present antigens from tumor cells and efficiently stimulate both CD4+ and CD8+ T-cell responses.[32] In addition to boosting adaptive immunity, DCs are also particularly adept at stimulating innate lymphocytes such as NK or NKT cells.[33–36] Direct study of patients and specific manipulation of the immune system is needed to harness the promise of the immune system to combat and prevent cancer.

[*Competing interests*: The author declares that he has no competing financial interests.]

REFERENCES

1. MITSIADES, C.S. *et al.* 2004. Focus on multiple myeloma. Cancer Cell **6:** 439–444.
2. KYLE, R.A. *et al.* 2002. A long-term study of prognosis in monoclonal gammopathy of undetermined significance. N. Engl. J. Med. **346:** 564–569.
3. ZHAN, F. *et al.* 2002. Global gene expression profiling of multiple myeloma, monoclonal gammopathy of undetermined significance, and normal bone marrow plasma cells. Blood **99:** 1745–1757.
4. FONSECA, R., *et al.* 2002. Genomic abnormalities in monoclonal gammopathy of undetermined significance. Blood **100:** 1417–1424.
5. BOON, T. & P. VAN DER BRUGGEN. 1996. Human tumor antigens recognized by T lymphocytes. J. Exp. Med. **183:** 725–729.
6. GILBOA, E. 1999. The makings of a tumor rejection antigen. Immunity **11:** 263–270.
7. PARDOLL, D. 2003. Does the immune system see tumors as foreign or self? Annu. Rev. Immunol. **21:** 807–839.
8. HOUGHTON, A.N., J.S. GOLD & N.E. BLACHERE. 2001. Immunity against cancer: lessons learned from melanoma. Curr. Opin. Immunol. **13:** 134–140.
9. HOUGHTON, A.N. 1994. Cancer antigens: immune recognition of self and altered self. J. Exp. Med. **180:** 1–4.
10. SOGN, J.A. 1998. Tumor immunology: the glass is half full. Immunity **9:** 757–763.
11. DHODAPKAR, M.V. *et al.* 2003. A reversible defect in natural killer T cell function characterizes the progression of premalignant to malignant multiple myeloma. J. Exp. Med. **197:** 1667–1676.
12. DHODAPKAR, K.M. *et al.* 2004. Invariant natural killer T cells are preserved in patients with glioma and exhibit antitumor lytic activity following dendritic cell-mediated expansion. Int. J. Cancer **109:** 893–899.
13. DUNN, G.P. *et al.* 2002. Cancer immunoediting: from immunosurveillance to tumor escape. Nat. Immunol. **3:** 991–998.
14. DHODAPKAR, M.V. *et al.* 2003. Expression of cancer-testis antigens (MAGE-A1, -A3, -A4, CT-7 and NY-ESO-1) in malignant gammopathies is heterogeneous and correlates with site, stage and risk status of disease. Cancer Immunity **3:** 9–16.
15. DHODAPKAR, M.V., J. KRASOVSKY & K. OLSON. 2002. T Cells from the tumor microenvironment of patients with progressive myeloma can generate strong, tumor-specific cytolytic responses to autologous, tumor-loaded dendritic cells. Proc. Natl. Acad. Sci. USA **99:** 13009–13013.
16. DHODAPKAR, K.M. *et al.* 2002. Antitumor monoclonal antibodies enhance cross-presentation of cellular antigens and the generation of myeloma-specific killer T cells by dendritic cells. J. Exp. Med. **195:** 125–133.
17. DHODAPKAR, K.M. *et al.* 2005. Selective blockade of inhibitory Fc{gamma} receptor enables human dendritic cell maturation with IL-12p70 production and immunity to antibody-coated tumor cells. Proc. Natl. Acad. Sci. USA **102:** 2910–2915.
18. NOONAN, K. *et al.* 2005. Activated marrow-infiltrating lymphocytes effectively target plasma cells and their clonogenic precursors. Cancer Res. **65:** 2026–2034.
19. DHODAPKAR, M.V. *et al.* 2003. Vigorous premalignancy specific effector T cell response in the bone marrow of patients with preneoplastic gammopathy. J. Exp. Med. **198:** 1753–1757.

20. YU, M., Q. ZHAN & O.J. FINN. 2002. Immune recognition of cyclin B1 as a tumor antigen is a result of its overexpression in human tumors that is caused by non-functional p53. Mol. Immunol. **38:** 981–987.
21. VLAD, A.M. *et al.* 2004. MUC1 immunobiology: from discovery to clinical applications. Adv. Immunol. **82:** 249–293.
22. SHANKARAN, V. *et al.* 2001. IFNgamma and lymphocytes prevent primary tumour development and shape tumour immunogenicity. Nature **410:** 1107–1111.
23. PREHN, R.T. 1994. Stimulatory effects of immune reactions upon growths of untransplanted tumors. Cancer Res. **54:** 908–914.
24. DANIEL, D. *et al.* 2003. Immune enhancement of skin carcinogenesis by CD4+ T cells. J. Exp. Med. **197:** 1017–1028.
25. COUSSENS, L.M. & Z. WERB. 2002. Inflammation and cancer. Nature **420:** 860–867.
26. RADISKY, D.C. & M.J. BISSELL. 2004. Cancer. Respect thy neighbor! Science **303:** 775–777.
27. ETZIONI, R. *et al.* 2003. The case for early detection. Nat. Rev. Cancer **3:** 243–252.
28. FINN, O.J. 2003. Premalignant lesions as targets for cancer vaccines. J. Exp. Med. **198:** 1623–1626.
29. BLATTMAN, J.N. & P.D. GREENBERG. 2004. Cancer immunotherapy: a treatment for the masses. Science **305:** 200–205.
30. STEINMAN, R.M. & M. DHODAPKAR. 2001. Active immunization against cancer with dendritic cells: the near future. Int. J. Cancer **94:** 459–473.
31. BANCHEREAU, J. *et al.* 2001. Immune and clinical responses in patients with metastatic melanoma to CD34(+) progenitor-derived dendritic cell vaccine. Cancer Res. **61:** 6451–6458.
32. HEATH, W.R. & F.R. CARBONE. 2001. Cross-presentation, dendritic cells, tolerance and immunity. Annu. Rev. Immunol. **19:** 47–64.
33. FERLAZZO, G. & C. MUNZ. 2004. NK cell compartments and their activation by dendritic cells. J. Immunol. **172:** 1333–1339.
34. FUJII, S.I. *et al.* 2002. Prolonged interferon-g producing NKT responses induced with a-galactosyl ceramide loaded dendritic cells. Nature Immunol. **3:** 867–874.
35. CHANG, D.H. *et al.* 2005. Sustained expansion of NKT cells and antigen-specific T cells after injection of {alpha}-galactosyl-ceramide loaded mature dendritic cells in cancer patients. J. Exp. Med. **201:** 1503-1517.
36. FUJII, S. *et al.* 2003. Detection and activation of human Valpha24+ natural killer T cells using alpha-galactosyl ceramide-pulsed dendritic cells. J. Immunol. Methods **272:** 147–159.

Evaluation of Anticyclin B1 Serum Antibody as a Diagnostic and Prognostic Biomarker for Lung Cancer

ANN MARIE EGLOFF,[a,b] JOEL WEISSFELD,[b] STEPHANIE R. LAND,[c] AND OLIVERA J. FINN[a]

[a]*Department of Immunology, University of Pittsburgh School of Medicine, Pittsburgh, Pennsylvania 15261, USA*

[b]*Department of Epidemiology, University of Pittsburgh Graduate School of Public Health, Pittsburgh, Pennsylvania 15261, USA*

[c]*Department of Biostatistics, University of Pittsburgh Graduate School of Public Health, Pittsburgh, Pennsylvania 15261, USA*

ABSTRACT: The primary aims of this study were to establish a high-throughput assay and analytic procedures that would allow us to assess with accuracy and reproducibility the presence of anti-cyclin B1 antibodies in a large cohort of subjects at-risk for development of lung cancer. The overall goal is to identify factors significantly associated with immune responses against this lung tumor antigen and to evaluate the relationship between anticyclin B1 antibodies and lung cancer risk in a prospective cohort. Successful cancer treatment relies on early detection. The immune system could respond to tumor antigens arising from altered host factors and provide an early readout for cancer presence. This study examines immune responses to the tumor antigen cyclin B1. Lung cancer patients have antibodies against cyclin B1. Unscheduled overexpression of this cell cycle regulator occurs early in tumorigenesis and might be detected by the immune system long before clinical diagnosis of cancer. Antibodies recognizing cyclin B1 were measured using semiautomated ELISAs in sera samples from subjects without detectable lung cancer enrolled in the Pittsburgh Lung Screening Study (PLuSS), a longitudinal study of long-term smokers over age 50. Factors significantly associated with antibody presence were identified using linear regression analysis. We have established a highly reproducible, semiautomated ELISA-based assay for the high-throughput assessment of serum antibody titers. Using this technology and a small subset of PluSS subjects, cyclin B1 antibody levels were found to be high in a small proportion of subjects tested. Regression analysis identified gender as well as age in women smokers to be significant determinants of cyclin B1 antibody levels, association not seen in male subjects. This work represents an important first step toward defining the importance of the presence of anticyclin B1 antibodies in an at-risk population and assessing the predictive value of serum cyclin B1 antibody as relates to lung cancer risk.

Address for correspondence: Olivera J. Finn, University of Pittsburgh School of Medicine, E1040 Biomedical Science Tower, Pittsburgh, PA 15261. Voice: 412-648-9816; fax: 412-648-7042.

ojfinn@pitt.edu

Ann. N.Y. Acad. Sci. 1062: 29–40 (2005). © 2005 New York Academy of Sciences.
doi: 10.1196/annals.1358.005

Keywords: tumor antigen; immune response; ELISA; smokers; regression analysis

INTRODUCTION

Despite improvements in imaging technologies and chemotherapeutic agents for lung cancer detection and treatment, respectively, cancer is the second leading cause of death in the United States after heart disease, and overall 5-year survival following diagnosis of lung cancer is only 10–15%.[1–3] Most diagnosed lung cancers are either regional or distant disease and have 5-year survival rates of 2–16%; localized lung cancers account for less than 20% of the lung cancers diagnosed and have 5-year survival rates of approximately 50%.[1] Advancing diagnosis of early lung cancer will be imperative for improving lung cancer outcomes. Current risk assessment for the development of lung cancer depends primarily upon information regarding smoking and occupational histories and presence of pulmonary problems.[4] Because currently employed methods for early-stage lung cancer detection are insufficient, we have undertaken the evaluation of a candidate biomarker for lung cancer early detection and prognosis, immune response to aberrantly expressed cyclin B1 protein.

Under normal conditions, cyclin B1 expression, protein accumulation and subcellular localization are tightly regulated throughout the cell cycle.[5,6] Several cancers, including lung cancers, have been found to express high levels of cyclin B1 protein, and the presence of high tumor cyclin B1 protein levels has been found to be a negative prognostic indicator in many cancers.[7–12] Cyclin B1 transcription is regulated in part by p53, and aberrant accumulation of cyclin B1 protein is dependent upon mutation of p53.[13–15] Aberrantly expressed cyclin B1 protein is found at high levels in the cytoplasm throughout the cell cycle where cyclin B1 can be proteolyzed and processed for presentation at the cell surface in the context of MHC molecules.[15]

Evidence strongly suggests that presentation of cyclin B1–derived peptides in quantities sufficient for recognition by the immune surveillance system is dependent upon high levels of aberrantly expressed cyclin B1 such as occurs only as a result of a pathological condition, and under normal conditions, cyclin B1 and cyclin B1–derived peptides are sequestered from the immune system. Cyclin B1–responsive T cells are present in many cancer patients, but not in healthy individuals.[15] As a result, serum anti-cyclin B1 antibodies are elevated in many patients with breast, liver, pancreatic, colon, and lung cancers relative to healthy individuals.[16–18]

Unscheduled overexpression of this cell-cycle regulator occurs early in tumorigenesis, and might be detected by the immune system long before clinical diagnosis of cancer is made. If this hypothesis is correct, a highly reproducible, high-throughput assay that can measure elevated levels of anticyclin B1 antibodies in sera of healthy individuals at high risk for developing lung cancer could be a useful tool for noninvasive diagnosis and early detection of lung cancer. If the presence of antibody has an effect on cancer progression, another hypothesis that needs to be tested, then this assay would also provide information helpful in evaluating the prognosis of an individual patient's disease.

We have established such an assay by making specific changes in a standard enzyme-linked immunosorbent assay (ELISA), and have begun to test the hypotheses just given using sera from the Pittsburgh Lung Screening Study (PLuSS), a longitudinal study of long-term smokers over age 50. We have also identified factors that significantly relate to anticyclin B1 serum antibody levels. The presence or absence of anticyclin B1 antibodies is documented in these screening study participants who will be followed forward through time for cancer events and other significant health outcomes. Thus, the PLuSS prospective study design with baseline blood collection prior to lung cancer diagnosis or treatment provides the opportunity for assessment of the predictive value of candidate serum biomarkers, including immune responses. We expect that significant findings using the PLuSS cohort will translate to other organ-site cancers also found to have accompanying high serum anticyclin B1 antibody levels.

MATERIALS AND METHODS

Study Population

The Pittsburgh Lung Screening Study (PLuSS) is an ongoing, longitudinal, multidetector computerized tomography (CT) screening study of men and women ages 50 to 79 years with long-term smoking histories and, therefore, at high risk for developing lung cancer. At the time of enrollment, each participant signed a consent form, answered a baseline questionnaire, submitted to a CT scan and lung function test, and donated blood. Blood samples, therefore, were collected prospectively/prediagnostically in persons who were not receiving or seeking clinical care for suspected lung cancer.

From 3600 PLuSS participants, a stratified sampling was created composed of 291 white subjects with requisite consent, sera, questionnaire, lung-function test, negative CT scan, and no interval cancer. Sampling fractions for the 291 white subjects were based on sex, age, smoking status (current smoker versus exsmoker), and severity of airflow obstruction, a measure of chronic obstructive pulmonary disease, (Gold 0–I versus Gold II+) (TABLE 1). The Global Initiative for Chronic Obstructive Lung Disease definitions were used for classifying severity of airflow obstruction.[19] Sera from all nonwhite subjects meeting the inclusion/exclusion criteria ($n = 74$) and the 291 samples previously described constituted the PLuSS stratified sample set ($n = 365$). Ten percent of these samples were assigned a second random unique iden-

TABLE 1. Stratum-specific sample numbers

		Female			Male			
	Age	50–59	60–69	70–79	50–59	60–69	70–79	
Smoking status	Lung function							Totals
Current smoker	Gold 0–I	13	13	11	12	12	7	68
Current smoker	Gold II+	13	12	13	13	13	12	76
Ex-smoker	Gold 0–I	13	13	13	13	13	12	77
Ex-smoker	Gold II+	13	13	11	13	13	7	70
Totals		52	51	48	51	51	38	291

tifier and duplicated within the sample set as internal controls. Laboratory personnel were masked regarding all subject information until the completion of laboratory procedures.

Plasma samples from healthy anonymous donors were maintained in the Finn laboratory. Information regarding age, sex, and smoking status of normal blood donors was not available. Benign lung disease subject plasma samples were selected from those used in a previously published study to represent the range of anticyclin B1 antibody levels found in plasma from subjects with benign lung disease.[16]

Immunoassay

Enzyme-linked immunosorbant assays (ELISAs) were performed as previously described with slight modification.[16] Purified recombinant human cyclin B1 protein at a concentration of 1 µg/µL in protein storage buffer (50% glycerol, 10 mM dithiolthreitol, 1X PBS), purchased from Santa Cruz Biotechnology Inc. (Santa Cruz, CA), was diluted 1:50 with PBS, 1 µg of diluted cyclin B1 protein was applied to each well of 96-well microtiter plates, and incubated overnight at 4°C. Plates were washed with PBS and blocked with 2.5% bovine serum albumin (BSA) in PBS for one hour at room temperature. After blocking, excess blocking agent was removed, and sera, diluted in 2.5% BSA in PBS, were added and incubated for 1 hour at room temperature. Sera were diluted 1:250 for analysis unless otherwise indicated. Plates were washed with 0.1% Tween 20 in PBS, and alkaline phosphatase-labeled polyvalent goat anti-human IgM, IgG, IgA (Sigma-Aldrich, St. Louis, MO), diluted in PBS containing 2.5% BSA, was added to wells and incubated for 1 hour at room temperature. Wells were washed, 100 µL of alkaline phosphatase substrate buffer (Sigma-Aldrich) was added, and plates were incubated 1 hour at room temperature in the dark. Reactions were stopped by the addition of 50 µL of 0.5 M NaOH, and absorbance at 405 nm was measured using a MRX Revelation plate reader (Thermo Labsystems, Chantilly, VA). Background absorbance was also determined for all sera using wells without antigen. Cyclin B1–specific reactivity (Delta) was calculated by subtracting absorbance in wells with cyclin B1 antigen (AG) from absorbance in the absence of antigen (NO). For soluble cyclin B1 ELISA competition assays, diluted sera were incubated with soluble cyclin B1 at various concentrations for 15 minutes prior to addition to ELISA plate wells. Incubations containing reduced quantities of soluble cyclin B1 were supplemented with protein storage buffer to ensure that buffer components were equivalent for all competition reactions. All other procedures were as described earlier. The PLuSS stratified samples were analyzed in duplicate. Liquid transfers and washes were performed using a Velocity11 VPrep pipetting station (Velocity11, Menlo Park, CA).

Statistical Methods

Nonparametric Spearman's correlations and linear curve-fitting equations were calculated using the SPSS statistical software. Univariate and multivariable linear regression analysis was performed using the statistical software STATA v8.1 with natural log-transformed cyclin B1–specific serum reactivity, ln(Delta), as the outcome variable.

Age, sex, race, current smoking status, and lung function category were tested in univariate regression models for significance ($P \leq .05$). Multiple regression analyses were performed to determine the significance of variables after controlling for the effects of parameters found to be significant in univariate regression models. Variables found to be significant ($P \leq .05$) upon addition to the multivariable model were retained in the main effects model. Pair-wise interactions of variables in the main effects model were evaluated for significance ($P \leq .05$). Coefficient estimates, standard errors of coefficients, and the portion of total variance explained by the model (R^2) were recorded.

Samples were also stratified by sex, and univariate and multivariable linear regression analyses were performed for males and females separately using the procedures previously described.

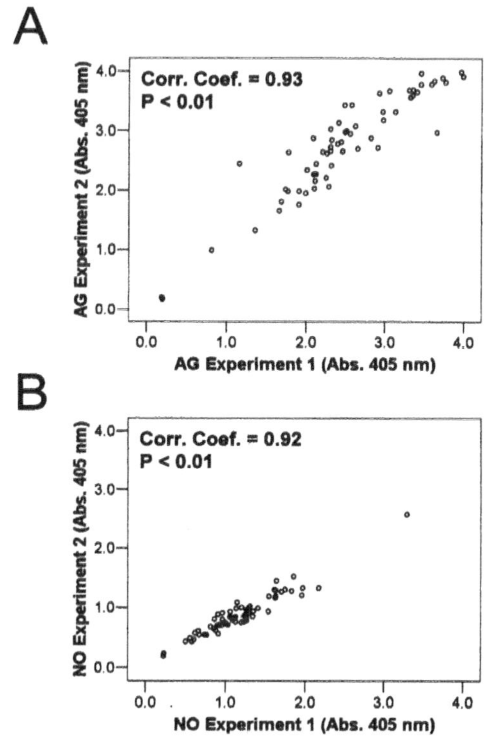

FIGURE 1. ELISA results using Velocity11 Vprep pipetting station were highly reproducible. Independent ELISAs to measure cyclin B1 reactivity in serum samples were performed using the Vprep. Means of triplicates for each sample are presented for (**A**) absorbance in wells containing cyclin B1 and (B) background reactivity from two independent experiments. Spearman's correlation coefficient and 2-tailed *P* value are given for each comparison. Sera were diluted 1:80 for these assays.

RESULTS AND DISCUSSION

Establishment of robotic ELISA platform

Serum samples were assayed by ELISA for cyclin B1–specific reactivity. Each sample served as its own control, and cyclin B1–specific reactivity for each sample was defined as reactivity in the presence of the cyclin B1 antigen minus the background reactivity in the absence of antigen. In ELISA experiments, including the addition of soluble competing cyclin B1 in varying quantities, serum cyclin B1 reactivity was titrated to approximately background levels (data not shown). Thus, the soluble cyclin B1–competable fraction of the serum cyclin B1 reactivity was the difference (Delta) between reactivity in the presence of cyclin B1 and reactivity in the absence of cyclin B1. Delta, therefore, was a measure of cyclin B1–specific serum reactivity, and was used to evaluate all subsequent experiments.

All sera were assayed for anticyclin B1 reactivity using a semi-automated, ELISA-based platform, the Velocity11 Vprep pipetting station. Procedures for sera dilution and ELISA assays using the Vprep pipetting station were highly reproducible, as illustrated in FIGURE 1. Spearman's nonparametric correlation coefficients for cyclin B1–specific and background ELISA results for independent experiments were greater than 0.92 (FIG. 1).

Anticyclin B1 Antibody Levels Are Elevated in Some PLuSS At-Risk Subjects

In order to define the distribution of anticyclin B1 serum reactivity in the at-risk PLuSS population and identify possible contributing factors, 365 at-risk PLuSS subjects were tested for serum reactivity to cyclin B1. Age, sex, current smoking status, and lung function stratum-specific sample numbers are indicated in TABLE 1. Cyclin

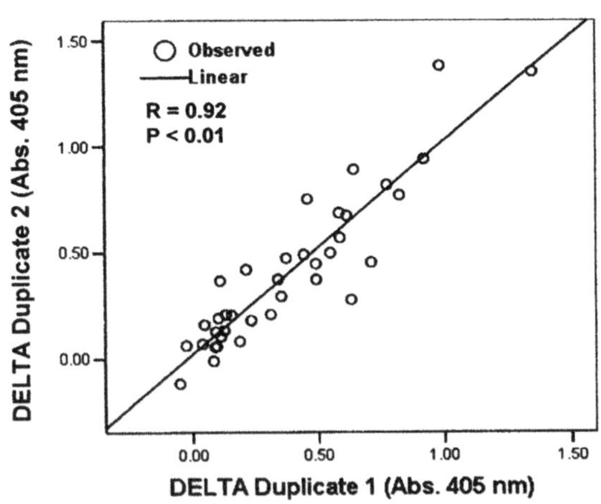

FIGURE 2. PLuSS stratified sample set internal duplicates indicate assay is reliable. Cyclin B1–specific ELISA assay results of internal duplicates (n = 37) are presented (○). Means of duplicate samples are presented. Linear regression of the data (Linear) produced a calculated regression coefficient of 0.918 ($R^2 = .84$).

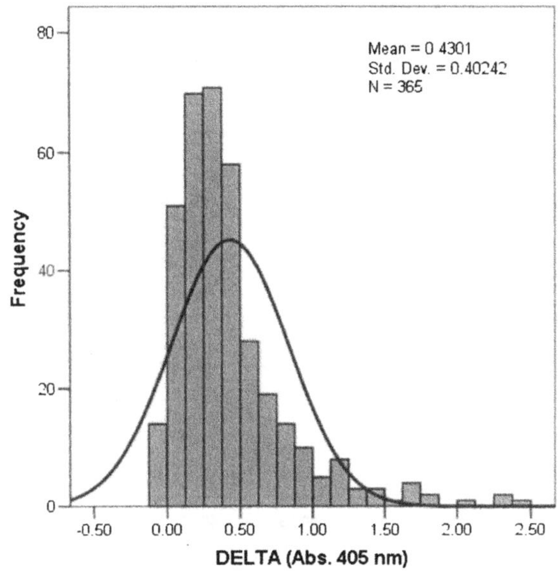

FIGURE 3. High levels of anticyclin B1 antibody are present in a minority of at-risk PLuSS subjects. Sera from the PLuSS stratified sample set were assessed for reactivity against recombinant cyclin B1 protein using ELISA. Histogram of cyclin B1–specific reactivity (Delta) is presented. Overlaid is the normal distribution curve.

B1 serum reactivity for samples in the PLuSS stratified set was evaluated using Velocity11 Vprep semiautomated ELISA protocols. Analysis of the duplicated samples distributed randomly throughout the sample set produced a linear regression coefficient of 0.92, indicating that the assay was robust to between plate variations (FIG. 2).

The distribution of reactivity to cyclin B1 in the PLuSS stratified sample set was skewed toward the higher values (FIG. 3). When stratified by age and sex, an increase in antibody levels in women, especially older women, was apparent (FIG. 4). Cyclin B1 reactivity in the majority of the PLuSS stratified sample is similar to the normal healthy and benign lung disease controls (Fig. 4). However, positive outliers were observed in every age by sex stratum.

All at-risk subjects in the PLuSS stratified sample were screened and found to be free of CT-detectable lung cancer. Therefore, the expected incidence of lung cancer cases among the PLuSS at-risk population is expected to be less than the incidence for unscreened individuals of similar age and with comparable smoking histories, and estimated to be 3 to 4 cases per year per 1000 subjects. For the at-risk stratified set of 365 samples, this translates into approximately 5 to 7 new lung cancer cases over the next 5 years. Positive outliers for cyclin B1 reactivity are apparent in the PLuSS at-risk sample set. Defining positive samples as those subjects with anticyclin B1 values greater than 2 SD above the combined normal and benign lung disease sample mean, 27 positive samples were identified. Defining positive samples as having anticyclin B1 values greater than 2 SD above the mean for each age by sex sub-

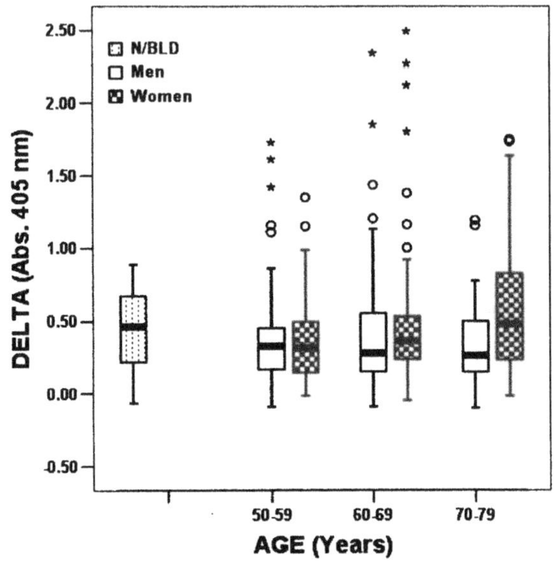

FIGURE 4. Anticyclin B1 antibody levels by age and sex. Cyclin B1 ELISA results of the PLuSS sera were grouped by subject age and sex. Age strata are as follows: (1) 50–59 years, (2) 60–69 years, and (3) 70–79 years. Medians, interquartile ranges (IQR), outliers (1.5–3 IQR, O), and extreme cases (>3 IQR, ∗) are indicated for age strata and sex. Range of reactivity for healthy and benign lung disease subject samples (N/BLD, $n = 8$) is indicated. Averages of duplicate cyclin B1–specific reactivity (Delta) are presented.

group, 19 positive samples were identified. Eighteen samples were defined as positive using both criteria. The specific criteria for defining clinically meaningful thresholds for the presence of antibodies are expected to be refined as more PLuSS samples are analyzed and as the availability of substantial numbers of age-matched, nonsmoking control subject sera increases. For our current purposes of examining the correlations between the presence/absence of cyclin B1–specific antibodies and lung cancer risk, these definitions suffice.

Regression Analysis Indicates Anticyclin B1 Antibody Levels Are Significantly Related to Sex

The PLuSS at-risk sample set was stratified by age, sex, and current smoking status and included white and nonwhite subjects, allowing the investigation of the relationships of these parameters with cyclin B1 serum reactivity. In all regression analyses, the natural log-transformation of cyclin B1–specific reactivity, Ln(Delta), was used as the outcome variable in order to produce models with normally distributed residuals. Univariate linear regression analyses indicated that only sex (P = .013) was significantly related to anticyclin B1 serum antibody levels and that age (P = .070) approached significance. Female sex and older age were associated with increased antibody levels. Race (P = .565), current smoking status (P = .153), and degree of airway restriction (P = .148) were not significant in univariate models. In a model containing sex and age, the significance of each parameter was nearly equal to the respective univariate model significance. An age-by-sex interaction parameter was significant ($P = .011$). Race, current smoking status, and lung function were all not significant after adjusting for age and sex effects.

Stratified Regression Analyses Indicate that Significantly Associated Factors Differ for Men and Women

Because evidence suggests that lung cancer risk factors and disease survival differ for men and women, a separate analysis for females and males was also performed.[1,3] The rationale for a stratified analysis by sex was also supported by the finding that sex was a significant parameter when modeling the full PLuSS stratified sample set.

When stratified by sex, age was significant only for females, and airway obstruction approached significance for females ($P = .056$) in univariate models (TABLE 2); increasing age and higher degree of airway obstruction were associated with increased antibody levels. After controlling for the effects of age, degree of airway obstruction approached significance for women ($P = .075$) (TABLE 2). Race and current smoking status were not significantly associated with anticyclin B1 antibody levels in women in univariate models or in models adjusted for age. Age, race, current smoking status, and degree of airway obstruction were all not significantly related to anticyclin B1 antibody levels in men (TABLE 2). For all models tested, the vari-

TABLE 2. Regression analysis of cyclin B1–specific serum reactivity stratified by sex[a]

Stratification	Female				Male			
Model Parameter(s)	Coefficient Estimate[b]	Standard Error[c]	P	R^{2d}	Coefficient Estimate	Standard Error	P	R^2
Age	0.0247	0.0074	.001	.056	–0.0072	0.0104	.486	.00
Racestratum[e]	–0.0159	0.1466	.913	.000	0.1534	0.2031	.451	.00
Smokenow[f]	0.1974	0.1229	.110	.014	0.0649	0.1568	.679	.00
Goldstratum[g]	0.2371	0.1234	.056	.014	0.0611	0.1563	.696	.00
Age	0.0263	0.0077	.001	.059	–0.0057	0.0107	.589	.00
Racestratum	0.1151	0.1477	.437		0.1280	0.2089	.541	
Age	0.0243	0.0074	.001	.067	–0.0079	0.0105	.449	.00
Smokenow	0.1822	0.1200	.131		0.0810	0.1584	.610	
Age	0.0240	0.0074	.001	.072	–0.0074	0.0104	.480	.00
Goldstratum	0.2159	0.1205	.075		0.0645	0.1566	.681	

[a]Linear regression analysis results using the natural log-transformed cyclin B1–specific serum reactivity as the dependent variable, ln(Delta), for females and males separately.

[b]Estimates for linear regression parameter coefficients.

[c]Standard errors of parameter coefficients.

[d]Proportion of variance explained by the model.

[e]White = 1; nonwhite = 2.

[f]Current smoker = 1; exsmoker = 2.

[g]Gold 0–I = 1; Gold I–II = 2.

ability explained by the models was small compared to the variability between subjects.

Anticyclin B1 antibody levels were found to be significantly higher for women than men, especially for older women. The effects of sex and age for women are also illustrated in FIGURE 4. This trend could be related to the general increase in antibodies found among older women that is not known to be related to cancer incidence. The nearly significant association of degree of airway obstruction with increased antibody levels only in women could also reflect this phenomenon. Airway obstruction is generally the result of airway injury and inflammatory responses.[20] It is likely that in older women especially the threshold for eliciting immune responses to tissue injury is decreased relative to men. This heightened immune response in women could manifest both as an immune response contributing to airway obstruction and increased antibody responses to aberrantly expressed cyclin B1 protein. The indications of an association between women and increased anticyclin B1 antibody levels, and age, and possibly airway obstruction, as factors associated with increased antibody levels only in women, is interesting in light of evidence that suggests that lung cancer susceptibility and survival rates differ for women and men.[1,3]

Race and current smoking status were not significantly associated with serum cyclin B1 reactivity in any of the models tested (TABLE 2). Twenty percent of our at-risk samples were from nonwhite subjects, therefore, our studies may have been underpowered to detect significant differences in cyclin B1 reactivity related to race. The lack of significant association of current smoking status and antibody levels suggests that cyclin B1 antibody responses are not an indicator of recent, general lung irritation, or injury. Further analysis will be required to investigate fully the relationships between serum antibody levels, these parameters, and the development of clinically detectable lung cancer.

Several hypotheses are to be tested using PLuSS samples, and the outcomes, though they will not be evident for several years, are expected to be of great interest. The first hypothesis is whether those participants with elevated cyclin B1–specific antibody but no CT-detectable lung cancer will develop lung cancer at higher rates than those with lower cyclin B1–specific antibody levels. A significant difference would suggest that tumor-specific antibodies signal the presence of cancer before the cancer has progressed sufficiently to be detected using current technologies. This would be of great utility given the importance of early detection to successful treatment. Another possible scenario is that the levels of tumor-specific antibodies are a measure of the strength of the immune response to a developing cancer. Elevated tumor-specific antibodies in this scenario would indicate a robust, responsive immune system, and therefore would be expected to correlate with increased longevity of a person diagnosed with lung cancer, reduced rate of disease recurrence, or reduced detectable cancer incidence in individuals without clinically detectable lung cancer. Only with this type of longitudinal study, which implements baseline blood collection, can one effectively address these hypotheses and analyze the predictive power of measurable biological markers.

SUMMARY

Successful cancer treatment relies on early detection. The immune system, which surveys the body, could respond to tumor antigens arising from altered host factors and provide an early readout for cancer presence. This study examines the immune response to tumor antigen cyclin B1. Unscheduled overexpression of this cell-cycle regulator occurs early in tumorigenesis and might be detected by the immune system long before clinical diagnosis of cancer is made. A stratified sample of PLuSS subjects without detectable cancers was analyzed for determinants of cyclin B1 antibody levels.

Cyclin B1 antibody levels were higher in some subjects from the PLuSS stratified at-risk sample compared to independently sampled healthy subjects, subjects with benign lung disease, and the majority of PLuSS subjects tested. Regression analysis of the PLuSS stratified serum samples identified sex as an important determinant of antibody levels, with women having generally higher titers of anticyclin B1 antibody than men. In women, but not men, age was significantly associated with cyclin B1–specific antibody levels, and degree of airway obstruction approached significance as a determinant of cyclin B1 antibody levels only in women. However, in all models presented, variability that could be attributed to all significant parameters was small relative to the amount of variability across subjects. This work represents an important step toward defining anticyclin B1 antibody levels for an at-risk population and assessing the predictive value of serum cyclin B1 antibody as it relates to lung cancer risk.

[*Competing interests*: The authors declare that they have no competing financial interests.]

REFERENCES

1. JEMAL, A., T. MURRAY, E. WARD, *et al.* 2005. Cancer statistics, 2005. CA: Cancer J. Clin. **55:** 10–30.
2. EZZATI, M. & A.D. LOPEZ. 2004. Regional, disease specific patterns of smoking-attributable mortality in 2000. Tob. Control **13:** 388–395.
3. FU, J B., T.Y. KAU, R.K. SEVERSON, *et al.* 2005. Lung cancer in women: analysis of the national Surveillance, Epidemiology, and End Results database. Chest **127:** 768–777.
4. HUMES, H.D. 2000. Kelley's Textbook of Internal Medicine. Lippincott Williams & Wilkins. Philadelphia.
5. CLUTE, P. & J. PINES. 1999. Temporal and spatial control of cyclin B1 destruction in metaphase. Nature Cell Biol. **1:** 82–87.
6. PORTER, L.A. & D.J. DONOGHUE. 2003. Cyclin B1 and CDK1: nuclear localization and upstream regulators. Prog. Cell Cycle Res. **5:** 335–347.
7. YOSHIDA, T., S. TANAKA, A. MOGI, *et al.* 2004. The clinical significance of Cyclin B1 and Wee1 expression in non-small-cell lung cancer. Ann. Oncol. **15:** 252–256.
8. TAKENO, S., T. NOGUCHI, R. KIKUCHI, *et al.* 2002. Prognostic value of cyclin B1 in patients with esophageal squamous cell carcinoma. Cancer **94:** 2874–2881.
9. ARINAGA, M., T. NOGUCHI, S. TAKENO, *et al.* 2003. Clinical implication of cyclin B1 in non-small cell lung cancer. Oncol. Rep. **10:** 1381–1386.
10. SORIA, J.C., S.J. JANG, F.R. KHURI, *et al.* 2000. Overexpression of cyclin B1 in early-stage non-small cell lung cancer and its clinical implication. Cancer Res. **60:** 4000-4004.
11. MURAKAMI, H., M. FURIHATA, Y. OHTSUKI, *et al.* 1999. Determination of the prognostic significance of cyclin B1 overexpression in patients with esophageal squamous cell carcinoma. Virchows Archiv. **434:** 153–158.
12. LI, J.Q., A. KUBO, F. WU, *et al.* 2003. Cyclin B1, unlike cyclin G1, increases significantly during colorectal carcinogenesis and during later metastasis to lymph nodes. Int. J. Oncol. **22:** 1101–1110.

13. INNOCENTE, S.A., J.L. ABRAHAMSON, J.P. COGSWELL, *et al.* 1999. p53 regulates a G2 checkpoint through cyclin B1. Proc. Natl. Acad. Sci. USA **96:** 2147–2152.
14. YU, M., Q. ZHAN & O.J. FINN. 2002. Immune recognition of cyclin B1 as a tumor antigen is a result of its overexpression in human tumors that is caused by non-functional p53. Mol. Immunol. **38:** 981–987.
15. KAO, H., J.A. MARTO, T.K. HOFFMANN, *et al.* 2001. Identification of cyclin B1 as a shared human epithelial tumor-associated antigen recognized by T cells. J. Exp. M. **194:** 1313–1323.
16. SUZUKI, H., D.F. GRAZIANO, J. MCKOLANIS, *et al.* 2005. T cell-dependent antibody responses against aberrantly expressed cyclin B1 protein in patients with cancer and premalignant disease. Clin. Cancer Res. **11:** 1521–1526.
17. KOZIOL, J.A., J.Y. ZHANG, C.A. CASIANO, *et al.* 2003. Recursive partitioning as an approach to selection of immune markers for tumor diagnosis. Clin. Cancer Res. **9:** 5120–5126.
18. COVINI, G., E.K. CHAN, M. NISHIOKA, *et al.* 1997. Immune response to cyclin B1 in hepatocellular carcinoma. Hepatology **25:** 75–80.
19. TOBIN, M.J. 2003. Chronic obstructive pulmonary disease, pollution, pulmonary vascular disease, transplantation, pleural disease, and lung cancer in AJRCCM 2002. Am. J.Respir Crit. Care Med. **167:** 356–370.
20. HOGG, J.C., F. CHU, S. UTOKAPARCH, *et al.* 2004. The nature of small-airway obstruction in chronic obstructive pulmonary disease.[see comment]. N. Engl. J. Med. **350:** 2645–2653.

Manipulating the Local Tumor Microenvironment with Poxviruses Expressing Costimulatory Molecules

HOWARD L. KAUFMAN

Departments of Surgery and Pathology, Columbia University, New York, New York 10032, USA

ABSTRACT: The identification of tumor-associated antigens and new insights into the molecular and cellular basis of tumor immunology have generated a variety of vaccine strategies. Although promising in animal models, data from early-phase clinical trials have not been encouraging. These studies have documented the ability of vaccines to prime T cells, but these responses have not correlated with therapeutic effectiveness. Because the location of T-cell activation and effector activity may impact T-cell function significantly, attention has been placed on the tumor microenvironment. There is now evidence that T-cell responses may be altered in the setting of established tumor growth. To alter the balance between local immune responses and tumor growth, a vaccine regimen using direct intratumoral delivery of poxvirus vaccines expressing co-stimulatory molecules was developed. An initial series of clinical trials has documented the safety profile of this approach and has suggested that local and systemic immunity can be induced. Herein, we review the general rationale for this approach, discuss the results of ongoing clinical trials, and highlight critical questions that can be addressed in well-designed preclinical and clinical studies.

KEYWORDS: costimulation; immunotherapy; poxviruses; vaccines; tumor microenvironment

INTRODUCTION

The promise of developing vaccines for the treatment or prevention of cancer has been recognized for many years. Significant advances have been made toward achieving this goal through the identification of tumor-associated antigens, a better understanding of how tumors are recognized and rejected, and the generation of relevant murine models to rapidly study vaccine candidates. Despite these advances, clinical trials have yielded disappointing results when vaccines have been evaluated, although many of these studies have targeted patients with advanced disease.[1] Nonetheless, many clinical trials have reported the induction of antigen-specific T-cell

Address for correspondence: Howard Kaufman, M.D., Columbia University Medical Center, 177 Fort Washington Avenue, MHB 7SK, New York, NY 10032. Voice: 212-342-6042; fax 212-342-0234.

hlk2003@columbia.edu

Ann. N.Y. Acad. Sci. 1062: 41–50 (2005).
doi: 10.1196/annals.1358.007

responses after vaccination, even if these responses have not correlated with objective clinical responses.[2] The ability to identify specific T cells through tetramer and fluorescence-activated cell sorting (FACS) analysis has provided a powerful tool for monitoring vaccine-induced T cells over time. These studies now suggest that even when robust T-cell responses are present, the cells may be ineffective once they enter the local tumor microenvironment.[3] The dampening of immunity within the local microenvironment represents an important mechanism for survival by established tumors.

The molecular mechanisms through which tumors suppress T-cell responses are not completely known and may include several distinct pathways. In contrast to viral infections, characterized by the production of local proinflammatory cytokines, tumors do not always exhibit signs of acute inflammation.[4] The lack of production of specific immunomodulatory molecules by tumor cells or surrounding stromal components may help maintain a locally suppressive environment for T-cell activation and effector function. Although our understanding of the causes for local immunosuppression in cancer are incomplete, there are already a variety of strategies that are targeting the local tumor microenvironment in an attempt to shift the balance back in favor of effective immune responses (TABLE 1). To address this, our group has concentrated on the development of poxviruses as vectors for local delivery of immunomodulatory molecules. The potential for poxvirus-mediated inflammation and the ability to express multiple eukaryotic genes makes these viruses ideal vectors for gene delivery and activation of local host immunity. Herein, we will discuss the rationale for local vaccination with poxvirus vectors, with an emphasis on the delivery of costimulatory molecules.

POXVIRUSES IN VACCINE DEVELOPMENT

Poxviruses are among the largest known mammalian viruses and are composed of a linear double-stranded DNA backbone surrounded by a complex envelope. The initial classification of the poxviruses was based on their host range and morphology, and later updated by results of DNA restriction mapping. The most widely studied poxvirus is vaccinia virus, used for smallpox prevention, and unique among poxviruses in that it exhibits a broad host range. Vaccinia virus is a minor human pathogen, and vaccination with vaccinia is associated with a low incidence of skin and central nervous system manifestations, generally restricted to immunocompromised hosts. The mechanisms underlying the host antivaccinia immune response have been the subject of intense investigation, and the virus can induce both neutralizing antibody titers as well as vaccinia-specific T-cell responses.[5]

Vaccinia virus can be used as an expression vector for both prokaryotic and eukaryotic genes.[6] In contrast to retroviruses and other small viruses, vaccinia virus can accommodate large DNA fragments without disrupting viral replication or gene expression. An additional advantage of vaccinia virus is that the life cycle of the virus is confined to the cytoplasm of infected cells and there is no risk of nuclear integration or cell transformation. Recombinant viruses are usually stable and have been shown to generate humoral and cellular immune responses against foreign transgene products.[7] The molecular approach to constructing recombinant vaccinia vectors has been well established.[8] The first poxviruses expressing human tumor-associated

TABLE 1. Selected immunomodulatory molecules for local tumor treatment

Class	Molecule	Reference
Cytokines	Interleukin-2	42
	GM-CSF	40
	Anti-IL-10 antibody	43
Chemokines	CCL16 (MCP-1)	44
	CCL21 (SLC)	45
Costimulatory molecules	B7.1	37
	B7.1, ICAM-1, and LFA-3 (TRICOM)	39
Toll-like receptor agonists	Imiquimod	46
	CpG	43
Viruses	Vaccinia virus	37,38
	Fowlpox virus	41
	Adenovirus	47
Radiation	Fractionated external beam therapy	48

antigens were reported around 1990 and included vectors expressing the p97 melanoma antigen and the carcinoembryonic antigen (CEA), with evidence that these vaccines could induce antigen-specific immunity and therapeutic responses in animal models.[9–11]

Based on the results of animal studies, several clinical trials were conducted using vaccinia virus vectors expressing tumor-associated antigens, such as CEA and prostate-specific antigen (PSA). Collectively, these trials demonstrated that vaccination was well tolerated, induced low-level T-cell responses in a minority of patients, and had little therapeutic benefit.[12–14] The reasons for the lack of clinical effect could be related to the low immunogenicity of the vaccine, the development of strong neutralizing antibody titers against the virus, the advanced stage of disease, and the presence of host immunosuppressive factors. The immunogenicity of the virus and generation of neutralizing antibodies have been addressed through the development of vaccines employing nonreplicating poxviruses, the use of heterologous prime-boost schedules, and the inclusion of potent immunomodulatory molecules as adjuvants to vaccination. The selection of appropriate patients for vaccination and overcoming host immunosuppression are the subject of ongoing investigation.

Whereas strong antibody titers are helpful for viral clearance, the rapid containment of viral replication may preclude effective immunity against foreign transgenes encoding weak antigens, such as tumor-associated antigens.[15,16] Because the appearance of antibodies depends on viral replication, nonreplicating poxvirus vectors have been developed. These vectors induce abortive infection of permissive cells, resulting in prolonged transgene expression and lower antibody titers.[17] There are two general classes of nonreplicating poxviruses that have been used for recombinant vaccine development: the avipoxviruses, including fowlpox virus and canarypoxvirus (ALVAC); and attenuated vaccinia viruses, such as NYVAC and modified vaccinia Ankara (MVA).[18] Similar to vaccinia virus, these vectors have been tested for safety in phase I clinical trials and appear to be well tolerated. Interestingly, both animal studies and early-phase clinical trials support the use of a heterologous prime-boost treatment schedule using vaccinia virus priming, followed by booster vaccinations with nonreplicating poxviruses.[19,20] The mechanism underlying this effect is not clear, and further research is needed to understand this and optimize the selection of the most appropriate vectors for clinical use.

The immunogenicity of poxviruses can also be altered by the expression of additional genes that influence the type or quality of immune response. This has been documented by coexpression of surrogate tumor antigens with defined cytokines and chemokines.[21] For example, we have reported previously that vaccinia viruses expressing murine interleukin-2 (IL-2) and IL-12 induced significantly better antitumor responses in mice compared with the same viruses without cytokines.[21] Others have demonstrated improved response using poxviruses expressing granulocyte-macrophage colony-stimulating factor (GM-CSF), and the combination of poxvirus vaccines and adjuvant recombinant cytokine treatment is now in clinical trials.[22,23] In addition to cytokines, a number of other immunomodulatory molecules are available for enhancing the immunogenicity of poxvirus vaccines (see TABLE 1).

COSTIMULATORY MOLECULES

Activation of naive T cells requires an antigen-dependent signal provided by T-cell receptor (TCR) recognition of cognate peptide bound to MHC complexes on antigen-presenting cells (APCs) and target cells. This signal alone is not sufficient for cell activation and may target such T cells for tolerance. To initiate T-cell activation, a second antigen-independent signal is required. These costimulatory signals are provided by a series of cell-surface expressed molecules on APCs that bind to defined ligands on the surface of T cells and mediate cell-cycle progression and cytokine production. Following activation of T cells, additional ligands are recruited to the cell surface, where they mediate cell-cycle arrest and downregulate T-cell activation. The costimulatory system thus acts as a type of rheostat to regulate the control of T-cell function.

B7.1 (C80), one of the best-characterized costimulatory molecules, is expressed on professional APCs, and binds to CD28 and CTLA-4 on T cells. In the setting of TCR engagement, CD28 signaling provides a positive stimulatory signal to responding T cells, resulting in proliferation and IL-2 secretion, whereas CTLA-4 exerts a negative regulatory signal.[24,25] Tumors may evade detection by T cells in part through downregulating costimulatory molecule expression.[26,27] Replacing the missing molecules has been shown to restore T-cell recognition and immune-mediated tumor clearance in animal models.[28] This system has also been manipulated to enhance immunogenicity by coexpressing B7.1 with defined tumor antigens, with improved therapeutic responses in murine models.[28,29] The availability of multiple costimulatory molecules has also led to the generation of viral constructs expressing multiple costimulatory molecules. Vaccinia and fowlpox viruses were used to express CEA with a triad of costimulatory molecules (TRICOM) consisting of B7.1, intercellular adhesion molecule 1 (ICAM-1), and lymphocyte function associated antigen 3 (LFA-3), which proved to be superior in priming T cells *in vitro* and inducing tumor regression in normal and CEA transgenic mice.[30–32]

Based on these preliminary results, vaccinia viruses expressing human B7.1 and the three TRICOM costimulatory molecules were generated. Because tumor antigens may not always be defined and may be modulated during tumor progression, we sought to evaluate these vectors as intratumoral vaccines, whereby autologous tumors would be able to present endogenous antigen in the context of high levels of costimulatory molecule expression. Our clinical investigation focused on malignant melanoma, as these tumors often are characterized by the presence of infiltrating T lymphocytes and are readily accessible for vaccination. Furthermore, vaccinia virus provides additional danger signals and induces a proinflammatory environment at the site of injection. The lytic nature of vaccinia infection might also result in cross-presentation of melanoma antigens, further augmenting the antitumor immune response. To test these hypotheses, we proposed a series of sequential phase I clinical trials to evaluate the local effects of vaccinia virus expressing B7.1 or TRICOM in patients with metastatic melanoma. The studies were designed to evaluate both the effects of local vaccination and the influence of local administration on systemic immunity.

MEASURING THE EFFECTS OF INTRATUMORAL VACCINATION

Although local vaccination is feasible in the clinic, it is important to monitor immune response at the site of vaccine administration, as well as the systemic components of the antitumor immune response. This measurement depends on validated assays for profiling and monitoring the molecular and cellular changes within the tumor microenvironment and in systemic compartments. This is challenging, because repeated biopsy procedures could influence the natural history of individual lesions and could preclude an accurate picture of the host-immune interaction within individual lesions. Fine-needle aspiration of lesions over time provides a method for collecting small samples of tissue for study, and can be used to extract RNA for serial gene-expression profiling to monitor response to treatment. This technique is complicated by the limited amount of RNA, but can be overcome by amplification methods that allow sufficient material for quantitative reverse transcription polymerase chain reaction (RT-PCR) or cDNA gene array.[33] This technique has been used by others who have reported a correlation between genetic profiles and clinical responses to immunotherapy.[34,35] In these studies several specific cytokines and pro-inflammatory mediators involved in T-cell recognition, monocyte function, and chemoattraction of specific effector cells were increased in melanoma lesions from patients responding to immunotherapy. These studies suggested that immune responsiveness might be predetermined by favorable changes in the tumor microenvironment.

Although genetic profiling and quantitative PCR technology can help us to understand changes at the molecular level within tumors, evidence of systemic immunity is complicated by the lack of defined antigens in this system. Circulating antibody titers and T-cell responses to vaccinia virus can be used to determine the extent of systemic vaccination, but assaying antitumor immunity requires the generation of autologous tumor cells or the use of known melanoma antigens. Because we did not want to disrupt established lesions, we collected peripheral blood lymphocytes (PBLs) and adopted an interferon-γ ELISPOT assay using two common melanoma antigens, gp100 and Melan-A/MART-1. This assay has been validated in previous clinical trials and has been useful for monitoring systemic immune responses in vaccine trials.[36]

CURRENT CLINICAL TRIAL RESULTS

A standard dose-escalation phase I clinical trial of recombinant vaccinia virus expressing B7.1 (rV-B7.1) was initiated in patients with unresectable metastatic melanoma.[37] The trial enrolled 12 patients at two vaccine doses. Patients were treated with monthly injections of vaccine into accessible cutaneous, subcutaneous, or lymph node tumor lesions over three months. Before the first vaccine administration, blood was collected for baseline immune evaluation and toxicity studies. Additional blood was collected two weeks after each vaccination. In addition, before each vaccine administration fine-needle aspirates of the tumor were collected for RNA isolation and PCR analysis. The results of this trial have been published elsewhere.[38] The approach was found to be well tolerated with only low-grade injection-site reactions and fatigue/myalgia reported. Three patients developed vitiligo, and there were two objective clinical responses. Evidence of systemic immunity was documented by an increase in gp100– and Melan-A–specific T cells after vaccination. All patients developed antivaccinia antibody titers and vaccinia-specific T cells. Local tumor immunity was monitored by quantitative real-time PCR, and we observed an association between local interferon-γ and clinical responses, although the sample size was too small to make meaningful conclusions.

A separate dose-escalation phase I clinical trial using vaccinia virus expressing TRICOM (rV-TRICOM) has recently completed enrollment.[39] The results from this trial are similar to those of the rV-B7.1 trial, with the same safety profile and objective clinical response rate. The reasons for this are not entirely clear, based on the preclinical data with these vectors, but the trials were not randomized and so direct comparisons cannot be made.

CRITICAL QUESTIONS

The completion of two clinical trials employing intratumoral vaccination of a vaccinia virus expressing B7.1 or a triad of costimulatory molecules (TRICOM) has yielded intriguing results, suggesting that this approach can induce meaningful clinical responses. Although these studies were designed to evaluate safety and feasibility, the induction of local and systemic immunity coupled with objective clinical responses suggest this may be a powerful strategy for tumor immunotherapy. These studies, however, raise a number of interesting questions. First, the role of antigen in this system is not clear, because antigen-specific immune responses could be detected in PBL samples but no antigen was present in the vaccine. Although it is likely that autologous tumor cells expressing melanoma-associated antigens were the source of antigen in these responses, there is murine data suggesting that intratumoral vaccination with antigen-expressing poxviruses can enhance the therapeutic benefit of this approach.[40] Second, the role of virus in this system is not well defined, although every patient was able to mount an immune response against vaccinia virus. We plan to address the possibility that nonreplicating vectors may be better by a randomized trial comparing recombinant fowlpox viruses expressing B7.1 or TRICOM.[41] Animal data further support the superiority of using a vaccinia prime and fowlpox virus boost strategy that has yet to be tested directly in the clinic.[40] Third, these trials employed direct intratumoral vaccination without prior systemic immunization. This assumes that there is already an established local T-cell response that can be enhanced by local vaccination, or that naive T cells can be primed at the tumor site or in regional draining nodal basins. These possibilities require further investigation, but animal experiments suggest that therapeutic responses are maximal when systemic vaccination precedes local vaccination.[40] The role of adjuvant cytokines and other immunomodulatory molecules also was not addressed in this study; these molecules may be useful for further augmenting both clinical and immunological responses. Finally, the use of local aspirates for molecular monitoring was validated in these studies, but the question of which markers to follow remains unanswered. At present, there are many biomarkers that could be selected for monitoring local and systemic antitumor immunity.

CONCLUSIONS

Vaccines for the immunotherapy of cancer have shown promise in animal models, but no therapeutic benefit has been seen in clinical trials. Although vaccination can initiate antigen-specific T-cell responses, the stimulated T cells have not been documented to find local sites of tumor growth or to mediate tumor regression. Evaluation of the local tumor microenvironment has suggested that tumor-reactive T cells may be present, but become tolerized and are unable to mediate effector function due to tumor and host suppressive factors. The loss of costimulatory molecule expression at the site of tumor growth may be one mechanism that limits local T-cell activity. To provide potent costimulatory signals we have evaluated vaccinia virus vectors expressing B7.1 or a triad of costimulatory molecules (TRICOM) as a direct intratumoral vaccine in patients with metastatic melanoma. The approach was feasible with an acceptable safety profile. There was evidence of both local and systemic immune responses, although the exact mechanism of this immune response could not be elucidated in these trials. Of note was the regression of tumor in some patients, suggesting potential clinical activity. These results support further investigation of local vaccination strategies as a general method for targeting the tumor microenvironment to overcome host immunosuppression. Unresolved issues relating the role of antigen, viral vectors, optimal immunomodulatory adjuvants, prime-boost schedules, and sequencing of systemic and local vaccination will be important for future clinical trial design.

ACKNOWLEDGMENTS

This work was supported by grants RO1 093696 from the NIH, T98052 from the Doris Duke Charitable Foundation, and The Dana Foundation.

[*Competing interests*: The authors declare that they have no competing financial interests.]

REFERENCES

1. ROSENBERG, S.A., J.C. YANG & N.P. RESTIFO. 2004. Cancer immunotherapy: moving beyond current vaccines. Nature Med. **10:** 909–915.
2. DISIS, M.L., T.A. GOOLEY, K. RINN, *et al.* 2002. Generation of T-cell immunity to the HER-2/neu protein after active immunization with HER-2/neu peptide-based vaccines. J. Clin. Oncol. **20:** 2624–2632.
3. ZIPPELIUS, A., P. BATARD, V. RUBIO-GODOY, *et al.* 2004. Effector function of human tumor-specific CD8 T cells in melanoma lesions: a state of local functional tolerance. Cancer Res. **64:** 2865–2873.
4. BALKWILL, F., K.A. CHARLES & A. MANTOVANI. 2005. Smoldering and polarized inflammation in the initiation and promotion of malignant disease. Cancer Cell **7:** 211–217.
5. BELYAKOV, I.M., P. EARL, A. DZUTSEV, *et al.* 2003. Shared modes of protection against poxvirus infection by attenuated and conventional smallpox vaccine viruses. Proc. Natl. Acad. Sci. USA **100:** 9458–9463.
6. PANICALI, D. & E. PAOLETTI. 1982. Construction of poxviruses as cloning vectors: insertion of the thymidine kinase gene from herpes simplex virus into the DNA of infectious vaccinia virus. Proc. Natl. Acad. Sci. USA **79:** 4927–4931.
7. MOSS,. B. 1996. Genetically engineered poxviruses for recombinant gene expression, vaccination, and safety. Proc. Natl. Acad. Sci. USA **93:** 11341–11348.
8. MACKETT, M., G.L. SMITH & B. MOSS. 1984. General method for production and selection of infectious vaccinia virus recombinants expressing foreign genes. J. Virol. **49:** 857–864.
9. ESTIN, C.D., U.S. STEVENSEN, G.D. PLOWMAN, *et al.* 1988. Recombinant vaccinia virus vaccine against the human melanoma antigen p97 for use in immunotherapy. Proc. Natl. Acad. Sci. USA **85:** 1052–1056.
10. KAUFMAN, H.L., J. KANTOR & J.A. SCHLOM. 1991. A recombinant vaccinia virus expressing human carcinoembryonic antigen (CEA). Int. J. Cancer **48:** 900–907.
11. Kantor, J., K. Irvine, S. Abrams, *et al.* 1992. Anti-tumor activity and immune responses induced by a recombinant vaccinia-carcinoembryonic antigen (CEA) vaccine. J. Natl. Cancer Inst. **84:** 1084–1091.
12. MARSHALL, J. 2003. Carcinoembryonic antigen-based vaccines. Semin. Oncol. **30:** 30–36.
13. ZHU, M.Z., J. MARSHALL, D. COLE, *et al.* 2000. Specific cytolytic T-cell responses to human CEA from patients immunized with recombinant avipox-CEA vaccine. Clin. Cancer Res. **6:** 24–33.
14. EDER, J.P., P.W. KANTOFF, K. ROPER, *et al.* 2000. A phase I trial of a recombinant vaccinia virus expressing prostate-specific antigen in advanced prostate cancer. Clin. Cancer Res. **6:** 1632–1638.
15. BACHMANN, M.F., U.H. ROHRER, U. STEINHOFF, *et al.* 1994. T Helper cell unresponsiveness: rapid induction in antigen-transgenic and reversion in non-transgenic mice. Eur. J. Immunol. **24:** 2966–2973.
16. MCELRATH, M.J., L. COREY, D. BERGER, *et al.* 1994. Immune responses elicited by recombinant vaccinia-human immunodeficiency virus (HIV) envelope and HIV envelope protein: analysis of the durability of responses and effect of repeated boosting. J. Infect. Dis. **169:** 41–47.
17. PAOLETTI, E. 1996. Applications of pox virus vectors to vaccination: an update. Proc. Natl. Acad. Sci. USA **93:** 11349–11353.
18. ANTOINE, G., F. SCHEIFLINGER, F. DORNER & F.G. FALKNER. 1998. The complete genomic sequence of the modified vaccinia Ankara strain: comparison with other orthopoxviruses. Virology **244:** 365–396.

19. HODGE, J.W., J.P. MCLAUGHLIN, J.A. KANTOR & J. SCHLOM. 1997. Diversified prime and boost protocols using recombinant vaccinia virus and recombinant non-replicating avian pox virus to enhance T-cell immunity and antitumor responses. Vaccine **15:** 759–768.
20. MARSHALL, J.L., R.J. HOYER, M.A. TOOMEY, *et al.* 2000. Phase I study in advanced cancer patients of a diversified prime-and-boost vaccination protocol using recombinant vaccinia virus and recombinant nonreplicating avipox virus to elicit anti-carcinoembryonic antigen immune responses. J. Clin. Oncol. **18:** 3964–3973.
21. KAUFMAN, H.L., K. FLANAGAN, C.S. LEE, *et al.* 2002. Insertion of interleukin-2 (IL-2) and interleukin-12 (IL-12) genes into vaccinia virus results in effective anti-tumor responses without toxicity. Vaccine **20:** 1862–1869.
22. AARTS, W.M., J. SCHLOM & J.W. HODGE. 2002. Vector-based vaccine/cytokine combination therapy to enhance induction of immune responses to a self-antigen and antitumor activity. Cancer Res. **62:** 5770–5777.
23. ROCHLITZ, C., R. FIGLIN, P. SQUIBAN, *et al.* 2003. Phase I immunotherapy with a modified vaccinia virus (MVA) expressing human MUC1 as antigen-specific immunotherapy in patients with MUC1-positive advanced cancer. J. Gene Med. **5:** 690–699.
24. CARRENO, B.M. & M. COLLINS. 2002. The B7 family of ligands and its receptors: new pathways for costimulation and inhibition of immune responses. Annu. Rev. Immunol. **20:** 29–53.
25. ALEGRE, M.L., K.A. FRAUWIRTH & C.B. THOMPSON. 2001. T-cell regulation by CD28 and CTLA-4. Nat. Rev. Immunol. **1:** 220–228.
26. DUNN, G.P., A.T. BRUCE, H. IKEDA, *et al.* 2002. Cancer immunoediting: from immunosurveillance to tumor escape. Nat. Immunol. **3:** 991–998.
27. OCHSENBEIN, A.F. 2002. Principles of tumor immunosurveillance and implications for immunotherapy. Cancer Gene Ther. **9:** 1043–1055.
28. TOWNSEND, S.E. & J.P. ALLISON. 1993. Tumor rejection after direct costimulation of CD8+ T cells by B7-transfected melanoma cells. Science **259:** 368–370.
29. CHEN, L., S. ASHE, W.A. BRADY, *et al.* 1992. Costimulation of antitumor immunity by the B7 counterreceptor for the T lymphocyte molecules CD28 and CTLA-4. Cell **71:** 1093–1102.
30. HODGE, J.W., H. SABZEVARI, A.G. YAFAL, *et al.* 1999. A triad of costimulatory molecules synergize to amplify T-cell activation. Cancer Res. **59:** 5800–5807.
31. GROSENBACH, D.W., J.C. BARRIENTOS, J. SCHLOM & J.W. HODGE. 2001. Synergy of vaccine strategies to amplify antigen-specific immune responses and antitumor effects. Cancer Res. **61:** 4497–4505.
32. HODGE, J.W., A.N. RAD, D.W. GROSENBACH, *et al.* 2000. Enhanced activation of T cells by dendritic cells engineered to hyperexpress a triad of costimulatory molecules. J. Natl. Cancer Inst. **92:** 1228–1239.
33. WANG, E., L.D. MILLER, G.A. OHNMACHT, *et al.* 2000. High-fidelity mRNA amplification for gene profiling. Nat. Biotechnol. **18:** 457–459.
34. WANG, E., L.D. MILLER, G.A. OHNMACHT, *et al.* 2002. Prospective molecular profiling of melanoma metastases suggests classifiers of immune responsiveness. Cancer Res. **62:** 3581–3586.
35. PANELLI, M.C., E. WANG, G. PHAN, *et al.* 2002. Gene-expression profiling of the response of peripheral blood mononuclear cells and melanoma metastases to systemic IL-2 administration. Genome Biol. **3:** RESEARCH0035.
36. KEILHOLZ, U., J. WEBER, J.H. FINKE, *et al.* 2002. Immunologic monitoring of cancer vaccine therapy: results of a workshop sponsored by the Society for Biological Therapy. J. Immunother. **25:** 97–138.
37. KAUFMAN, H.L., W. CONKRIGHT, J. DIVITO, *et al.* 2000. A phase I trial of intra-lesional rV-B7.1 vaccine in the treatment of malignant melanoma. Human Gene Ther. **11:** 1065–1082.
38. KAUFMAN, H.L., G. DERAFFELE, J. MITCHAM, *et al.* 2005. Targeting the local tumor microenvironment by vaccinia virus expressing B7.1 for the treatment of melanoma. J. Clin. Invest. **115:** 1903–1912.

39. KAUFMAN, H.L., G. DERAFFELE, J. DIVITO, *et al.* 2001. A phase I trial of intra-lesional rV-TRICOM vaccine in the treatment of malignant melanoma. Human Gene Ther. **12:** 1459–1480.
40. KUDO-SAITO, C., J. SCHLOM & J.W. HODGE. 2004. Intratumoral vaccination with diversified subcutaneous/intratumoral vaccination with recombinant poxviruses encoding a tumor antigen and multiple costimulatory molecules. Clin. Cancer Res. **10:** 1090–1099.
41. KAUFMAN, H.L., K. CHEUNG, Z. HASKALL, *et al.* 2003. Intra-lesional rF-B7.1 versus rF-TRICOM vaccine in the treatment of metastatic cancer. Human Gene Ther. **14:** 803–827.
42. RADNY, P., U.M. CAROLI, J. BAUER, *et al.* 2003. Phase II trial of intralesional therapy with interleukin-2 in soft-tissue melanoma metastases. Br. J. Cancer **89:** 1620–1626.
43. GUIDUCCI, C., A.P. VICARI, S. SANGALETTI, *et al.* 2005. Redirecting *in vivo* elicited tumor infiltrating macrophages and dendritic cells towards tumor rejection. Cancer Res. **65:** 3437–3446.
44. TSUCHIYAMA, T., S. KANEKO, Y. T.NAKAMOTO, *et al.* 2003. Enhanced antitumor effects of a bicistronic adenovirus vector expressing both herpes simplex virus thymidine kinase and monocyte chemoattractant protein-1 against hepatocellular carcinoma. Cancer Gene Ther. **10:** 260–269.
45. FLANAGAN, K., R.T. GLOVER, H. HORIG & H.L. KAUFMAN. 2004. Local delivery of recombinant vaccinia virus expressing secondary lymphoid chemokine (SLC) results in a CD4+ T cell dependent antitumor response. Vaccine **22:** 2894–2903.
46. POWELL, A.M., R. RUSSELL-JONES & R.J. BARLOW. 2004. Topical imiquimod immunotherapy in the management of lentigo maligna. Clin. Exp. Dermatol. **29:** 15–21.
47. YANG, S.C., S. HILLINGER, K. RIEDL, *et al.* 2004. Intratumoral administration of dendritic cells overexpressing CCL21 generates systemic antitumor responses and confers tumor immunity. Clin. Cancer Res. **10:** 2891–2901.
48. CHAKRABORTY, M., S.I. ABRAMS, C.N. COLEMAN, *et al.* 2004. External beam radiation of tumors alters phenotype of tumor cells to render them susceptible to vaccine-mediated T-cell killing. Cancer Res. **64:** 4328–4337.

CD154 Gene Therapy for Human B-Cell Malignancies

DAVORKA MESSMER AND THOMAS J. KIPPS

Moores Cancer Center, University of California, San Diego, La Jolla, California 92093, USA

ABSTRACT: Patients with chronic lymphocytic leukemia cells (CLL) who received a one-time bolus infusion of autologous leukemia cells transduced with adenovirus encoding recombinant CD154 experienced acute and long-term reductions in leukemia cell counts and lymph-node size. This was associated with increases in the numbers of leukemia-specific CD4$^+$ T cells and high serum-levels of IL-12 and IFN-γ. CD40-ligation induces CLL cells to express the proapoptotic molecule Bid and death receptors CD95 (Fas) and DR5, rendering CLL B cells first resistant and then sensitive to Fas-mediated apoptosis. Increasing sensitivity to Fas-mediated apoptosis was also due to differential expression of pro- and antiapoptotic proteins at early versus late time points after activation. Additional treatment with inhibitors to the X-linked inhibitor to apoptosis (XIAP) rendered the CD40-activated cells sensitive to Fas-mediated apoptosis even at early time points after CD40-activation, suggesting that XIAP inhibitors might enhance the effectiveness of CD154-based immune-gene therapy strategies for patients of B-cell malignancies.

KEYWORDS: leukemia; antigen presentation; immune activation; gene therapy

INTRODUCTION

Tumor immunotherapy harnesses the immune system to kill tumor cells. The premise of this approach is that immune-targeted tumor killing can be achieved without effecting healthy cells. Tumor immunotherapy encompasses passive immunotherapy as well as active immunotherapy, such as that used in tumor vaccines.

Passive immunotherapy involves transfer of monoclonal antibodies to patients. It is passive in that it does not require the patient to elicit an immune response against tumor-associated antigens (TAAs). Rather this approach relies on the use of monoclonal antibodies that recognize antigens that distinguish normal from malignant tissue or that react with differentiation antigens found only on the tumor cells and the normal cells from which they arise. Though truly tumor-specific antigens are rare, differentiation antigens commonly are expressed by tumor cells, providing targets for monoclonal antibodies that can be used in immune therapy. This is particularly the case when such antigens are expressed only on cells that are not vital to the pa-

Address for correspondence: Thomas J. Kipps, Moores Cancer Center, University of California San Diego, 3855 Health Science Dr., Number 0820, La Jolla CA 92093-0820. Voice: 858-534-4500, Fax: 858-534-5620.

tkipps@ucsd.edu

Ann. N.Y. Acad. Sci. 1062: 51–60 (2005). © 2005 New York Academy of Sciences.
doi: 10.1196/annals.1358.008

tient at the time of therapy or that are overexpressed by the tumor cells relative to that found on their presumed normal cell counterparts. Such monoclonal antibodies are relatively well tolerated and therapeutically effective. Chimeric and humanized monoclonal antibodies directed against TAAs have shown activity as monotherapy in the treatment of hematological malignancies and have been used as important adjuvants to improve the activity of standard anticancer drug therapy.[1,2]

Active immunotherapy requires the patient to elicit an immune response against TAA expressed by the tumor cell. TAAs provide the basis for antigen-specific vaccines in the form of protein, peptides, or DNA, generally used in conjunction with an adjuvant to bolster the immune response against TAAs, which typically are only weakly antigenic.

There are several limitations associated with active immunotherapy: (1) Truly tumor-specific TAAs have not been identified for most tumors, requiring the use of tumor-cell lysates or whole tumor cells as a vaccine; (2) cancer patients, in particular those with lymphoid leukemias or lymphomas, generally have impaired immune systems and respond weakly even to conventional vaccines; (3) although tumors may be eliminated by immune surveillance,[3,4] most clinically detectable tumors actually are found to induce immune tolerance to their TAAs.[5–7] One of the major challenges for tumor immunotherapeutic approaches is to break this immune tolerance for tumor cells so as to elicit immune responses that are therapeutically effective.[6]

Strategies to overcome immune tolerance to TAAs must cause the activation of antigen-presenting cells (APCs) to states in which they induce potent antitumor immune responses. While earlier approaches involved mixing tumor cells with strong adjuvants, such as *bacillus Calmette-Guerin* or *Corneabacterium parvum*, more recent approaches have involved transduction of tumor cells with genes encoding molecules that can stimulate the immune response. These genes include major histocompatibility complex (MHC) genes, cytokine genes, or genes encoding membrane-associated immune costimulatory molecules, such as CD80. The central premise of these approaches is that conversion of tumor cells into APCs will enable them to induce antitumor immune responses.

In the case of B-cell chronic lymphocytic leukemia (CLL), the tumor cell is derived from cells that can function as APCs. However, CLL cells are very ineffective APCs despite expressing high levels of class I and class II molecules of the major histocompatibility complex. This poor APC-function is underscored by the observation that CLL B cells are ineffective even at stimulating normal allogeneic T cells in mixed lymphocyte reactions.[8,9] The poor APC activity of CLL cells has been attributed in part to the fact that they lack expression of important immune costimulatory molecules, such as CD80 and CD86, that are critical for effective T-cell activation.[10–12]

The poor APC activity of CLL cells can be reversed via CD40-ligation. CD40–CD40 ligand (CD154) interactions play a critical role in immune activation. CD40-ligand (CD154) is a member of the tumor necrosis factor (TNF) family of ligands and class II membrane glycoproteins.[13–16] CD154 is expressed transiently on activated T cells. Cross-linking CD40 on nonleukemia or CLL B cells significantly enhanced their capacity to present alloantigen and, in the case of CLL cells, CLL-associated antigens. This was in part attributed to increased expression of CD80 and CD86.[8,17,18] Since CLL B cells are the most abundant APC-population in CLL patients, conversion of CLL cells into potent APC may induce immune responses against leukemia-associated antigens (LAAs) because of their potential capacity to break immune tolerance to such LAA. An additional benefit is that CD154 also can activate dendritic cells (DCs), thereby enhancing the capacity of these cells to activate immune responses.

TRANSDUCTION OF CLL CELLS WITH AD-CD154

To extend these findings into a strategy for immunotherapy of CLL, we constructed replication defective adenovirus vectors using serotype 5 adenovirus in which the E1 region of the virus genome was replaced with the gene encoding either human or mouse CD154 flanked in the 5′ direction with a heterologous cytomegalovirus promoter, and in the 3′ direction with a bovine polyadenylation signal (Ad-CD154). Since soluble mouse CD154 binds human CD40[19] and mouse CD154 was found to be expressed more effectively on human B leukemias and lymphomas than human CD154,[20,21] the mouse CD154 was used in these studies. This also allowed us to distinguish the transgene product from endogenously expressed human CD154 in transduced human cells.[21]

We examined whether transduction of CLL cells with either vector could induce changes in the leukemia B-cell phenotype, as observed with CD40 cross-linking with antibody, that would facilitate T-cell immune recognition. CLL B cells transduced with Ad-CD154 expressed surface CD154 by 24 h after infection that reached maximum plateau levels by 48 h after transduction. Expression of CD154 enhanced the expression of CD54, CD80, CD86, CD58, CD70, and CD95 on the transduced CLL B cells. Furthermore, CD27, which impairs the antigen-presenting capacity of leukemia cells, was down-regulated. In addition, transduced CLL cells caused transactivation of nontransduced bystander leukemia B cells and up-regulation of CD54 and CD86. Ad-CD154-transduced leukemia cells were effective activators of allogeneic T cells in mixed lymphocyte reactions. We observed increased expression of CD69, increased secretion of IFN-γ, and increased T-cell proliferation. The T cells activation was overall more potent than that caused by CLL cells activated with an anti-CD40 monoclonal antibody. Furthermore, Ad-CD154-transduced CLL cells were capable of inducing MHC class I-dependent cytotoxic T lymphocyte (CTL) responses against autologous, but not allogeneic, leukemia cells.[21]

CD154 GENE THERAPY TRIAL FOR CLL

Since our *in vitro* studies suggested that Ad-CD154 could potentially elicit a therapeutic antileukemia response, we performed a phase-I dose-escalation study, assessing the safety of a single intravenous injection of autologous Ad-CD154-transduced leukemia cells to CLL patients (FIG. 1).[22] We investigated the immunological and clinical responses to infusion of Ad-CD154–CLL cells into eleven patients with progressive, intermediate, or high-risk CLL. Patients received infusion of transduced CLL cells on average 44+/– 23 days after leukapheresis. Patients were divided into groups that received injections of different amounts of leukemic cells, 3×10^8, 1×10^9, or 3×10^9 cells. Approximately half the CLL cells in all three groups expressed the transgene before injection. Expression of CD154 was detected

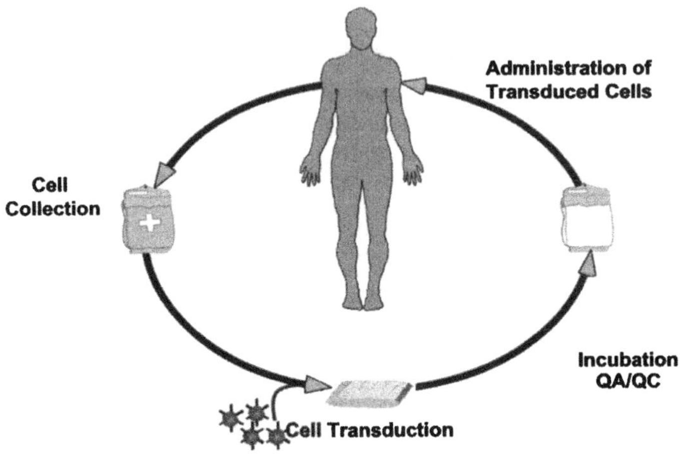

FIGURE 1. Ad-CD154 gene therapy of CLL. Patients underwent leukapheresis, after which their blood mononuclear cells were isolated and infected for 24 h with high titer replication-defective Ad-CD154. Following infection, cells were washed and frozen for storage. Before freezing an aliquot was tested for bacterial culture to ensure sterility. Autologous frozen cells were thawed, washed, and administered as a single intravenous bolus infusion over approximately 10 min.

in blood mononuclear cells of patients in all groups for at least 8 h after the infusion. An acute reduction in leukemic cells in blood was observed in all groups (FIG. 2a). The blood lymphocyte counts of two of the three patients in group 1 decreased by 68% and 87% from pretreatment values within 48 h after infusion. These two patients also had sustained reduction within 2 to 4 weeks after treatment. Similar responses were observed in the other groups as well. Blood lymphocyte counts after therapy were below pretreatment values in all patients. Patients in all three groups also experienced reduction in lymph node size 1 to 4 weeks after treatment, which was sustained for 3 months or more in most cases (FIG. 2b). Treatment was well tolerated, and the observed clinical abnormalities and flulike symptoms were transient. We did not observe any autoimmune side effects, such as autoimmune thrombocytopenia or hemolytic anemia, or dose-limiting toxicity.

These clinical responses were associated with biological effects in both the T- and the B-cell compartment. As observed in our *in vitro* studies, increased or *de novo* expression of CD80, CD86, CD54, and CD95 was observed on bystander nontransduced CLL cells *in vivo* for several days after a one-time bolus infusion of autologous Ad-CD154-transduced leukemia cells. Patients experienced a greater than 240% increase in absolute blood $CD4^+$ T-cell counts within 1 to 4 weeks of treatment. In particular, treatment increased the numbers of leukemia-specific T cells, as evident by increased IFN-γ secretion observed in autologous ELISPOT assays measured 4 weeks after treatment. In addition, treated patients had high plasma levels of the Th1-type cytokines IL-12 and IFN-γ after infusion. T-cell responses against autologous CLL cells, as evidenced by increased IFN-γ secretion as well as

T-cell proliferation in an autologous MLR, were observed even at 6 months after treatment, indicating the development of memory antileukemia immune responses.[22] Long-term follow-up studies showed that although the number of blood leukemic cells increased after a one-time injection of Ad-CD40L-transduced cells, repeated injections resulted in a stabilized and reduced leukemia cell counts and disease stabilization. This was associated with increased numbers of $CD3^+$ T cells after each injection and the development of antibodies against CLL-associated cell surface antigens.

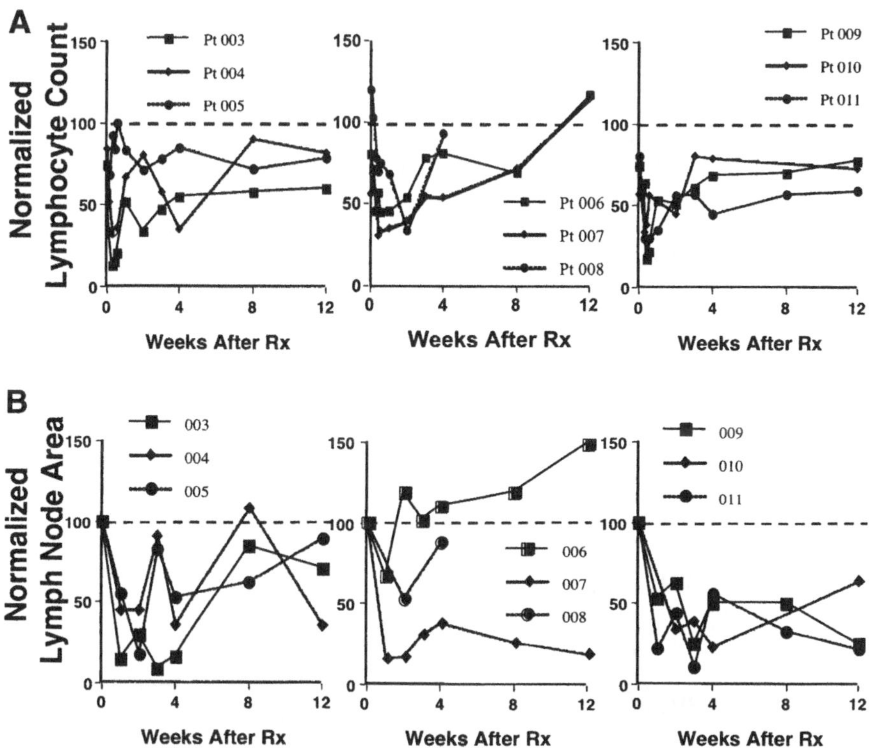

FIGURE 2. Measurement of absolute lymphocyte count and lymph-node size in CLL patients after infusion of autologous Ad-CD154-transduced CLL cells. Patients Pt 003-005 received approximately 3×10^8, patients Pt 006-008 received 1×10^9, and patients Pt 009-011 received 3×10^9 autologous transduced CLL cells. (**A**) Complete blood counts and manual differential were performed from patients (Pt 003-Pt 011) at the indicated time points after infusion at day 0. Data shown are lymphocyte counts normalized with respect to the lymphocyte counts before leukapheresis (100%). (**B**) The lymph-node area was assessed by nodal palpitation in two dimensions in the right and left cervical, supraclavicular, and axillary lymph nodes. Data shown are from the largest lymph node in each of the right and left nodal regions at the day of infusion was followed over time. The data shown are normalized lymph-node area, which represents the sum lymph-node area from the largest lymph node at a particular time as a fraction of the sum area on the day of infusion.

MECHANISMS OF LEUKEMIC CELL DEATH IN AD-CD154 GENE THERAPY

The induced expression of the cell-death receptors, such as Fas (CD95), on bystander CLL cells probably contributed to the observed acute declines in leukemic cell counts following Ad-CD154 gene therapy. Although *in vitro* CD40-activated CLL cells initially are resistant to CD95-mediated apoptosis, CLL cells become increasingly sensitive to CD95-mediated apoptosis over time. This sensitivity was associated with progressive declines in Flice-inhibitory protein (FLIP) and progressive increases in levels of Fas-associated death-domain protein (FADD) and DAP3 following CD40 activation. Thus, ligation of CD40 on CLL cells induces a series of events that shifts the balance of anti- and proapoptotic proteins that eventually sensitizes the leukemia cells to death induced by ligation of the nascent death receptors (FIGS. 3 and 4). Although sole ligation of CD95 was not sufficient to induce apoptosis of newly activated CLL cells, $CD4^+$ CTLs were able to kill newly activated CLL cells via a CD95-dependent pathway.[23]

CD40 activated CLL cells also express DR5, a receptor for TNF-related apoptosis-inducing ligand (TRAIL), which is expressed on activated $CD4^+$ CTL. Activated blood $CD4^+$ CTLs of patients with CLL were found to coexpress both CD178 and TRAIL. Increased DR5 and CD95 expression also was observed on CLL cells of patients treated 24 h earlier via infusion of Ad-CD154-transduced, autologous CLL cells. Simultaneous cross-linking of these death receptors on CD40-activated CLL cells via TRAIL and Fas-ligand (CD178) acted synergistically to induce caspase-dependent apoptosis *in vitro* and possibly *in vivo* within 24 h after CD40-activation.

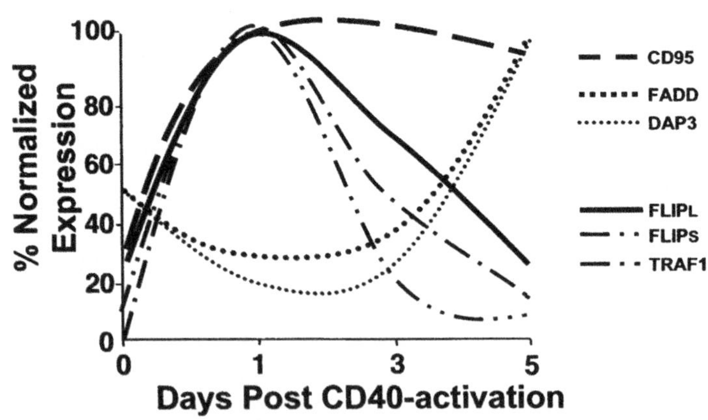

FIGURE 3. Temporal expression of apoptosis regulatory proteins in CLL cells after CD4-activation. CLL cells were cultured for 24 h on HeLa cells expressing CD154. The CLL cells were then separated from HeLA cells and cultured in their absence for the indicated period of time. CLL cells were harvested before (day 0) and at days 1, 2, and 3 after CD40 activation. Lysates were prepared for Western blot analysis, and data shown are protein levels normalized to actin bands. Relatively constant: Bcl-2, Bcl-X_L, XIAP, Bad, caspase-8.

CD154 *in vitro* and *in vivo* also induced CLL cells to express the proapoptotic protein, BH3 interacting domain death agonist (Bid). Bid can facilitate cross talk between mitochondrial-dependent, apoptosis-inducing pathways and death receptors, such as DR5. CD40-ligation causes increased expression of Bid, CD95, and DR5 in CLL cells, which together can act synergistically to induce caspase-dependent cell death. The expression of Bid has been associated with sensitivity to anticancer drugs.[24,25] Thus, the temporal events induced by CD40-activation could render CLL cells first resistant and then sensitive to antileukemic drugs.[26,27] If CD40 activation is combined with other treatments at optimal time points, more efficient tumor killing might be achieved.

We further found that the initial resistance to CD95-mediated apoptosis was due in part to high-level expression of the X-linked inhibitor of apoptosis protein (XIAP) by CLL cells (FIG. 5). We examined whether we could inhibit XIAP in CLL cells using a novel XIAP inhibitor, an analog of a recently described phenylurea-based compound 1540-14. This compound can dissociate XIAP from the effector caspase-

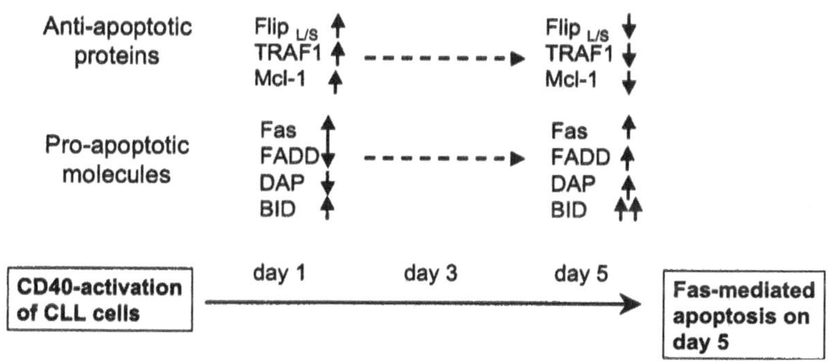

FIGURE 4. Model for apoptosis induction in CD40-activated CLL cells. Summary of changes in levels of pro- and antiapototic proteins in CLL cells after CD40-ligation.

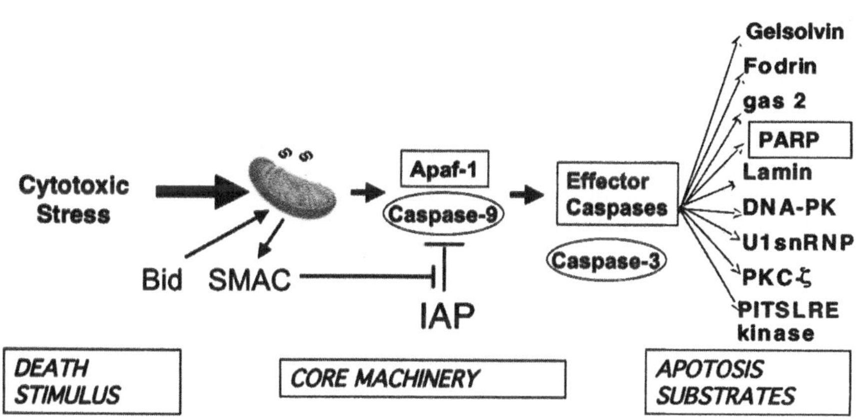

FIGURE 5. Schematic of programmed cell death.

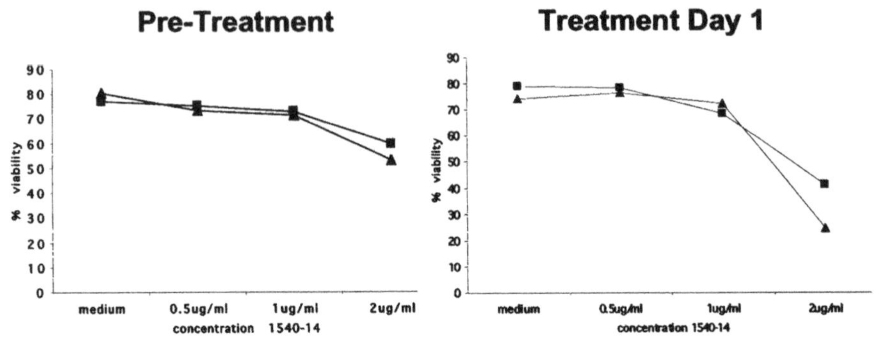

FIGURE 6. XIAP inhibitors increase the sensitivity of CLL cells from Ad-CD154-treated patients to CD95-mediated apoptosis. CLL cells were isolated from peripheral blood before and 24 h after infusion of autologous Ad-CD154 transduced CLL cells. In contrast to the CLL cells isolated prior to treatment, the CLL cells isolated from patients after the infusion of Ad-CD154 expressed CD95. After isolation, the CLL cells were cultured in a medium containing 1540-14 (squares) of the anti-CD95 monoclonal antibodty, CH11, and 1540-14 (triangles) at different concentrations of 1540-14. Viability of CLL cells was accessed after 24 h by flow cytometry using 3,3′-dihexyloxacarbocyanine and propidium iodide. Data shown are relative viability compared to CLL cells cultured in medium only. Addition of CH11 alone did not reduce the viability of CLL cells pre- or posttherapy.

3, thereby restoring caspase-3 activity. Furthermore, this compound does not compete with the natural XIAP inhibitor, Smac/DIABLO, in restoring caspase activity.[28] Cells isolated from patients one day after infusion of Ad-CD154-transduced CLL cells were found to have enhanced sensitivity to apoptosis when treated with 1540-14 (FIG. 6). A key event in the latent sensitivity to Fas-mediated apoptosis could be the degradation of Bid into tBid, which links the death-receptor pathway to the mitochondrial apoptotic pathway.[29–32] CLL cells ordinarily lack expression of Bid; however, Bid is expressed after CD40-activation. At day one after CD40-activation, CLL cells show reduced Bid levels when treated with an agonistic CD95 antibody. This is even more pronounced at day 3 after activation. CD95-mediated degradation of Bid was caspase dependent. Treatment of CD40-stimulated CLL cells with 1540-14 induced high-level activation of caspase-8 and -3 and cleavage of poly(adenosine diphosphate [ADP]-ribose) polymerase following CD95 ligation. CLL cells of Ad-CD154-treated patients might have encountered cells that express CD178 and TRAIL *in vivo,* which primed them for apoptosis. These results indicate that XIAP inhibitors might enhance the effectiveness of Ad-CD154 therapy.

ACKNOWLEDGMENTS

This work was funded in part by funds provided by the Dana Foundation and the PO1 grant for the CLL Research Consortium (2 PO1 CA081534) awarded to one of the authors (T.J.K.) for the CLL Research Consortium. We thank Andrew Graves for assistance with the graphics.

[*Competing interests*: The authors declare that they have no competing financial interests.]

REFERENCES

1. HUHN, D., C. VON SCHILLING, M. WILHELM, *et al.* 2001. Rituximab therapy of patients with B-cell chronic lymphocytic leukemia. Blood **98:** 1326–1331.
2. GRILLO-LOPEZ, A.J., C.A. WHITE, B.K. DALLAIRE, *et al.* 2000. Rituximab: the first monoclonal antibody approved for the treatment of lymphoma. Curr. Pharm. Biotechnol. **1:** 1–9.
3. BURNET, F.M. 1970. The concept of immunological surveillance. Prog. Exp. Tumor Res. **13:** 1–27.
4. THOMAS, L. 1959. Discussion of Cellular and Humoral Aspects of the Hypersensitivity. Hoeber-Harper. New York. 5.WILLIMSKY, G. & T. BLANKENSTEIN. 2005. Sporadic immunogenic tumours avoid destruction by inducing T-cell tolerance. Nature **437:** 141–146.
5. WILLIMSKY, G. & T. BLANKENSTEIN. 2005. Sporadic immunogenic tumours avoid destruction by inducing T-cell tolerance. Nature **437:** 141–146.
6. ZOU, W. 2005. Immunosuppressive networks in the tumour environment and their therapeutic relevance. Nat. Rev. Cancer **5:** 263–274.
7. EMENS, L.A., R.T. REILLY & E.M. JAFFEE. 2005. Breast cancer vaccines: maximizing cancer treatment by tapping into host immunity. Endocr. Relat. Cancer **12:** 1–17.
8. YELLIN, M.J., J. SINNING, L.R. COVEY, *et al.* 1994. T lymphocyte T cell-B cell-activating molecule/CD40-L molecules induce normal B cells or chronic lymphocytic leukemia B cells to express CD80 (B7/BB-1) and enhance their costimulatory activity. J. Immunol. **153:** 666–674.
9. WOLOS, J.A. & F.R. DAVEY. 1980. Function of lymphocyte subpopulations in chronic lymphocytic leukemia. Activity in the allogeneic and autologous mixed lymphocyte reaction. Cancer **45:** 893–898.
10. SCHULTZE, J., L.M. NADLER & J.G. GRIBBEN. 1996. B7-mediated costimulation and the immune response. Blood Rev. **10:** 111–127.
11. LENSCHOW, D.J., T.L. WALUNAS & J.A. BLUESTONE. 1996. CD28/B7 system of T cell costimulation. Annu. Rev. Immunol. **14:** 233–258.
12. GREENFIELD, E.A., K.A. NGUYEN & V.K. KUCHROO. 1998. CD28/B7 costimulation: a review. Crit. Rev. Immunol. **18:** 389–418.
13. ARMITAGE, R.J., W.C. FANSLOW, L. STROCKBINE, *et al.* 1992. Molecular and biological characterization of a murine ligand for CD40. Nature **357:** 80–82.
14. NOELLE, R.J., M. ROY, D.M. SHEPHERD, *et al.* 1992. A 39-kDa protein on activated helper T cells binds CD40 and transduces the signal for cognate activation of B cells. Proc. Natl. Acad. Sci. USA **89:** 6550–6554.
15. YANG, Y. & J.M. WILSON. 1996. CD40 ligand-dependent T cell activation: requirement of B7-CD28 signaling through CD40. Science **273:** 1862–1864.
16. GREWAL, I.S., H.G. FOELLMER, K.D. GREWAL, *et al.* 1996. Requirement for CD40 ligand in costimulation induction, T cell activation, and experimental allergic encephalomyelitis. Science **273:** 1864–1867.
17. RANHEIM, E.A. & T.J. KIPPS. 1993. Activated T cells induce expression of B7/BB1 on normal or leukemic B cells through a CD40-dependent signal. J. Exp. Med. **177:** 925–935.
18. VAN DEN HOVE, L.E., S.W. VAN GOOL, P. VANDENBERGHE, *et al.* 1997. CD40 triggering of chronic lymphocytic leukemia B cells results in efficient alloantigen presentation and cytotoxic T lymphocyte induction by up-regulation of CD80 and CD86 costimulatory molecules. Leukemia **11:** 572–580.
19. LANE, P., T. BROCKER, S. HUBELE, *et al.* 1993. Soluble CD40 ligand can replace the normal T cell-derived CD40 ligand signal to B cells in T cell-dependent activation. J. Exp. Med. **177:** 1209–1213.
20. CANTWELL, M.J., W.G. WIERDA, I.S. LOSSOS, *et al.* 2001. T cell activation following infection of primary follicle center lymphoma B cells with adenovirus encoding CD154. Leukemia **15:** 1451–1457.

21. KATO, K., M.J. CANTWELL, S. SHARMA & T.J. KIPPS. 1998. Gene transfer of CD40-ligand induces autologous immune recognition of chronic lymphocytic leukemia B cells. J. Clin. Invest. **101:** 1133–1141.
22. WIERDA, W.G., M.J. CANTWELL, S.J. WOODS, *et al.* 2000. CD40-ligand (CD154) gene therapy for chronic lymphocytic leukemia. Blood **96:** 2917–2924.
23. CHU, P., D. DEFORCE, I.M. PEDERSEN, *et al.* 2002. Latent sensitivity to Fas-mediated apoptosis after CD40 ligation may explain activity of CD154 gene therapy in chronic lymphocytic leukemia. Proc. Natl. Acad. Sci. USA **99:** 3854–3859.
24. KIM, R., K. TANABE, Y. UCHIDA, *et al.* 2002. Current status of the molecular mechanisms of anticancer drug-induced apoptosis. The contribution of molecular-level analysis to cancer chemotherapy. Cancer Chemother. Pharmacol. **50:** 343–352.
25. SAX, J.K., P. FEI, M.E. MURPHY, *et al.* 2002. BID regulation by p53 contributes to chemosensitivity. Nat. Cell Biol. **4:** 842–849.
26. ROMANO, M.F., A. LAMBERTI, P. TASSONE, *et al.* 1998. Triggering of CD40 antigen inhibits fludarabine-induced apoptosis in B chronic lymphocytic leukemia cells. Blood **92:** 990–995.
27. DE TOTERO, D., P.L. TAZZARI, M. CAPAIA, *et al.* 2003. CD40 triggering enhances fludarabine-induced apoptosis of chronic lymphocytic leukemia B-cells through autocrine release of tumor necrosis factor-alpha and interferon-gama and tumor necrosis factor receptor-I-II upregulation. Haematologica **88:** 148–158.
28. SCHIMMER, A.D., K. WELSH, C. PINILLA, *et al.* 2004. Small-molecule antagonists of apoptosis suppressor XIAP exhibit broad antitumor activity. Cancer Cell **5:** 25–35.
29. BECATTINI, B., S. SARETH, D. ZHAI, *et al.* 2004. Targeting apoptosis via chemical design: inhibition of bid-induced cell death by small organic molecules. Chem. Biol. **11:** 1107–1117.
30. DENG, Y., Y. LIN & X. WU. 2002. TRAIL-induced apoptosis requires Bax-dependent mitochondrial release of Smac/DIABLO. Genes Dev. **16:** 33–45.
31. LI, S., Y. ZHAO, X. HE, *et al.* 2002. Relief of extrinsic pathway inhibition by the Bid-dependent mitochondrial release of Smac in Fas-mediated hepatocyte apoptosis. J. Biol. Chem. **277:** 26912–26920.
32. SUN, X.M., S.B. BRATTON, M. BUTTERWORTH, *et al.* 2002. Bcl-2 and Bcl-xL inhibit CD95-mediated apoptosis by preventing mitochondrial release of Smac/DIABLO and subsequent inactivation of X-linked inhibitor-of-apoptosis protein. J. Biol. Chem. **277:** 11345–11351.

The Challenge of Analyzing the Proteome in Humans with Autoimmune Diseases

STEVEN M. CHAN AND PAUL J. UTZ

Department of Medicine, Division of Immunology and Rheumatology, Stanford University School of Medicine, Stanford, California 94305, USA

Abstract: Analysis of blood samples from patients suffering from autoimmune diseases remains a mainstay in the clinic for initial diagnosis, prognostication, and clinical decision making. In particular, testing for the presence of serum autoantibodies has proved to be one of the most useful confirmatory assays for many different diseases. Recent genomic and transcript profiling studies have implicated certain cytokines, surface receptors, signaling pathways, and cell types in the pathogenesis of inflammatory diseases. The next obvious step is to delve into the much more complex level that follows the genome and transcriptome—the expressed proteome. This review focuses on several proteomics technologies being applied and/or developed by our laboratory for the study of autoimmunity, cancer, and cardiovascular disease, all of which are known to be associated with defects in immunity and inflammation. The findings of other participants in the recent Human Immunology Conference hosted by the Dana Foundation and the New York Academy of Sciences (May 17 & 18, 2005) are included. In particular, major pitfalls in the study of the human proteome are pointed out, and important areas for immediate investigation to move the field forward as rapidly as possible are proposed.

Keywords: proteomics; protein arrays; autoimmunity; signaling; autoantibodies

INTRODUCTION

Proteomics is the comprehensive study of the proteins expressed in a cell, tissue, biological fluid, or organism. We and others hypothesize that comparison of the proteome in healthy and diseased blood cells or biological fluids will provide insights into autoimmune disease pathogenesis, and will also identify useful biomarkers and, ultimately, surrogate markers that can be used in the clinic. Relatively few methods have emerged that appear promising for this purpose, in particular mass spectrometry, cytokine profiling using a variety of techniques, MHC-tetramer arrays, lysate and autoantigen microarray profiling, and polychromatic phospho-flow cytometry.[1] Initial studies using these techniques in inbred animal models of autoimmunity have been very successful, and have argued strongly for similar studies in human beings. Unfortunately, human patients are genetically diverse, are exposed to different envi-

Address for correspondence: Paul J. Utz, Stanford University of Medicine, CCSR Building, Room 2215A, 269 Campus Dr., Stanford, CA 94305. Voice: 650-724-5421; fax: 650-723-7509. pjutz@stanford.edu

Ann. N.Y. Acad. Sci. 1062: 61–68 (2005). © 2005 New York Academy of Sciences. doi: 10.1196/annals.1358.009

ronmental and dietary conditions, have relatively long disease courses that make them difficult to study over time, are highly mobile, and are treated with different therapeutic regimens at different medical centers. Moreover, current proteomics assay platforms are not standardized, nor do reference samples exist with which to disseminate many of these assays. This has meant that few centers are capable of properly analyzing samples from patients with rare autoimmune diseases and patients enrolled in clinical trials.

In this chapter we describe three techniques presented at the Human Immunology Conference that are being used by our lab—autoantigen microarrays for antibody profiling, lysate microarrays for profiling of signaling pathways, and phospho-flow cytometry for studying signaling events in single cells—focusing on pitfalls associated with each platform. We conclude by identifying areas for future investigation that need to be addressed for proteomics to succeed in the coming decade.

AUTOANTIGEN MICROARRAY TECHNOLOGY FOR ANTIBODY PROFILING

Protein microarrays have generated much excitement over the past five years because of their potential to profile protein levels and their posttranslational modifications at a scale that has never before been possible. It has been the hope of the research community that protein microarrays will impact the field of proteomics in much the same way that DNA microarrays have impacted genomics. Although the concept of using microarrays to profile proteins quantitatively is straightforward, progress in protein profiling microarrays has been slower than originally anticipated. A dearth of high-quality capture reagents (e.g., monoclonal antibodies) of high affinity and low cross-reactivity that bind analytes in their native conformation in solution is the major obstacle that currently faces the field.[2,3] In contrast, "protein function" microarrays have made significant strides in recent years and will likely become the dominant protein microarray platform in the near future. Protein function microarrays essentially consist of a large number of purified proteins and peptides arrayed on a planar surface. A seminal paper by MacBeath and Schreiber in 2000 described a series of elegant proof-of-principle experiments demonstrating the potential of protein function microarrays to screen for novel protein–protein interactions, kinase substrates, and protein targets of small molecules.[4]

Joos, Robinson, and others adapted protein microarray technology for the study of autoimmunity with the construction of a connective tissue–disease autoantigen microarray using a conventional DNA microarrayer.[5–7] Autoantigen microarrays consist of purified proteins, synthetic peptides, nucleic acids, carbohydrates, and lipids that are deposited in a spatially addressable manner on chemically derivatized glass microscope slides. The arrays are probed with serum or other biological fluids (e.g., synovial fluid, cerebrospinal fluid) from autoimmune patients or animals. Bound antibodies are subsequently detected using fluorescently tagged secondary antibodies. The fluorescence intensity of each spot thus corresponds to the titer of the specific autoantibody present in the original biological sample. Because potentially thousands of antigens can be printed on a single slide, antigen microarrays represent a powerful platform for high-throughput profiling of serum autoantibodies.

Although the technology is still in its developmental stages, and many technical hurdles must be overcome before it is sufficiently reliable for routine clinical and research applications, our group and others have generated promising data demonstrating its utility in autoimmunity research. In the following sections, we review recent work on antigen microarrays and speculate on potential applications of this technology.

APPLICATIONS OF ANTIGEN MICROARRAYS

Although the precise role of autoantibodies in the pathogenesis of many autoimmune diseases is not clear, and in some cases is controversial, it has been known for many years that serum autoantibodies have important diagnostic value, especially for connective tissue diseases. The main problem with relying on autoantibodies alone for establishing a diagnosis is that most autoantibodies have shown poor sensitivity and/or specificity for their associated diseases. It is our hypothesis that it is the profile of multiple autoantibody reactivities, not reactivity to a single autoantigen, that will provide a diagnostic test with the highest sensitivity and specificity. Autoantigen microarrays can be used to test this hypothesis based on the pattern of reactivity to potentially thousands of unique whole antigens, as well as epitopes contained within individual antigens. More important, we believe that it may be possible to screen for patients who are likely to develop disease by monitoring their autoantibody profiles before clinical manifestation of symptoms. This is important because interventions can be administered to those patients to prevent or delay the disease. A recent study by Quintana *et al.* showed that the profile of autoantibody reactivity using a diabetes autoantigen microarray could distinguish male nonobese diabetic (NOD) mice that were susceptible to cyclophosphamide-induced diabetes from those that were resistant.[8] Importantly, the autoantibody profiles were obtained from mice before the appearance of disease manifestations, indicating that microarray profiling may be valuable as a screening tool for patients with an increased likelihood of disease development. Indeed, autoantibodies are frequently found in systemic lupus erythematosus (SLE), rheumatoid arthritis (RA), and type 1 diabetes (T1D) patients many years before the onset of clinical symptoms.[9–12] Whether microarray profiling of autoantibodies has a higher positive predictive value than any single autoantibody test alone remains to be determined. This line of reasoning can be extended to prognostication in human patients with an established autoimmune diagnosis. Let us take SLE as an example. Although up to 75% of SLE patients develop some form of renal disease, the severity of renal involvement varies widely between patients, ranging from minimal deposition of immune complexes in the mesangium to severe glomerulonephritis (GN) leading to nephrotic syndrome and/or renal insufficiency. Although antibodies to C1q and autoantibodies of certain isotypes (e.g., IgG3) have been linked to lupus nephritis, there is currently no prognostic marker that is used clinically to predict renal disease in an individual SLE patient.[13,14] Can autoantibody microarray profiling aid in the prognostic classification of lupus patients? Precisely this question is being addressed in our laboratory using lupus autoantigen microarray analysis in pediatric lupus patients, and in adult patients enrolled in clinical trials testing novel therapeutics.

Recent work from our laboratory and the Robinson laboratory has expanded further the potential application of antigen microarrays for guiding therapy of autoimmune diseases and infectious diseases such as human immunodeficiency virus infection (HIV).[15] Our lab is interested in the development of DNA vaccines for antigen-specific tolerizing therapy.[16] However, the diversity of autoantigens being targeted in any given autoimmune disease poses a challenge to selecting the appropriate antigens for inclusion in the DNA vaccine. We hypothesize that autoantigen microarrays can help guide this selection process by profiling the autoantibody response. To test this hypothesis, a "myelin proteome" microarray was constructed to profile the evolution of autoantibody responses in experimental autoimmune encephalomyelitis (EAE), a mouse model for multiple sclerosis (MS). Based on the autoantibody profile generated, autoantigen targets were selected and included in expression vectors for immunization. The resulting DNA vaccine was successful in treating established EAE. Furthermore, using the myelin proteome microarray, we were able to show reduced epitope spreading in vaccinated mice.[16] This study highlights the potential use of autoantigen microarrays to aid the design of patient-tailored therapies and to monitor patient responses to therapies. Studies currently are being performed in our laboratory to determine whether this new therapeutic paradigm will work in human patients. This work has led to an ongoing phase I/II trial (Bayhill Therapeutics, Palo Alto, CA) of a tolerizing DNA plasmid–encoding myelin basic protein (MBP) in human MS patients, who are being monitored using antigen microarray technology for profiling autoantibodies. Similar monitoring studies in SLE, primary biliary cirrhosis (PBC), and vasculitis patients treated with Rituximab and other investigational drugs also are underway.

REVERSE-PHASE PROTEIN LYSATE MICROARRAYS

Reverse-phase protein (RPP) microarrays were described originally by the Petricoin and Liotta groups in a paper showing activation of prosurvival pathways (e.g., phosphorylation of Akt) in the transition from normal prostate epithelium to prostate intraepithelial neoplasia, and then to invasive prostate cancer.[17] Before we delve into the technical aspects of RPP microarrays, it is helpful to distinguish first between "forward-phase" and "reverse-phase" approaches, and to discuss why RPP arrays have unique advantages over other array formats for protein profiling, especially for the study of signaling networks, which often are dysregulated in cells involved in the initiation and maintenance of autoimmunity.

As noted earlier, the lack of specific monoclonal antibodies for binding native proteins in solution poses a challenge to the development of conventional protein profiling arrays, in which the capture reagents are immobilized on the array surface. One can view the forward-phase approach as an array of miniaturized immunoprecipitation (IP) reactions that occur proximal to the array surface. Based on our own experience, past literature, and information supplied by commercial vendors, we estimate that only about 20% of commercially available antibodies that target intracellular proteins can be used for IP experiments. It is important to note that this estimate applies only to conventional antibodies. We estimate that the fraction of phosphorylation-specific antibodies that can be used for IP reactions is less than 10%. In contrast, close to 100% of these antibodies should bind to their antigen with high affinity when the antigen is denatured and immobilized on a membrane, as in Western blotting. The forward-phase approach is complicated further by the issue of detection. Direct labeling of the protein sample with fluorescent "tags" is one approach that has been tried by several groups. However, the tags can interfere sterically with antibody binding if they are located within binding epitopes. Furthermore, the efficiency of protein labeling reactions is notoriously variable, making quantitative comparisons between samples difficult. Currently, the "sandwich immunoassay" approach appears to be the best option for forward-phase microarrays. However, antibody pairs are not available for many intracellular proteins. This led us to explore reverse-phase protein microarrays, in which the samples are immobilized on the array surface. The arrays are then probed with specific antibodies that are either phosphorylation-state–dependent or –independent. Bound antibodies are detected using secondary antibodies conjugated to horseradish peroxidase (HRP), followed by a tyramide-based amplification step that deposits biotin molecules adjacent to the HRP signal. A fluorescent signal is generated by incubating the arrays with fluorophore-conjugated streptavidin. The main advantage of this technique is that thousands of samples can be analyzed simultaneously on the same platform, greatly increasing throughput and simplifying quantitative analysis between samples. Furthermore, an exceedingly small amount of sample is required for printing the arrays, thus permitting the analysis of rare and valuable patient samples. Importantly, most if not all commercially available antibodies should work in this format, unlike forward-phase approaches. A clear limitation to this approach is that only one analyte can be measured on a single array. To partially overcome this limitation, arrays can be printed in a multisector format (arrays of arrays), allowing for up to 16 analytes to be analyzed on a single slide. Although this number is still orders of magnitude smaller than the number of probes on a DNA microarray, it is not as limiting as one might think if the analysis is focused on one functional class of proteins (e.g., signal transduction proteins or apoptosis-related proteins). A particularly successful application of RPP microarrays has been the profiling of phosphorylation states of signaling proteins with the use of phospho-antibodies.[18] This has been possible only within the last few years with the availability of an expanding collection of well-characterized phospho-specific antibodies. Indeed, the use of RPP microarrays for the analysis of phospho-signaling networks in immune-related cells has been the focus of our research.[18,19]

POLYCHROMATIC FLOW CYTOMETRY FOR STUDYING SIGNALING PATHWAYS IN SINGLE CELLS

Fluorescence-activated cell sorting (FACS) has revolutionized the study of immunology. FACS has allowed the discovery and characterization of antigen-specific T and B lymphocytes, and has identified subsets of cells that have important functional roles in the immune system. In 2002, Perez and Nolan reported a comprehensive demonstration of intracellular staining of cells with phospho-specific antibodies.[20] In this platform, cell populations are identified by using monoclonal antibodies specific for various cell-surface proteins. Each of the antibodies is conjugated to a spectrally resolvable fluorophore. A complex mixture of cells can be analyzed, as one can gate on different cell-surface markers. Cells are then fixed and permeabilized using protocols developed in the Nolan lab. The cells are stained using antibodies that recognize intracellular proteins, including cytokines, chemokines, structural proteins, apoptosis-specific proteins, and, more important, signaling molecules such as kinases and their substrates. Monoclonal antibodies recognizing phospho-specific epitopes in particular were used in their original study. Perez and Nolan showed the simultaneous detection of several different kinase families, including mitogen-activated protein kinases (P38 MAPK, P44/42 MAPK, and JNK), kinases associated with cell survival (AKT/PKB), and a T-cell activation kinase (TYK2). Signaling was measured in peripheral blood mononuclear cells (PBMCs) following a variety of different physiologic stimuli. Human memory cells as well as naive lymphocytes were exposed to cytokines, and the signaling pathways were studied using five different differentiation markers to analyze the cell populations. Finally, hierarchical signaling nodes were studied in an attempt to order the activation of each of the kinases. This important paper showed that polychromatic flow-cytometric analysis of signaling pathways could be performed at a single-cell level, with obvious implications for the study of human samples, particularly from patients with autoimmune disease.

An elegant extension of this study was performed looking at cancer cells. Irish and colleagues applied the same technology to the study of acute myeloid leukemia (AML) samples.[21] The hypothesis being tested was that differences in signaling could segregate patients into those who may or may not respond to therapy, and also might correlate with clinical outcome regardless of therapy. Cancer cells were obtained from patients through collaboration with investigators in Norway. Cells were frozen and then analyzed using phospho-specific FACS. Cells were thawed and exposed to various cytokines before staining with antibodies directed against phosphorylated STAT molecules, as well as other signaling proteins. The results obtained through genetic analysis as well as disease outcome correlated well with unique cancer network profiles that were obtained by FACS.

The Nolan lab has now initiated studies in collaboration with our lab and the Robinson lab as part of our NHLBI proteomics contract. We are studying the natural history of the autoimmune response in three different mouse models of lupus, and in the collagen-induced arthritis (CIA) model of rheumatoid arthritis. We are analyzing subsets of B cells, T cells, and dendritic cells obtained from mice at different ages, and correlating results with pathologic specimens obtained at the same time points. Autoantibody profiling also is being studied in these animals. Samples are being obtained after stimulation with various cytokines and chemokines, and ligation of cell-surface receptors. The initial goal is to replicate published data demonstrating defects in T-cell receptor and other signaling pathways in these autoimmune diseases. Ultimately, we hope to identify novel alterations in signaling pathways. The second stage of the study is to identify changes in the signaling proteome in response to therapeutic interventions, using mice treated with standard therapies that are used currently in clinical practice in humans. These regimens include treatment with oral steroids and cyclophosphamide, exposure to a lipid-lowering class of drugs (statins), and treatment with a variety of proprietary inhibitors of LFA-1. DNA vaccine studies also are being analyzed using this approach, although MHC-tetramers that would allow the study of antigen-specific immune responses do not yet exist for lupus or rheumatoid arthritis. These studies have been extended to the study of human samples, described in more detail in this issue by Perez.[22]

CRITICAL PROBLEMS THAT MUST BE SOLVED

Proteomics studies in animal models of autoimmunity form the basis for the next step—the study of human patients. However, animal models, particularly rodent models, are highly biased, as the animals are inbred, and in some cases complete Freund's adjuvant (CFA) is used to initiate disease, markedly enhancing antibody production and T-cell activation above physiologic levels. A number of important limitations in using proteomics to study autoimmunity were identified by attendees at the Dana Foundation meeting: (1) Handling and storage of clinical samples need to be optimized and standardized. Freeze/thaw protocols need to be validated fully, particularly for the study of human blood cells. (2) The enormous volume of data generated by proteomics platforms such as mass spectrometry and protein arrays will require creative advances in bioinformatics. (3) Inter- and intra-assay normalization for autoantibody profiling remains to be resolved, a task that is of the highest priority for the future. (4) Improvements in technologies, particularly more reproducible methods for printing proteins, and better methods for performing and quantitating mass spectrometry, are required. (5) The generation of high-affinity, non–cross-reactive antibodies is perhaps the biggest challenge facing future development of reverse-phase protein microarrays. Without prior protein separation, the accuracy of the results depends solely on the specificity of the antibodies that are used. (6) Newly developed detection technologies using alternative fluorophores need to be validated further. Fluorophores that emit in the infrared range permit scanning at higher wavelengths. (7) Finally, the development of reagents such as MHC-tetramers for studying human antigen-specific immune responses may fundamentally alter our understanding of autoimmune disease pathogenesis.

ACKNOWLEDGMENTS

One of the authors (S.C.) is funded by the Stanford Medical Scientist Training Program and the Floren Family Foundation. The other author (P.J.U.) is the recipient of a Donald E. and Delia B. Baxter Foundation Career Development Award and was supported by the Dana Foundation, the Northern California Chapter of the Arthritis Foundation, the Stanford Program in Molecular and Genetic Medicine (PMGM), NIH Grants P30 DK56339 (Stanford Digestive Disease Center), DK61934, AI50854, AI50865, AR49328, and NHLBI Proteomics Contract N01-HV-28183 during the period when many of these technologies were first developed. We thank members of the Utz lab for development of proteomics technologies, some of which are described in this review.

[*Competing interests*: P.J. Utz states the following conflict of interest disclosures, all directly relevant to proteomics technology described in this manuscript: In the past three years he has served as a consultant to Becton Dickinson Biosciences (San Jose, CA) and Genentech, Inc. (South San Francisco, CA). He is a member of the Scientific Advisory Board of Monogram Biosciences (South San Francisco, CA), XDx, Inc. (South San Francisco, CA), Centocor (Horsham, PA), MedImmune (Gaithersberg, MD), and Biogen/IDEC (Cambridge, MA). He is a cofounder and consultant at Bayhill Therapeutics (Palo Alto, CA), which is using antibody microarray profiling in a human MS trial.]

REFERENCES

1. Utz, P.J. 2005. Protein arrays for studying blood cells and their secreted products. Immunol. Rev. **204:** 264–282.
2. Haab, B.B., M.J. Dunham & P.O. Brown. 2001. Protein microarrays for highly parallel detection and quantitation of specific proteins and antibodies in complex solutions. Genome Biol. **2:** RESEARCH0004.
3. Nielsen, U.B. *et al.* 2003. Profiling receptor tyrosine kinase activation by using Ab microarrays. Proc. Natl. Acad. Sci. USA **100:** 9330–9335.
4. MacBeath, G. & S.L. Schreiber. 2000. Printing proteins as microarrays for high-throughput function determination. Science **289:** 1760–1763.
5. Joos, T. *et al.* 2000. A microarray enzyme-linked immunosorbent assay for autoimmune diagnostics. Electrophoresis **21:** 2641–2650.
6. Robinson, W.H. *et al.* 2002. Autoantigen microarrays for multiplex characterization of autoantibody responses. Nat. Med. **8:** 295–301.
7. Schena, M. *et al.* 1995. Quantitative monitoring of gene expression patterns with a complementary DNA microarray. Science **270:** 467–470.
8. Quintana, F.J. *et al.* 2004. Functional immunomics: microarray analysis of IgG autoantibody repertoires predicts the future response of mice to induced diabetes. Proc. Natl. Acad. Sci. USA **101**(Suppl. 2): 14615–14621.
9. Rantapää-Dahlqvist, S. *et al.* 2003. Antibodies against cyclic citrullinated peptide and IgA rheumatoid factor predict the development of rheumatoid arthritis. Arthritis Rheum. **48:** 2741–2749.
10. Hagopian, W. *et al.* 1995. Glutamate decarboxylase, insulin, and islet cell autoantibodies and HLA typing to detect diabetes in a general population-based study of Swedish children. J. Clin. Invest. **95:** 1505–1511.
11. Arbuckle, M.R. *et al.* 2003. Development of autoantibodies before the clinical onset of systemic lupus erythematosus. N. Engl. J. Med. **349:** 1526–1533.
12. Scofield, R.H. 2004. Autoantibodies as predictors of disease. Lancet **363:** 1544–1546.
13. Utz, P.J. 2004. Multiplexed assays for identification of biomarkers and surrogate markers in SLE. Lupus **13:** 304–311.
14. Seelen, M.A., L.A. Trouw & M.R. Daha. 2003. Diagnostic and prognostic significance of anti-C1q antibodies in systemic lupus erythematosus. Curr. Opin. Nephrol. Hypertens. **12:** 619–624.
15. De Vegvar, H. *et al.* 2003. Microarray profiling of antibody responses against simian-human immunodeficiency virus: postchallenge convergence of reactivities independent of host histocompatibility type and vaccine regimen. J. Virol. **77:** 11125–11138.
16. Robinson, W. *et al.* 2003. Protein microarrays guide tolerizing DNA vaccine treatment of autoimmune encephalomyelitis. Nat. Biotech. **21:** 1033–1039.
17. Paweltz, C. 2001. Reverse phase protein microarrays which capture disease progression show activation of pro-survival pathways at the cancer invasion front. Oncogene **20:** 1981–1989.
18. Chan, S. *et al.* 2004. Protein microarrays for multiplex analysis of signaling pathways. Nat. Med. **10:** 1390–1396.
19. Ermann, J. & C. Fathman. 2002. Autoimmune diseases: genes, bugs and failed regulation. Nat. Immunol. **2:** 759–761.
20. Perez, O. & G. Nolan. 2002. Simultaneous measurement of multiple active kinase states using polychromatic flow cytometry. Nat. Biotech. **20:** 155–162.
21. Irish, J. *et al.* 2004. Single cell profiling of potentiated phospho-protein networks in cancer cells. Cell **118:** 217–228.
22. Perez, O. 2005. Appreciating the heterogeneity in autoimmune disease: multiparameter assessment of intracellular signaling mechanisms. Ann. N.Y. Acad. Sci. **1062:** 155–164.

The Immune Response to BCG Vaccination of Newborns

WILLEM A. HANEKOM

South African Tuberculosis Vaccine Initiative (SATVI), Institute of Infectious Diseases and Molecular Medicine, University of Cape Town, Cape Town, South Africa

ABSTRACT: The aim of this study is to identify immune correlates of protection against tuberculosis induced by the current vaccine, Bacille Calmette Guerin (BCG). This knowledge should be valuable for developing and testing novel tuberculosis vaccines. Blood from 5675 10-week-old South African infants, routinely vaccinated with BCG at birth, was collected, processed, and stored. Subsequently, infants who have developed tuberculosis disease—"not protected by the vaccine"—and infants who have remained healthy despite exposure to adults with tuberculosis—"protected by the vaccine"—have been identified. Recall immune responses to mycobacterial antigens in whole blood samples from the infants have been elicited; the next step will be to retrieve stored blood of "unprotected" and "protected" infants and compare immunity induced by BCG in the two groups. To guide the immune analysis, various pilot studies are being conducted to characterize the vaccination-induced host response. Preliminary results indicate that BCG does indeed induce a potent CD8 T-cell response, with cytokine-producing or cytotoxic potential, in infants. An induction of FoxP3 mRNA expression in some mycobacteria-stimulated whole-blood samples is also being found, which suggests the presence of BCG-induced regulatory CD4 T cells. Finally, stimulation of whole blood with mycobacterial antigens has resulted in a consistent pattern of cytokine release: significant numbers of infants make either large amounts of the effector cytokine interferon-γ, or large amounts of the regulatory cytokine interleukin-10, but not both. Tests will, therefore, be made to determine whether CD8 or regulatory CD4 T-cell responses, as well as "outlier" cytokine responses, are associated with vaccination-induced protection against tuberculosis.

KEYWORDS: tuberculosis; vaccination; bacille Calmette-Guérin (BCG); CD8 T cell; CD4 T cell; cytokines; FoxP3 mRNA; interferon-γ; interleukin-10

VACCINATION-INDUCED PROTECTION AGAINST TUBERCULOSIS

The World Health Organization (WHO) declared tuberculosis (TB) a global health emergency in 1993.[1] The situation is no less urgent today: one-third of the world's population is infected with *Mycobacterium tuberculosis*, 8.8 million developed TB disease in 2002 alone; 1.8 million died.[2] Control of the epidemic remains

Address for correspondence: Willem A. Hanekom, SATVI, Institute of Infectious Diseases and Molecular Medicine, UCT Health Sciences Faculty, Wernher & Beit S2.01, Anzio Road, Observatory, 7925 Cape Town, South Africa.Voice: +27-21-406-6080; fax. +27-21-406-6081.
Willem@rmh.uct.ac.za

Ann. N.Y. Acad. Sci. 1062: 69–78 (2005). © 2005 New York Academy of Sciences.
doi: 10.1196/annals.1358.010

difficult, because TB control programs often lack adequate resources, prevalent human immunodeficiency virus (HIV) infection increases risk of disease, and multidrug resistance is emerging. An effective vaccine that prevents lung TB would be an attractive and sustainable long-term intervention.

Mycobacterium bovis Bacille Calmette Guérin (BCG) remains the only available vaccine against TB. This vaccine offers variable, mostly poor, protection against pulmonary TB.[3] Yet, adults with lung disease spread the pathogen. Further, although BCG is safe in the normal host, it may cause disease in HIV-infected persons.[4,5] There is, therefore, an urgent need for new vaccines that may better prevent lung TB, and may be safer in immune-compromised hosts.

Worldwide, five novel TB vaccines will have entered clinical trials by the end of 2005 (U. Furth, personal communication, 2004). At the South African Tuberculosis Vaccine Initiative (SATVI) in Cape Town, South Africa, we will commence clinical trials of a modified vaccinia virus Ankara–expressing antigen 85A (MVA85A), a novel vaccine designed for use as a boost after BCG prime.[6,7] The testing of any reasonable vaccine candidate is urgent, given the scope of the TB epidemic. However, success is unlikely unless a better understanding of the host response to TB and to BCG can be incorporated into vaccine design and clinical testing. This is the objective of our studies.

To date, immunological studies at SATVI have focused on BCG vaccination of newborns. Most of the world's newborns receive BCG soon after birth, because the vaccine affords ~80% protection against severe childhood TB, that is, miliary disease and meningitis.[3] Severe childhood TB is therefore a clinical setting in which we can determine which immune components induced by BCG are associated with protection. This is the aim of our largest project. To guide immune analysis of this study, we are conducting multiple pilot studies to characterize the host response to the vaccine. In a complementary project, we are determining whether BCG is immunogenic in HIV-infected infants; this is one study in a range aimed at assessing the risks and benefits of this WHO-recommended practice.

A CASE-CONTROL STUDY TO DETERMINE BCG-INDUCED IMMUNE CORRELATES OF PROTECTION AGAINST CHILDHOOD TB

To determine infant immune correlates of protection against TB, we have already collected, processed, and stored blood from 5675 infants who were routinely vaccinated with BCG at birth. The infants were enrolled at SATVI's rural vaccine evaluation site in the Cape Town region. In this area, TB is rife: the disease incidence in children <5 years old is in excess of 2000 per 100,000 per year (G.D. Hussey, personal communication, 2004).

Blood was collected at 10 weeks of age, as pilot studies have suggested that the BCG-immune response is quantitatively greater at this age, compared with later ages. Blood collection in infants <10 weeks of age was not deemed practical.

Among enrolled infants, we have subsequently identified children who, over the first four years of life, have developed TB disease. We presume that these children have not been protected by BCG vaccination ($n = 105$). Correspondingly, we have identified children who have remained healthy despite exposure to adults with TB. We presume that these children have been protected by BCG ($n = 100$). Our immediate plan is to retrieve stored blood of "unprotected" and "protected" infants, and to compare immunity induced by BCG. This will allow identification of immune components associated with protection against TB.

WHICH IMMUNE COMPONENTS MAY BE ASSOCIATED WITH BCG-INDUCED PROTECTION AGAINST TB?

Our approach to immune analysis in the immune-correlates study will be fourfold.

First, we will focus on immunity currently viewed to be important in protection against TB, based on clinical and experimental evidence.[8–11] We will therefore analyze T helper type-1 CD4 T-cell immunity, as infants with abnormal genes for interleukin-12 (IL-12) or interferon-γ (IFN-γ) receptors manifest severe disease from avirulent mycobacteria,[12–14] and HIV-associated CD4 T-cell depletion markedly increases the risk of TB or *M. avium* disease.[15] We will also characterize the BCG-induced CD8 T-cell response (see below).

Second, we will determine how this conventional T-cell immunity is regulated. Our hypothesis is that BCG has the potential to induce specific regulatory CD4 T cells (Tregs), which modulate conventional vaccination-induced responses (see below).

Third, we propose that current knowledge of mycobacterial immunity, and how this is regulated, needs to be expanded, and that novel genes involved in BCG-induced protection will be described with DNA microarray analysis. Functional aspects of these genes will be characterized.

Fourth, although T-cell responses are important in protection against TB, recent clinical and experimental evidence point toward a role of antibodies in protection against TB as well.[16,17] We will therefore examine whether antibodies induced by BCG or passively (transplacentally) transferred from a vaccinated infant's mother play a role in vaccination-induced protection against TB.

HOW SHOULD WE MEASURE THE HOST IMMUNE RESPONSE IN A RURAL, UNDERDEVELOPED SETTING?

Measuring vaccination-induced immunity in a rural vaccine evaluation setting, particularly in large numbers of small infants, is challenging. Our group has optimized various whole-blood assays to investigate immunity induced by BCG[18] (FIG. 1). Very small blood volumes are required, and results are sensitive, specific, and reproducible. We have chosen short-term whole-blood assays for various reasons. First, a "snapshot" of immunity present at the time of blood collection, in an entire immune compartment (peripheral blood), is measured. Second, very small blood volumes are required. Third, immediate stimulation of whole blood increases sensitivity of the measured T-cell response by approximately 30%, compared with stimulation of cryopreserved peripheral blood mononuclear cells (PBMCs). Fourth, assay backgrounds are lower than those of PBMC-based assays, increasing sensitivity even more.

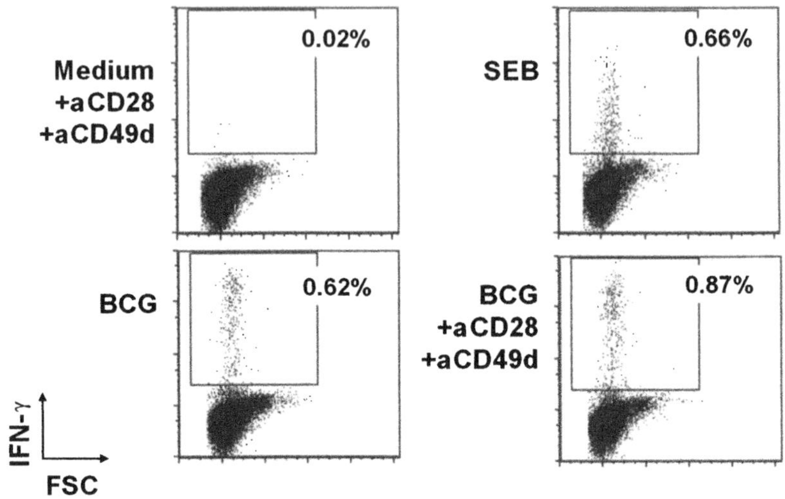

FIGURE 1. Results from a whole-blood assay for the flow cytometric detection of mycobacteria-specific, IFN-γ–expressing, CD4 T cells. Whole blood from a 10-week-old infant, routinely vaccinated with BCG at birth, was collected in heparinized 2-mL polypropylene tubes (Sarsted), and immediately incubated with BCG (SSI strain, prepared from the vaccine vial from Statens Serum Institut, 2.4×10^5 organisms per 200 μL blood), medium alone (negative control), or staphylococcal enterotoxin B (SEB, Sigma, positive control, 10 μg/mL), in the presence of the costimulatory antibodies anti-CD28 and anti-CD49d (BD Biosciences, 1 μg/mL), for 18 h. Brefeldin-A (Sigma, 10 μg/mL) was added for the last 5 h of incubation. Blood was harvested with EDTA (Sigma, 2 μM), and red cells were lysed and white cells fixed with FACS Lysing Solution (BD Biosciences). After cryopreservation in this solution, cells were thawed, washed, permeabilized (0.1% saponin, 0.1% bovine serum albumin, both Sigma, in PBS, Gibco) and incubated with fluorescence-conjugated antibodies (BD Biosciences). The frequency of IFN-γ–expressing CD4 T cells under the different conditions was determined by flow cytometry, as previously described.[18] Dot-plot results shown are gated on CD4 T cells.

An extremely important variable in successful completion of short-term whole-blood assays is immediate incubation of blood into the assay after collection. Our early experiments showed that delay in incubation of blood with the antigen whole viable BCG resulted in dramatic reduction of the frequency of CD4 T cells producing IFN-γ (FIG. 2). We have overcome this constraint with a novel system of blood processing, which starts with incubation of the blood immediately after collection (FIG. 3). All studies described below were conducted with this blood stimulation technique, which also allows isolation of white cells, mRNA, or plasma for analysis.

DOES BCG INDUCE CD8 T CELLS?

Mycobacteria do induce specific CD8 T-cell responses in humans,[9,19,20] and animal studies suggest that these responses are important for control of *Mycobacterium tuberculosis*.[21] However, traditionally, BCG has been thought to be a poor inducer

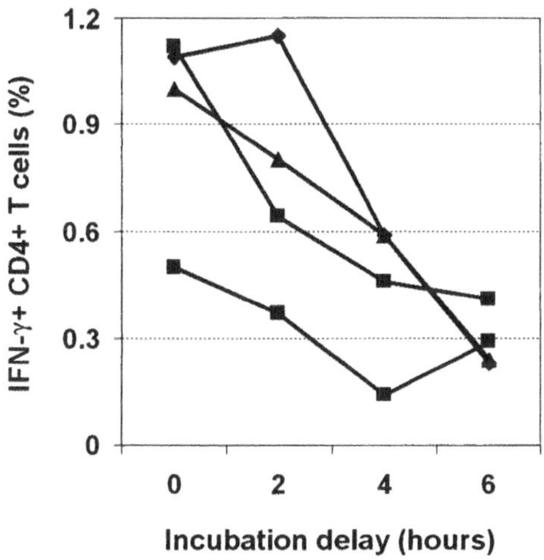

FIGURE 2. Effect of delay in blood processing, following collection, on a whole-blood intracellular cytokine assay performance. Whole blood from tuberculin skin test–positive persons was collected and either incubated immediately, or kept at room temperature for 2, 4, or 6 h before incubation. In each case, BCG was incubated with whole blood at 37°C for 18 h. The rest of the assay was completed as described in FIGURE 1. The frequency of IFN-γ–expressing CD4 T cells under the different conditions was determined by flow cytometry. Each line represents results from an individual participant.

of CD8 T-cell responses in humans.[11] We have therefore embarked on characterizing the CD8 T-cell response induced by BCG vaccination of newborns.

We have shown that 10 weeks after newborn vaccination, BCG-specific proliferating CD8 T cells are present in peripheral blood (FIG. 4). CD8 T-cell proliferation was quantitatively lower than that of CD4 T cells (FIG. 4). Similarly, although IFN-γ + CD8 T cells also have been detected, the frequency of specific CD8 T cells was lower than that of CD4 T cells (data not shown). We conclude that BCG does indeed induce functional CD8 T cells in infants.

Currently, we are examining functional aspects of specific CD8 T cells. We have shown upregulation of cell-specific expression of granzyme A, granzyme B, and perforin 72 h after incubation of PBMCs with BCG (data not shown). Similarly, degranulation potential of CD8 T cells has been shown by detection of cell-associated expression of the granule-specific molecules CD107a and CD107b[22] (data not shown). These preliminary results indicate that specific CD8 T cells with cytotoxic potential are indeed present after BCG vaccination.

DOES BCG INDUCE REGULATORY CD4 T CELLS?

Tregs may be critical for regulating the delicate balance between T-cell responses that efficiently control an infectious pathogen and exaggerated T-cell responses that may cause inflammation and tissue damage.[23,24] We hypothesize that BCG vaccination of newborns induces specific Tregs.

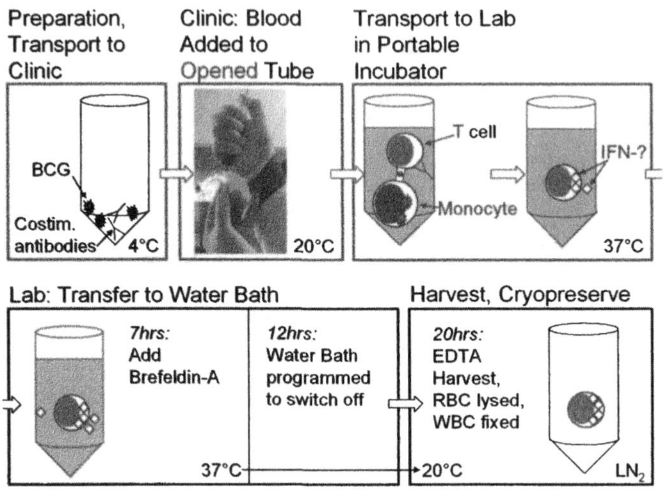

FIGURE 3. Optimized procedure for stimulating whole blood to determine the frequency of IFN-γ–expressing T cells, in field studies. Full assay details were reported recently.[18] Briefly, BCG is prepared, placed in polypropylene tubes with the costimulatory antibodies anti-CD28 and anti-CD49d, and transported at 2° to 8°C to clinics. Here, tubes are brought to room temperature. Blood, collected in a sodium-heparinized syringe, is added dropwise to an opened tube, up to a level marked on the side of the tube. The tube is closed and vortexed in the clinic, and placed in a portable 37°C incubator for transport to the laboratory. At the laboratory, tubes are transferred to a 37°C water bath (CO_2 is not required for this short-term assay). Brefeldin-A is added at 7 h. After 12 h, the optimal duration of stimulation with BCG, but a time point that often falls in the middle of the night, the preprogrammed water bath switches off. The temperature gradually drops to room temperature. After 20 h, the cells are harvested following incubation with EDTA. Red cells are lysed while white cells are fixed in a single step. The cells are pelleted, and cryopreserved in liquid nitrogen in a DMSO-containing solution.

In studies in progress, BCG stimulation of whole blood from 10-week-old infants vaccinated with BCG at birth results in a modest upregulation of mRNA expression of the Treg-specific transcription factor FoxP3 (FIG. 5). We will now also determine expression of this marker on a cell-specific level.

FoxP3 mRNA expression correlates with that of TGF-β, IL-10, and CTLA-4, putative effector molecules of Tregs (data not shown). These molecules may indeed inhibit conventional BCG-induced immunity, as neutralizing TGF-β, IL-10, and CTLA-4 results in a modest enhancement of IFN-γ production in purified protein derivative–stimulated whole blood (FIG. 6).

Currently, we are examining BCG-induced CD4 T-cell expression of these effector molecules and of the conventional/effector cytokine IFN-γ. However, on a soluble level, there is a consistent pattern of induction of IL-10 and IFN-γ production in plasma of BCG-stimulated whole blood: overall, expression of the two cytokines appears to correlate, suggesting a dynamic equilibrium between regulatory and conventional/effector immunity. However, some infants produce either excessive IL-10, or excessive IFN-γ, but not both (FIG. 7). This has led to the hypothesis that "outlier"

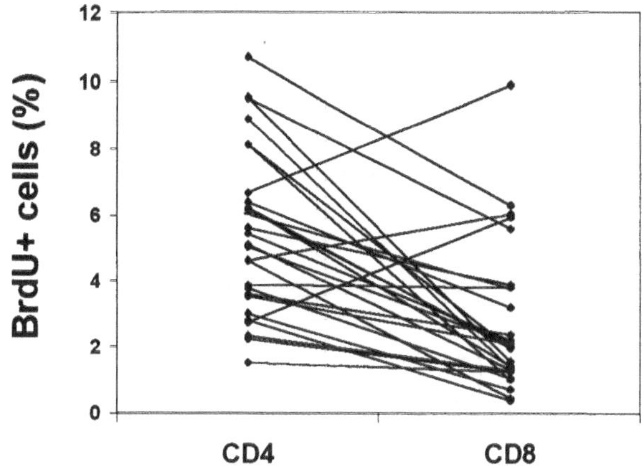

FIGURE 4. Proliferation of BCG-specific CD8 T cells from peripheral blood of infants vaccinated with BCG. Fifty microliters of blood, collected from 10-week-old infants routinely vaccinated with BCG at birth, was diluted to 500 μL in RPMI. The diluted blood was incubated at 37°C in 5% CO_2 for 6 days in the presence of BCG (SSI, at a multiplicity of infection of 0.5). On day 6, bromodeoxyuridine (BrdU, Sigma, 10 μM) was added for the final 4 h of incubation. Cells were harvested using EDTA (2 μM), lysed, fixed with FACS Lysing Solution (BD Biosciences), and cryopreserved. Fixed cells were thawed, permeabilized as described in FIGURE 1, and stained with fluorescence-conjugated antibodies (BD Biosciences) in the presence of DNAse. Flow cytometry was performed to determine the frequency of proliferating ($BrdU^+$) CD8 T cells.

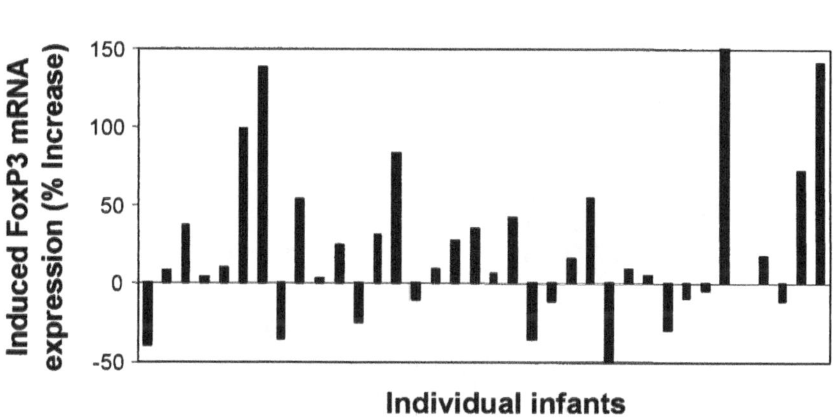

FIGURE 5. mRNA expression of FoxP3, a regulatory CD4 T cell–specific transcription factor, in BCG-stimulated whole blood of vaccinated infants. Whole blood from 10-week-old infants vaccinated with BCG at birth was incubated with BCG or with medium for 12 h at 37°C. Red cells were lysed and RNA isolated from white cells (QIAamp RNA Blood Minikit, Qiagen). mRNA expression of FoxP3 and of the housekeeping gene Hprt was determined by real-time PCR. The change in FoxP3 expression (corrected for Hprt), compared with this expression in the medium-stimulated blood, of each infant is shown.

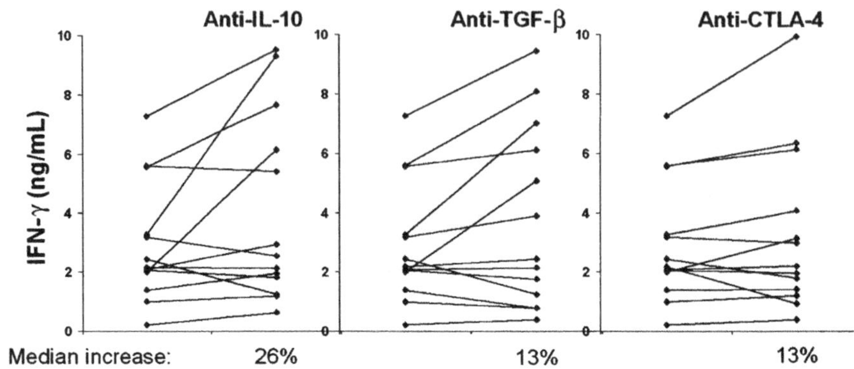

FIGURE 6. Effect of neutralization of putative effector molecules of regulatory CD4 T cells on mycobacteria-induced IFN-γ production in blood from vaccinated infants. Whole blood from 10-week-old infants, vaccinated with BCG at birth, was incubated at 37°C with purified protein derivative of *M. tuberculosis* (SSI, 25 μg/mL), with or without neutralizing antibodies against IL-10, TGF-γ, or CTLA-4. After 7 h, plasma was harvested. Plasma soluble IFN-γ was detected by ELISA (BD Biosciences). Each line represents results from plasma from an individual infant, without and with antibody neutralization.

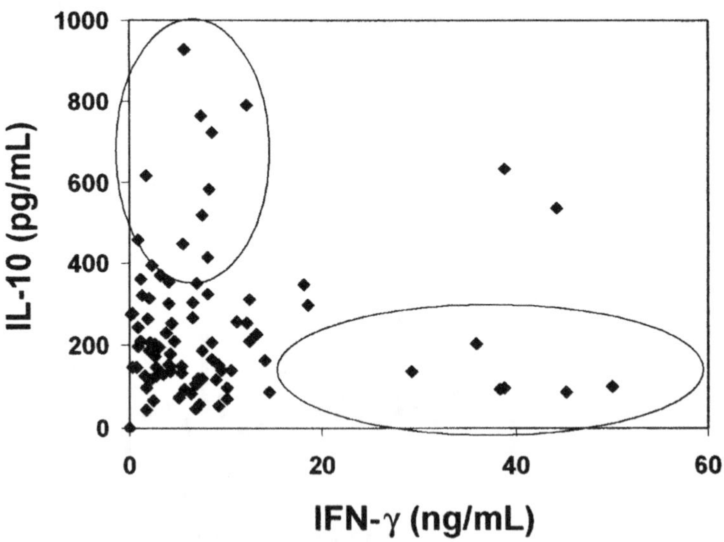

FIGURE 7. Plasma levels of the regulatory cytokine IL-10 and of the effector cytokine IFN-γ in BCG-stimulated blood from vaccinated infants. Whole blood from 10-week-old infants, vaccinated with BCG at birth, was incubated at 37°C with BCG (SSI). After 7 h, plasma was harvested. Plasma-soluble IL-10 and IFN-γ were detected by ELISA (BD Biosciences). Each *diamond* represents results from plasma from an individual infant. The results suggest that, in the majority, expression of the two cytokines correlate; however, some infants produce high levels of either IL-10 or IFN-γ (*circles*), but not both.

immune responses may be associated with aberrant vaccination-induced protection against TB.

FUTURE DIRECTIONS OF OUR RESEARCH

Our immediate focus is to complete the case-control study to determine BCG-induced immune correlates of protection. These immune markers will be validated as surrogates of protective immunity in studies to follow.

We have stored both whole blood stimulated with BCG, and unstimulated PBMCs, for analysis. Some PBMCs will be saved for studies of novel antigens that may be associated with protection against TB. Novel TB antigen discovery is a major component of a newly funded Gates Global Challenge Grant project focusing on biomarkers of protection against TB (principal investigator: Stefan Kaufmann).

Finally, immune regulation may also occur at the level of the innate immune response. We will now investigate the role of macrophages and dendritic cells in vaccination-induced protection. We will call back "unprotected" and "protected" infants, and collect more blood to investigate the role of these cells using newly optimized whole-blood assays. At the same time, we will investigate whether polymorphisms in toll-like receptors, critical pattern-recognition receptors of innate immune cells, are associated with BCG-induced protection against TB.

ACKNOWLEDGMENTS

Many persons have played central roles in the ongoing immunology projects of SATVI. The author wishes specifically to acknowledge Rose Ann Murray, Nazma Mansoor, Joanne Riley, Alana Keyser, Helen Fletcher, Virginia Davids, Sebastian Gelderbloem, Jane Hughes, Hoyam Gamieldien, Mzwandile Sidibana, Nazma Mansoor, Andrea Soares, Deon Minnies, Anthony Hawkridge, Adrian Hill, Larry Geiter, Gregory D. Hussey, and particularly Gilla Kaplan, from whose laboratory these immunology studies were commenced initially, and who remains a central collaborator in the projects.

[*Competing interests*: The author states that he has no competing financial interests.]

REFERENCES

1. WORLD HEALTH ORGANIZATION. 1993. Tuberculosis fact sheet. World Health Organization. Geneva.
2. WORLD HEALTH ORGANIZATION. 2002. Tuberculosis fact sheet. World Health Organization. Geneva.
3. FINE, P. 2000. BCG vaccines and vaccination. *In* Tuberculosis: A Comprehensive International Approach. L.B. Reichman & E.S. Hershfield, Eds.: 503–524. Marcel Dekker. New York.
4. CAMPOS, J.M. *et al.* 1996. Disseminated Bacillus Calmette-Guerin infection in HIV-infected children: case report and review. Pediatr. AIDS HIV Infect. **7:** 429–432.
5. HESSELING, A.C. *et al.* 2003. Danish bacille Calmette-Guerin vaccine-induced disease in human immunodeficiency virus-infected children. Clin. Infect. Dis. **37:** 1226–1233.

6. McShane, H. *et al.* 2005. Boosting BCG with MVA85A: the first candidate subunit vaccine for tuberculosis in clinical trials. Tuberculosis (Edinb.). **85:** 47–52.
7. McShane, H. *et al.* 2004. Recombinant modified vaccinia virus Ankara expressing antigen 85A boosts BCG-primed and naturally acquired antimycobacterial immunity in humans. Nat. Med. **10:** 1240–1244.
8. Boom, W.H. *et al.* 2003. Human immunity to M. tuberculosis: T cell subsets and antigen processing. Tuberculosis (Edinb.). **83:** 98–106.
9. Flynn, J.L. 2004. Immunology of tuberculosis and implications in vaccine development. Tuberculosis (Edinb.). **84:** 93–101.
10. Lewinsohn, D.M., D.A. Lewinsohn & J.E. Grotzke. 2003. TB vaccines at the turn of the century: insights into immunity to M. tuberculosis and modern approaches for prevention of an ancient disease. Semin. Respir. Infect. **18:** 320–338.
11. Kaufmann, S.H. & A.J. McMichael. 2005. Annulling a dangerous liaison: vaccination strategies against AIDS and tuberculosis. Nat. Med. **11:** S33–S44.
12. Casanova, J.L. & L. Abel. 2002. Genetic dissection of immunity to mycobacteria: the human model. Annu. Rev. Immunol. **20:** 581–620.
13. Doffinger, R. *et al.* 2002. Inherited disorders of IL-12- and IFNgamma-mediated immunity: a molecular genetics update. Mol. Immunol. **38:** 903–909.
14. Ottenhoff, T.H. *et al.* 2003. Human deficiencies in type-1 cytokine receptors reveal the essential role of type-1 cytokines in immunity to intracellular bacteria. Adv. Exp. Med. Biol. **531:** 279–294.
15. Pozniak, A. 2002. Mycobacterial diseases and HIV. J. HIV Ther. **7:** 13–16.
16. Casadevall, A. 2003. Antibody-mediated immunity against intracellular pathogens: two-dimensional thinking comes full circle. Infect. Immun. **71:** 4225–4228.
17. Glatman-Freedman, A. 2003. Advances in antibody-mediated immunity against Mycobacterium tuberculosis: implications for a novel vaccine strategy. FEMS Immunol. Med. Microbiol. **39:** 9–16.
18. Hanekom, W.A. *et al.* 2004. Novel application of a whole blood intracellular cytokine detection assay to quantitate specific T-cell frequency in field studies. J. Immunol. Methods **291:** 185–195.
19. Dong, Y. *et al.* 2004. HLA-A2-restricted CD8+-cytotoxic-T-cell responses to novel epitopes in Mycobacterium tuberculosis superoxide dismutase, alanine dehydrogenase, and glutamine synthetase. Infect. Immun. **72:** 2412–2415.
20. Kawashima, T. *et al.* 2003. Cutting edge: major CD8 T cell response to live bacillus Calmette-Guerin is mediated by CD1 molecules. J. Immunol. **170:** 5345–5348.
21. Serbina, N.V., V. Lazarevic & J.L. Flynn. 2001. CD4(+) T cells are required for the development of cytotoxic CD8(+) T cells during Mycobacterium tuberculosis infection. J. Immunol. **167:** 6991–7000.
22. Betts, M.R. *et al.* 2003. Sensitive and viable identification of antigen-specific CD8+ T cells by a flow cytometric assay for degranulation. J. Immunol. Methods **281:** 65–78.
23. Mittrucker, H.W. & S.H. Kaufmann. 2004. Mini-review: regulatory T cells and infection: suppression revisited. Eur. J. Immunol. **34:** 306–312.
24. Vigouroux, S. *et al.* 2004. Antigen-induced regulatory T cells. Blood **104:** 26–33.

Regulation of Acquired Immunity by $\gamma\delta$ T-Cell/Dendritic-Cell Interactions

NIRAJ SHRESTHA,[a] JAMES A. IDA,[a] A. STEVEN LUBINSKI,[b] MARIA PALLIN,[a] GILLA KAPLAN,[b] AND PATRICK A.J. HASLETT[a,c]

[a]*The Department of Microbiology and Immunology, University of Miami Miller School of Medicine, Miami, Florida 33136, USA*

[b] *The Public Health Research Institute, Newark, New Jersey, USA*

[c]*Miami Veterans Administration Medical Center, Miami, Florida, USA*

ABSTRACT: In humans, innate immune recognition of mycobacteria, including *Mycobacterium tuberculosis* and *Mycobacterium leprae*, involves toll-like receptor-2 (TLR-2), expressed on immature dendritic cells (DCs), and the T-cell $\gamma\delta$ receptor expressed by a subpopulation of T cells that utilize Vδ2 (Vδ2 T cells). To investigate modulatory relationships between these host-cell populations in a microbial context, *in vitro* experiments were performed with human DCs and Vδ2 T cells stimulated with model TLR-2 ligands and phosphoantigens, respectively. We observed that TLR-2–stimulated DCs enhanced interferon-γ (IFN-γ) production by Vδ2 T cells; conversely, activated Vδ2 T cells enhanced TLR-2–induced DC maturation via soluble factors including IFN-γ, which co-stimulated interleukin-12 (IL-12) p70 secretion by DCs. Exposure of DCs to activated Vδ2 T cells was critical for Th1 T-cell priming when TLR-2 stimulation was limiting. These results suggest that Vδ2 T cells may play an adjuvant role in priming protective antimycobacterial immunity when TLR-2 stimulation is lacking, as may occur if the infectious inoculum is small, or if the pathogen is an intrinsically weak activator of DCs.

KEYWORDS: $\gamma\delta$ T cells; dendritic cells; mycobacterium; tuberculosis; leprosy

INTRODUCTION

Immunity against intracellular pathogens such as *Mycobacterium tuberculosis* (*M.tb*) and *Mycobacterium leprae* depends upon the induction of pathogen-specific, IFN-γ–producing CD4$^+$ (Th1) T cells. However, effective Th1 immunity cannot be achieved without prior activation of the innate immune response. The mode and extent of innate immune activation are powerful determinants of CD4$^+$ T-cell differen-

Address for correspondence: Patrick A.J. Haslett, 1580 NW 10th Ave., BCRI 743, Miami, FL 33136. Voice: 305-243-2189; fax 305-243-7211.
phaslett@med.miami.edu

**Ann. N.Y. Acad. Sci. 1062: 79–94 (2005). © 2005 New York Academy of Sciences.
doi: 10.1196/annals.1358.011**

tiation into Th1, Th2, or regulatory phenotypes. Initial, direct recognition of unprocessed pathogen products/components is a function of dendritic cells, which act as sentinels in peripheral tissues, detecting microbes via germline-encoded (hence, "innate") receptors, such as members of the toll-like receptor (TLR) family.[1,2] Upon TLR-mediated activation, a maturation program is initiated in DCs, so that they migrate to regional lymph nodes, where processed, pathogen-derived antigens are presented to naive T cells. In the steady state, that is, in the absence of such pathogenic stimuli, dendritic cells constitutively present self antigens as a means of maintaining peripheral self-tolerance.[3,4] The latter process may involve the generation of self-reactive regulatory T cells.[5] Thus, initial discrimination between self and pathogen is an innate function of dendritic cells, which then prime adaptive T-cell responses for tolerance or immunity. Recent studies have begun to elucidate the mechanisms by which various pathogens may elicit different types of T-cell response by interacting with different TLRs on DCs.[6–8] Of the 10 known human TLRs, TLR-2 appears to be the receptor most relevant to mycobacterial infection,[9–15] binding lipoproteins such as the ***M.tb*** 19-kDa antigen, as well as several lipoproteins derived from *M. leprae,*[16] the bacillus that causes leprosy.

Direct recognition of unprocessed pathogen molecules, including those present in mycobacteria, is also a feature of a subset of human γδ T cells with antigen receptor variable regions encoded by Vγ9 and Vδ2 (Vδ2 T cells). In healthy adults, γδ T cells make up between 1 and 10% of peripheral blood T cells.[17] The Vδ2 T-cell population comprises a minor subset at birth, but expands over the first 5 to 10 years of life to form the majority of circulating γδ T cells.[18] Microbial activation of these cells is via the T-cell receptor; activation is mediated by low molecular-weight (<1 kDa) nonpeptide phosphoantigens, without a requirement for MHC, in a strictly conformation-dependent manner, akin to antigen recognition by immunoglobulin.[19] So far, γδ T cells with specificity for phosphoantigens have been described only in humans and other primates. Isopentenyl pyrophosphate (IPP), isolated from mycobacteria, was the first such phosphoantigen to be studied.[19] However, IPP is a ubiquitous product of the mevalonate pathway of isoprenoid synthesis and may therefore act as a self antigen. A clue to the mechanism for self versus pathogen discrimination by Vδ2 T cells came with the recent delineation of the alternative, largely prokaryotic 2-*C*-methyl-D-erythritol 4-phosphate pathway of isoprenoid synthesis.[20] Intermediates of this pathway are up to 10,000 times more potent than IPP in activating Vδ2 T cells. Therefore, the Vδ2 T-cell receptor functions to recognize microbial patterns, similarly to true innate receptors, discerning potential pathogens by the differential potency of their phosphoantigens.

In tuberculosis patients, Vδ2 T cells are frequently increased in number.[21,22] A protective role for Vδ2 T cells in this infection has been inferred from their rapid production of effector molecules, such as IFN-γ and tumor necrosis factor alpha (TNF-α).[23–26] Moreover, recent data in a rhesus macaque tuberculosis model indicate that the Vδ2 T-cell population is capable of an anamnestic response upon reexposure to mycobacterial antigens *in vivo*.[27] In addition to a possible a role for γδ T cells in host defense, data suggest that these cells may function to maintain epithelial homeostasis[28,29] and immune tolerance.[30] Because both DCs and Vδ2 T cells exist in the periphery, and can be directly activated by bacterial antigens, we hypothesized that a comodulatory relationship exists between these cell populations, which may influence priming of T cells that express the conventional αβ antigen receptor.

METHODS

Study Subjects

Peripheral venous blood was obtained from healthy adult volunteers. Written consent was obtained according to a protocol approved by the University of Miami Institutional Review Board.

Reagents

The following fluorescence-conjugated antibodies were used to stain cells for flow cytometric analysis: CD3 PerCP, CD4 FITC, pan γδTCR biotin/streptavidin APC, Vδ2 FITC, Vγ9 PE, CD25 PE, CD80 PE, CD83 PE, CD80 PE, CCR7 PE, IFN-γ PE, TNF-α FITC, and IL-10 PE (obtained from BD Pharmingen, San Diego, CA). For cytokine blockade, soluble IFN-γR1 and TNFR1 were obtained from R&D Systems, Minneapolis, MN. The following immune stimulatory ligands were purchased from Sigma Aldrich, St. Louis, MO: lipoteichoic acids (LTA) from *Streptococcus pyogenes*, *Staphylococcus aureus*, and *Bacillus subtilis* (TLR-2 ligands); isopentenyl pyrophosphate (IPP, ligand for Vδ2 T-cell receptor). *M.tb* whole-cell lysate, and *M.tb* triton-X114 detergent extract, which is enriched with mycobacterial TLR-2 stimulatory lipoproteins, were obtained from John Belisle, Colorado State University, via NIH, NIAID TB Research Materials and Vaccine Testing Contract, NO1 AI-75320. The synthetic TLR-2 stimulatory lipopeptide, Pam3Cys was purchased from EMC Microcollections, Tuebingen, Germany.

Preparation of Cell Populations

Peripheral blood mononuclear cells (PBMCs) were isolated from heparinized blood by differential centrifugation over Ficoll-Paque (Pharmacia, Piscataway, NJ).

Cell purification/enrichment was performed by either negative or positive selection with immmunomagnetic beads (Miltenyi Biotech, Auburn, CA), in accordance with the manufacturer's instructions. Purified "untouched" T-cell populations were isolated from PBMCs by negative selection. Naive $CD4^+$ T cells were purified further from these populations by depletion of $CD45RO^+$ memory cells, followed by positive selection of $CD4^+$ cells. Purified γδ T cells were obtained by positive selection from PBMCs. In some experiments, depletion of T cells, NK cells, and monocytes from PBMCs was performed with a cocktail of anti-CD2, anti-CD56, and anti-CD14 antibodies to yield an enriched mixture of peripheral blood DCs and B cells, which were then sorted into B-cell and bulk DC populations by positive selection of B cells. Purified cell populations were routinely >95% pure, as ascertained by flow cytometry. Depletion of monocyte/macrophages from PBMCs was achieved by incubating 1×10^7 PBMCs in 100-mm plastic petri dishes for 1 h at 37°C. Nonadherent cells were collected and found to be efficiently depleted of monocytes by flow cytometry.

Immature monocyte-derived DCs were generated from positively selected, purified $CD14^+$ monocyte precursors by culture in RPMI 1640 (Gibco-Invitrogen, Carlsbad, CA) containing 5% human Ab serum, recombinant human IL-4, 0.2 ng/mL (Endogen, Rockford, IL), and recombinant human GM-CSF, 1 ng/mL (Endogen).

Cytokine-matured DCs were generated by incubating immature DCs for 2 days in medium supplemented with TNF-α, 10 ng/mL (Alexis Biochemicals, San Diego, CA), IL-1β, 10 ng/mL (BD Biosciences-Pharmingen, San Diego, CA), and PG E_2, 1 μg/mL (Sigma-Aldrich, St. Louis, MO).

Short-term Vδ2 T-cell lines were obtained by stimulating PBMCs with 30 mM IPP. Cells were cultured in 24-well tissue culture plates at 1×10^6 PMBCs/mL/well in RPMI 1640 supplemented with 10% FBS (Hyclone, Logan, UT). Fresh medium containing 0.1 nM recombinant human IL-2 (Chiron, Emeryville, CA) was added on days 3 and 7 of 10-day cultures. Flow cytometry performed at day 10 showed that ~85% of cells expressed the Vδ2 T-cell receptor.

DC/Vδ2 T-Cell Coculture

Cocultures of Vδ2 T-cell lines and DCs were set up either with direct contact between the cell populations, or in a transwell system mounted in a 24-well tissue culture plate. Then 1×10^5 immature DCs were placed in the lower chamber, and 1×10^6 Vδ2 T cells in the upper, together with IPP and TLR-2 ligands, as indicated. After 48 h, supernatants were harvested for cytokine ELISA, the lower chamber removed, and the conditioned DCs were harvested for flow cytometric analysis, or washed twice before use as stimulators of naive allogeneic $CD4^+$ T cells.

Analysis of Intracellular Cytokines by Fluorescence-Activated Cell Sorting

Brefeldin A (Sigma Aldrich) 10 μg/mL, was added during the last 5 h of cell culture to block cytokine secretion. Harvested cells were first stained for surface markers before subsequent fixation with 4% paraformaldehyde and permeabilization in phosphate-buffered saline containing 0.1% saponin and 0.1% bovine serum albumin. Staining with anticytokine antibodies took place in 50 μL permeabilization buffer. Subsequently, cells were washed twice in permeabilization buffer, resuspended in PBS, and transferred to plastic tubes for analysis with an LSR-1 flow cytometer (Becton Dickinson). Flow cytometric data were analyzed with FlowJo software (Tree Star Inc., Ashland, OR).

Lymphocyte Proliferation Assays

Lymphocyte proliferation was measured by standard ^{3}H-thymidine incorporation assay to quantify DNA synthesis, as described previously.[31] Briefly, triplicate cultures of 1×10^5 T cells were stimulated with allogeneic DCs at various DC-to-T-cell ratios, and pulsed for the last 6 h of 72- to 120-hour cultures with 0.5 μCi ^{3}H-thymidine (NEN Products, Boston, MA). DNA was harvested onto fiber mats with an automatic cell harvester (Skatron, Stirling, VA), and β emission measured with a Wallac LKB liquid scintillation counter. In some experiments, T-cell proliferation was measured by flow cytometric analysis of dilution of the cytosolic dye, carboxyfluorescein diacetate succinimidyl ester (CFSE), which is partitioned between daughter cells upon cell division. The latter technique permitted the simultaneous assessment of intracellular cytokine expression, as described previously.[32] Briefly, naive $CD4^+$ T cells were suspended in RPMI 1640 at 5×10^7 cells/mL. An equal volume of 16 μM CFSE (Molecular Probes, Eugene, OR) in RPMI 1640 was added and the cells incubated for 10 min at 37°C in 5% CO_2. The cells were then washed twice in RPMI 1640 containing 10% human Ab serum, and set up in culture with the experimental stimuli. BFA was added to the cultures for the last 5 h of 72- to 96-hour cultures, following which cells were processed for intracellular cytokine analysis, as described before.

Cytokine ELISA

IL-12p70, IL-10, IFN-γ, IL-4, and TNF-α were measured by ELISA using paired antibody kits obtained from R&D Systems, Minneapolis, MN. Assays were performed on freshly collected culture supernatants, according to the manufacturer's instructions.

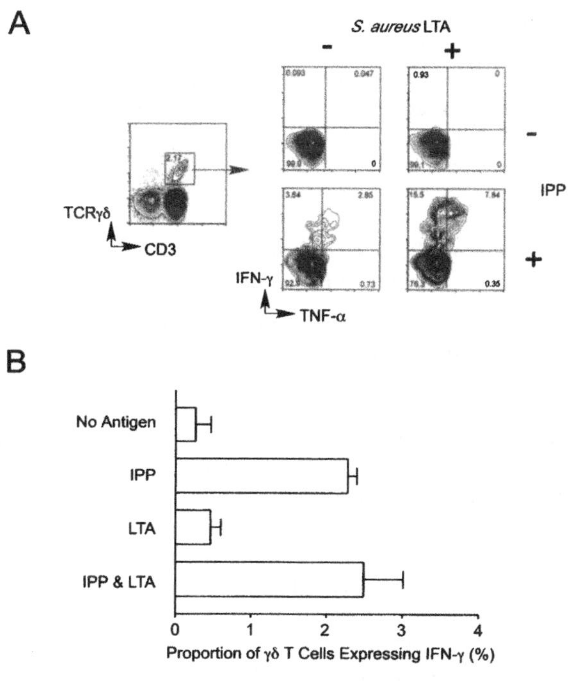

FIGURE 1. Costimulation of γδ T cells by TLR-2 ligand. (**A**) Intracellular cytokine expression by γδ T cells in PBMC cultures stimulated for 18 h with isopentenyl pyrophosphate (IPP), 30 μM, in the presence or absence of *S. aureus* lipoteichoic acid (LTA), 10 μg/mL, a TLR-2 ligand. Electronic gating strategy is shown. (**B**) Lack of effect of LTA on purified γδ T cells. Immunomagnetically purified γδ T cells were incubated with IPP ± LTA for 18 h, followed by intracellular detection of IFN-γ by flow cytometry. Mean results of three experiments shown.

RESULTS

TLR-2 Ligation Costimulates Vδ2 T-Cell Activation

To ascertain the effect of TLR-2 ligation on Vδ2 T-cell responses, PBMCs from healthy donors were stimulated with IPP, to activate Vδ2 T cells, in the presence or absence of different TLR-2 ligands. After overnight incubation, responsiveness was measured by flow cytometric evaluation of intracellular IFN-γ and TNF-α expression in γδ T cells. We found that the frequency of γδ T cells that expressed IFN-γ, or that were double-positive for IFN-γ and TNF-α, was increased when TLR-2 ligands were added to IPP. TLR-2 ligands alone did not stimulate significant cytokine responses in γδ T cells. Hence, TLR-2 ligation provided costimulation for γδ T-cell activation. FIGURE 1A shows a representative experiment, where *S. aureus* LTA was used as a model TLR-2 ligand. Therefore, TLR-2 ligation exerted a costimulatory effect on Vδ2 cytokine expression. Staining with specific antibodies confirmed that the IPP-stimulated cytokine-positive T cells were $V\delta2^+V\gamma9^+$ (not shown). Similar results were obtained with LTAs from *S. pyogenes* and *B. subtilis*, and *M.tb* whole cell lysate or triton X114 extracts (not shown).

TLR 2 gene expression has been reported in murine γδ T cells.[33] To test whether LTA costimulation was being delivered directly to γδ T cells, we performed experiments with purified γδ T cells. FIGURE 1B shows the result of a representative experiment, demonstrating that there was no costimulatory effect of *S. aureus* LTA when purified γδ T cells were stimulated with IPP. Similar negative results were obtained with short-term Vδ2 T-cell lines and purified bulk T cells (not shown). These observations indicate that an accessory cell is necessary for TLR-2 costimulation of Vδ2 T-cell responses.

TLR-2 Costimulation of Vδ2 T-Cell Activation Is Efficiently Mediated by Immature Dendritic Cells

Alveolar macrophages have been reported to have an accessory role in stimulating γδ T-cell responses to mycobacterial antigens.[34] We therefore compared the costimulatory activity of TLR-2 ligands on IPP-stimulated Vδ2 T-cell responses in bulk PBMCs and in PBMCs depleted of monocyte/macrophages by plastic adherence. FIGURE 2A shows the results of experiments performed with five different donors and with various TLR ligands. We observed that, in general, the costimulatory effect of TLR-2 ligation was enhanced, not abrogated, by monocyte depletion. We next performed experiments where purified candidate accessory cells, B cells, monocyte-derived immature dendritic cells, and dendritic cells directly isolated from PBMCs were combined with purified autologous T cells at a ratio of 1 accessory cell to 10 T cells, and cocultures stimulated with IPP ± TLR-2 ligands. A representative experiment is shown in FIGURE 2B, indicating that maximal γδ T-cell responses were elicited in the presence of TLR-2–stimulated dendritic cells. Interestingly, dendritic cells also enhanced the IPP-stimulated γδ T-cell response in the absence of TLR stimulation. When mature and immature DCs were compared, the costimulatory activity was only evident in immature DCs (FIG. 2C), in keeping with the known downregulation of TLR upon maturation of DCs.[35] Together, these experiments show that TLR-2 costimulation of Vδ2 T-cell responses requires accessory cell function, and that this is most efficiently provided by immature DCs.

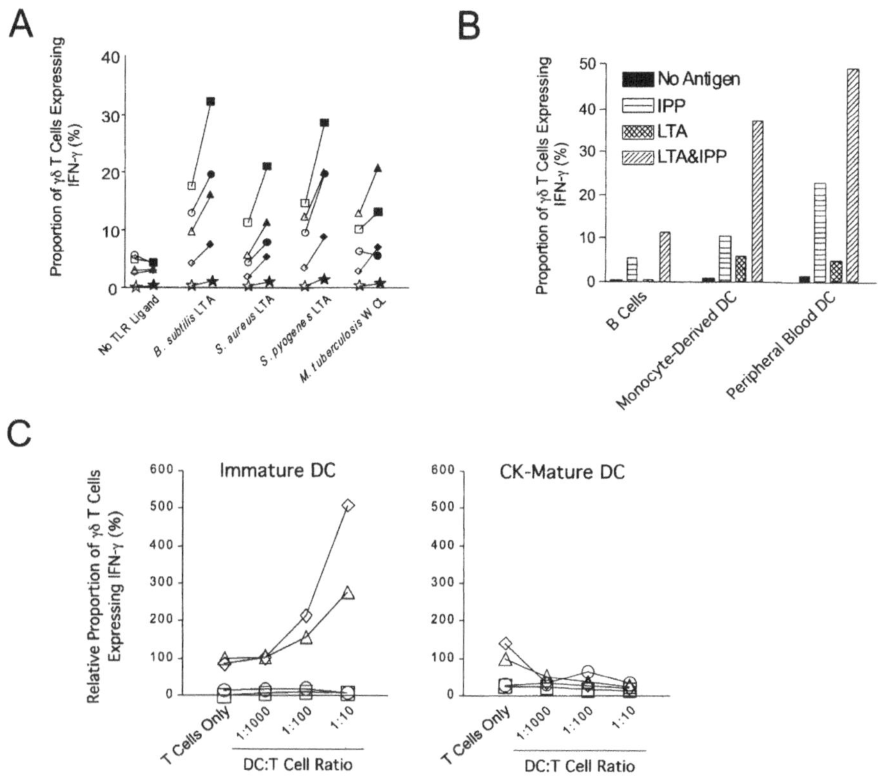

FIGURE 2. (**A**) Effect of monocyte depletion on γδ T-cell IFN-γ response. Data from experiments performed with five healthy donors are shown. *Open symbols*: whole PBMC; *solid symbols*: monocyte-depleted PBMCs. Each symbol represents an individual donor. (**B**) Dendritic cells are efficient promoters of LTA-enhanced IPP response by Vδ2 T cells. Purified T cells cocultured overnight with immunomagnetically purified B cells, monocyte-derived DCs or bulk blood DCs at a ratio of 10 T cells to 1 accessory cell. (**C**) Accessory role in TLR-2–mediated costimulation of Vδ2 T-cell IPP response performed by immature, not mature, monocyte-derived DCs. Purified T cells were cocultured with immature DCs or DCs that had been matured with a proinflammatory cytokine cocktail (CK-matured DCs) at the indicated ratios for 18 h. Intracellular IFN-γ in Vδ2 T cells measured by flow cytometry.

Activated Vδ2 T Cells Cause Partial Maturation of DCs

Because TLR-2–activated immature DCs were found to costimulate Vδ2 T cells, we next asked whether activation of Vδ2 T cells could reciprocally activate or induce maturation in DCs. We performed experiments with short-term Vδ2 T-cell lines generated by IPP stimulation of PBMCs with IL-2 supplementation, as described in METHODS. After 10 days, >85% of the cultured cells were Vγ9Vδ2 positive (not shown). The cells were washed twice and incubated overnight in the absence of IL-2 and IPP. Subsequently, the γδ T cells were incubated with immature DCs at a ratio of 10 Vδ2 T cells per DC. The cells were cocultured either with cell–cell contact, or

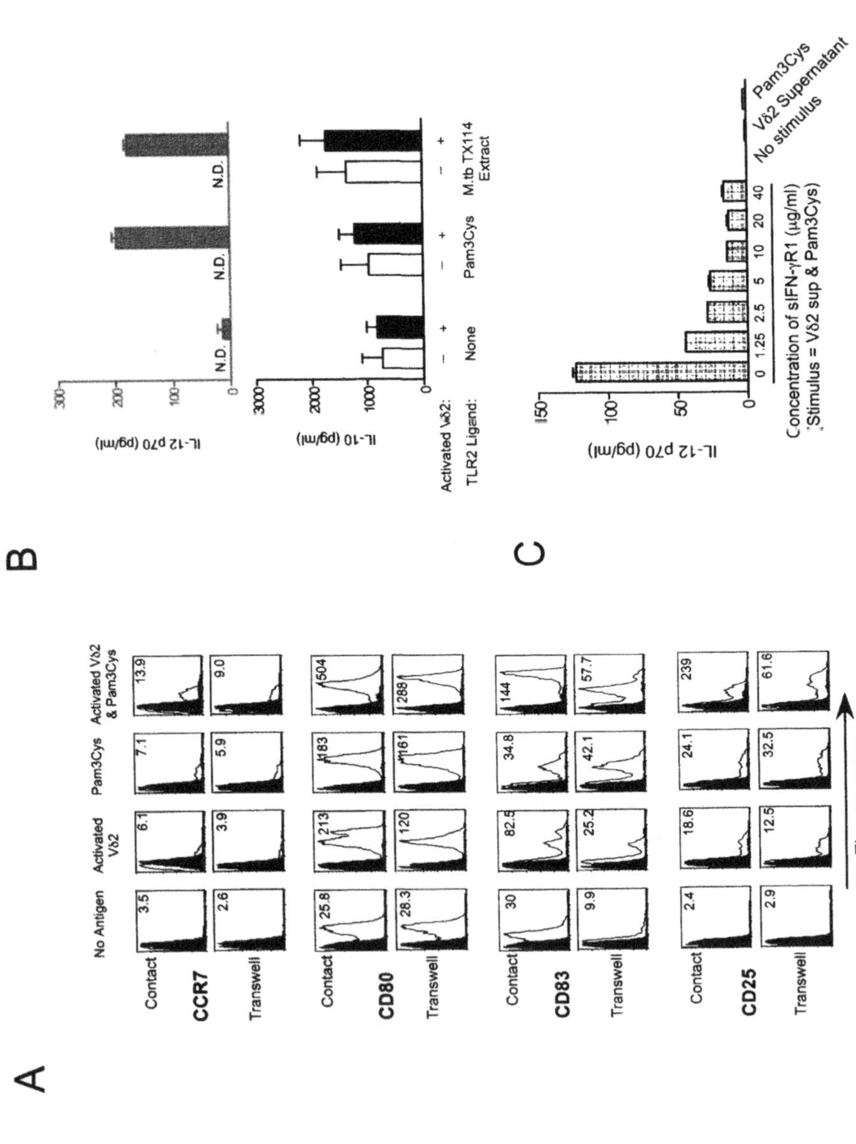

FIGURE 3. *See following page for legend.*

separated by a transwell membrane with 0.4 μm pores to allow free exchange of soluble factors between upper and lower chambers. Cocultures were stimulated with TLR-2 ligand, IPP, or both. After 48 h in culture, the cells were harvested, and DC maturation phenotype was assessed by cell-surface expression of CCR7, CD80, CD83, and CD25. FIGURE 3A shows that IPP-activated Vδ2 T cells stimulated partial DC maturation. We confirmed previous findings that TLR-2 ligation causes DC maturation,[12] and observed that the latter effect is enhanced by simultaneous Vδ2 T-cell activation. The effect of Vδ2 T-cell activation on DC maturation was similar whether the two cell populations were in contact or not (FIG. 3A). We noted the same effect on DC maturation with a variety of TLR-2 ligands, including *S. aureus* LTA, *M.tb* TX114 extract, and Pam3Cys, a synthetic lipoprotein that is a pure TLR-2 ligand. In the absence of IPP activation, Vδ2 T cells had no effect on DC maturation. Similarly, in the absence of Vδ2 T cells, IPP had no effect on DC maturation (not shown). These experiments indicate that activated Vδ2 T cells secrete a soluble factor that promotes DC maturation, and exerts an additive effect when combined with TLR-2 ligands.

IFN-γ Production by Activated Vδ2T Cells Provides Costimulation for TLR-2-Induced IL-12 p70 Production by DCs

Secretion of IL-12p70 and IL-10 by DCs are key determinants of T-cell differentiation at the time of the priming interaction between DCs and naive T cells. Therefore, we studied the effect of activated Vδ2 T cells and/or TLR-2 ligation on secretion of these cytokines by DCs. The results of a representative experiment are shown in FIGURE 3B. TLR-2 ligation and Vδ2 T-cell activation alone were insufficient to stimulate secretion of IL-12 p70, although this cytokine was consistently detectable when both stimuli were present. In contrast, Vδ2 T-cell activation did not influence IL-10 secretion. Similar costimulatory activity for IL-12 p70 production was observed whether Vδ2 T cells were activated in the transwell apparatus, or if supernatants from activated Vδ2 T-cell cultures were used (FIG. 3C).

Because IFN-γ has been reported to act as a costimulus for IL-12 p70 secretion by TLR-2 stimulated DCs,[36] we tested whether this cytokine was the costimulatory factor secreted by activated Vδ2 T cells. Supernatant from activated Vδ2 T cells was preincubated with sIFN-γR1 and then added to immature DCs, together with

FIGURE 3. (**A**) Effect of activated Vδ2 T cells ± Pam3Cys, a synthetic pure TLR-2 ligand, on DC maturation markers. Immature monocyte-derived DCs were cultured with short-term Vδ2 T cell lines at a DC-to-Vδ2 T-cell ratio of 1:10 for 48 h in the indicated conditions. The cell populations were either in contact or separated by a transwell membrane. DCs were harvested and flow cytometric analysis of the indicated cell surface molecules performed. *Inset numbers*: mean fluorescence intensity of the experimental population. *Shaded histograms*: isotype control. (**B**) Effect of Vδ2 T-cell activation ± TLR-2 ligand on IL-12p70 (*upper panel*) and IL-10 production in 48-h DC/Vδ2 T-cell cocultures. DC and Vδ2 T-cell lines were separated in a transwell system. Cytokines assayed by ELISA. (**C**) Effect of neutralization of IFN-γ in Vδ2 culture supernatants on IL-12p70 production by DCs. Supernatants of Vδ2 T-cell lines restimulated overnight with IPP were collected and preincubated for 1 h with the indicated concentrations of soluble IFN-γ receptor-1 (sIFN-γR1). Supernatants were added to immature DCs together with Pam3Cys, 5 μg/mL. Untreated Vδ2 supernatant or Pam3Cys alone elicited no IL-12p70 secretion by DCs.

Pam3Cys. FIGURE 3C shows concentration-dependent inhibition of IL-12 p70 production by blockade of IFN-γ, to a maximum of 88% inhibitory activity. Inhibition of TNF-α with sTNFR1 showed no inhibitory activity on IL-12 production (not shown). Hence, in this system, IFN-γ production by activated Vδ2 T cells accounted for the bulk of the costimulatory activity for IL-12 p70 production by TLR-2-stimulated DCs.

Activated Vδ2 T Cells Increase Th1 Polarization of DCs Simultaneously Activated by TLR-2 Ligand

We next examined the effect of DCs matured by these stimuli in priming purified allogeneic CD4+ T cells. Immature DCs (iDCs) were conditioned by exposure to TLR-2 ligand (TLR-2-DCs), IPP-activated Vδ2 T cells in a transwell system (Vδ2-DCs), or both stimuli (TLR-2-Vδ2-DCs). After 48 h, the Vδ2 T-cell population could be removed without contamination of the remaining DCs. DCs were then harvested, washed, and subsequently combined with purified naive allogeneic CD4+ T cells at various DC-to-T-cell ratios. As a reference standard for optimal maturation of DCs, some DCs were exposed to a cocktail of TNF-α, IL-1β, and PGE2 for 48 h (cytokine-DCs).[37,38] FIGURE 4A shows the resulting T-cell proliferation, measured by ^{3}H-thymidine incorporation after 5 days of culture. As expected, iDCs were the least stimulatory of proliferation, whereas cytokine-DCs were maximally stimulatory. TLR-2-DCs were intermediately potent, whereas exposure to activated Vδ2 T cells did not increase the capacity of DCs to stimulate T-cell proliferation, irrespective of exposure to TLR-2 ligand. Hence, the apparent upregulation of DC maturation phenotype by Vδ2 T-cell activation (FIG. 3A) did not correspond to an increase in stimulation of CD4+ T-cell proliferation. However, striking differences in T-cell function were apparent when T-cell cytokine production was examined. The Th1 and Th2 cytokines, IFN-γ and IL-4, respectively, were measured by ELISA in supernatants of DC/CD4+ T-cell coculture supernatants collected after 72 h of culture. FIGURE 4B shows the results of five consecutive experiments, performed with DC/T-cell cultures from different donor pairs. The expected donor-to-donor variation notwithstanding, the T-helper polarization pattern was consistent: iDCs stimulated a pure IL-4 response, as reported previously,[39] whereas a pure IFN-γ response was stimulated, with increasing efficiency, by cytokine-DCs, TLR-2-DCs, and TLR-2-Vδ2-DCs. Interestingly, Vδ2-DCs stimulated neither IFN-γ nor IL-4 secretion. Simultaneous evaluation of proliferation and IFN-γ expression by flow cytometry confirmed the additive effects of activated Vδ2 and TLR-2 ligand on Th1 priming of CD4 (FIG. 4C). These data suggest that exposure of DCs to activated Vδ2 T cells increases the sensitivity of DCs for Th1 priming by TLR-2 ligand. To test this hypothesis, we studied the Th1 priming function of DCs that had been stimulated with titrated concentrations of TLR-2 ligands in the presence of Vδ2T cells that had been activated or not with IPP. As before, Vδ2 T cells and DCs were separated by a transmembrane so that DCs could be harvested and washed without γδ T-cell contamination. FIGURE 4D shows that in the absence of Vδ2 T-cell activation, significant IFN-γ production by naive CD4+ T cells was stimulated by DCs that had been exposed to a minimum of 1.0 μg/mL of Pam3Cys, whereas in the presence of activated Vδ2 T cells, this threshold was reduced 100-fold to 0.01 μg/mL of Pam3Cys. Similar results were obtained when *M.tb* TX114 extract was used as a source of TLR-2 ligand (FIG. 4D).

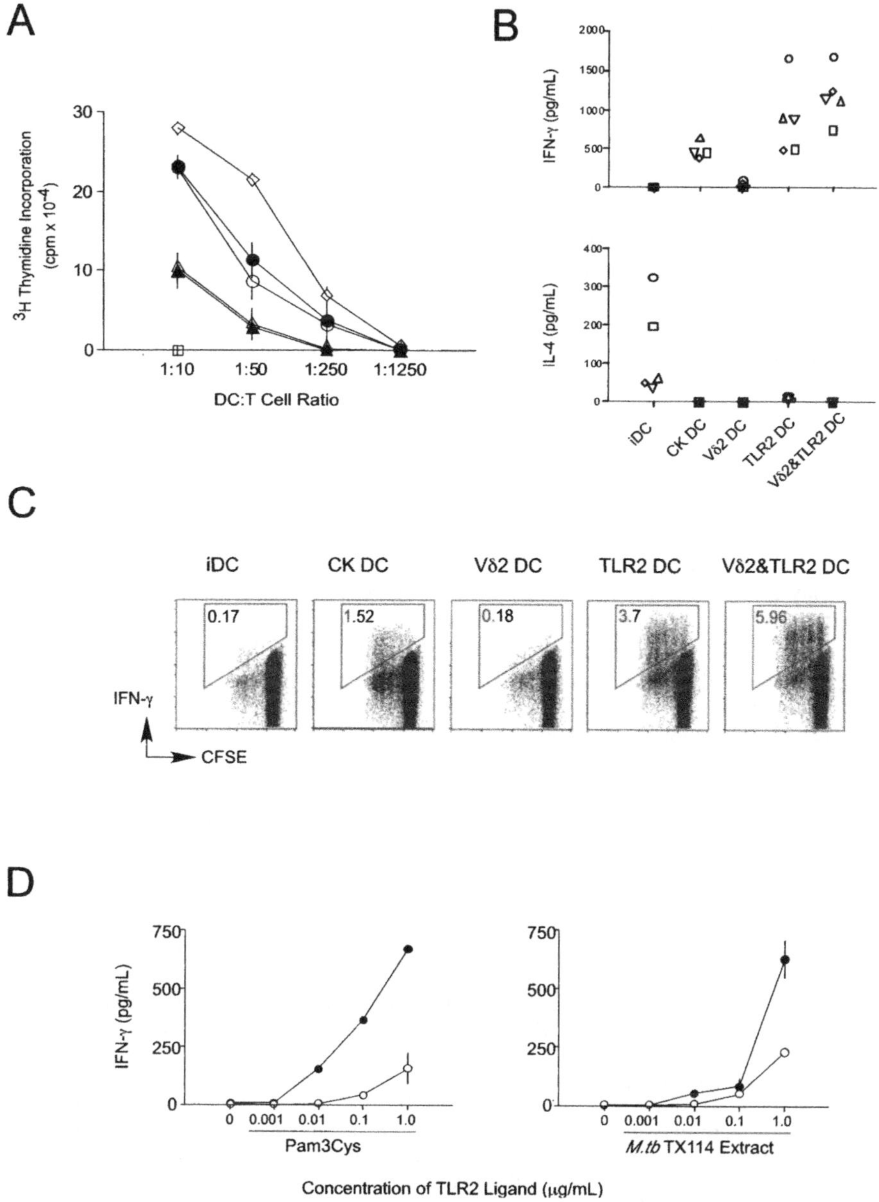

FIGURE 4. (**A**) Priming of allogeneic naive CD4$^+$ T cells by DCs conditioned by Vδ2 T cells ± Pam3Cys. CD4$^+$CD45RO$^-$ T cells were immunomagnetically purified and added to the various DC populations at the indicated ratios. Triplicate cultures of 1×10^5 T cells + DCs were pulsed with ^{3}H-thymidine for the last 6 out of 120 h. *Triangles*: immature DCs; *circles*: Pam3Cys-matured DCs; *diamonds*: cytokine-matured DCs; *open symbols*: DCs not exposed to activated Vδ2 T cells; *solid symbols*: DCs conditioned by activated Vδ2 T cells; *open squares*: T cells alone. (**B**) Production of Th1 (IFN-γ) and Th2 (IL-4) cytokines in

Together, these data suggest that IFN-γ, produced by activated Vδ2 T cells, acts as a costimulus for Th1 polarization by DCs, which is critical when the abundance of TLR-2 ligand for DC maturation is limiting.

DISCUSSION

In this study, we show that activated Vδ2 T cells can act as modulators of αβ $CD4^+$ T-cell function, with this activity critically mediated by DCs. A mutually costimulatory relationship was found between Vδ2 T cells and DCs that were activated directly by phosphoantigens and TLR-2 ligands, respectively. Thus, IFN-γ production by antigen-stimulated Vδ2 T cells was enhanced in the presence of TLR-2–stimulated DCs. Conversely, activated Vδ2 T cells enhanced DC maturation by TLR-2 ligands, as well as providing a key costimulus, largely IFN-γ, for the production of biologically active, heterodimeric IL-12 p70. We observed that activated Vδ2 T cells sensitized DCs to limiting concentrations of TLR2 ligand, thereby promoting effective priming of Th1 $CD4^+$ T cells.

The notion that γδ T cells might influence the priming of acquired immunity is supported by the recent finding that activated Vδ2 T cells express the lymph node–homing chemokine receptor, CCR7.[40] Indeed, it was recently reported that Vδ2 T cells may themselves act as antigen-presenting cells.[41] Our studies show that activated Vδ2 T cells induce modest expression of CCR7 on immature DCs, and enhance CCR7 expression induced by TLR-2 ligands. Together, these observations suggest that simultaneous exposure of these host-cell populations to pathogens such as *M.tb* may result in their coordinated migration to lymphoid tissues, where priming of $CD4^+$ T-cell responses takes place.

---

priming cultures of DCs and allogeneic naive $CD4^+$ T cells. Naive $CD4^+$ T cells were incubated with DCs for 72 h at a T-cell-to-DC ratio of 10:1. Cytokines in supernatants assayed by ELISA at 72 h. (iDC = immature DCs; CK DC = DCs matured in cytokine cocktail (TNF-α, IL-1β, and PG E_2); Vδ2 DC = DCs conditioned by 48 h exposure to activated Vδ2 T-cell line in transwell system; TLR2 DC = DCs matured in presence of Pam3Cys, 5 μg/mL; Vδ2&TLR2DC = DCs matured in the presence of both activated Vδ2 T cells and Pam3Cys). Results of five consecutive experiments performed with five different donor pairs are shown. Each symbol represents one experiment. (**C**) Simultaneous analysis of proliferation and single-cell IFN-γ production by $CD4^+$ T cells primed by DCs that had been conditioned as indicated. T cell to DC ratio = 10:1. Cells were harvested at 72 h. An electronic gate was set on $CD3^+$ cells. *Inset numbers*: percentage of T cells expressing IFN-γ. (**D**) Effect of activated Vδ2 T cells on Th1 polarizing of limiting concentrations of Pam3Cys (*left panel*) and TX114 lipoprotein extract of *M.tb* (*right panel*). Immature DCs were incubated for 48 h in the presence of graded concentrations of Pam3Cys or *M.tb* extract, with or without activated Vδ2 T-cell lines in a transwell apparatus. DCs were harvested, washed, and cocultured in duplicates with naive allogeneic $CD4^+$ T cells at a T-cell-to-DC ratio of 10:1. *Open symbols*: DCs treated in absence of Vδ2 T cells; solid *symbols*: DCs treated in presence of Vδ2 T cells. IFN-γ assayed in 72-h supernatants of $CD4^+$ T cell–DC cocultures.

We found that exposure of DCs to activated Vδ2 T cells in the absence of TLR stimulation resulted in partially matured DCs that failed to prime T cells to secrete IFN-γ production, but that abrogated the "default" Th2 cell priming exhibited by immature DCs, described previously.[39]

Two recent reports have also described the capacity of γδ T cells to promote DC maturation and IL-12 p70 production. One study, by Ismaili *et al.*, found that freshly isolated gd T cells could mature DCs as effectively as those activated by phosphoantigen, and that activated Vδ2 T cells alone were sufficient to induce IL-12 p70 production by DCs.[42] In contrast, we found that activation of Vδ2 T cells was necessary even for partial maturation of DCs, and that another signal, namely TLR-2 ligation, was necessary to stimulate IL-12 p70 secretion. Differences in methodology may account for this discrepancy; indeed, the positive selection technique of γδ T cells used by Ismaili *et al.* may have introduced additional activation stimuli, as acknowledged by the authors.[42] In another report, Leslie *et al.* looked at a different population of human γδ T cells that uses Vδ1 (Vδ1 T cells). It was shown that Vδ1 T-cell clones could be activated by iDCs in a CD1-dependent manner, in the absence of exogenous antigen, to provide a DC maturation stimulus, and a necessary costimulus for IL-12 p70 production in response to lipopolysaccharide (a TLR4 ligand).[43] In both the latter reports, IFN-γ produced by γδ T cells played a major role in costimulating IL-12 p70 production, consistent with the findings presented here.

Tuberculosis and leprosy are the two most important human mycobacterioses. Th1 $CD4^+$ T-cell immunity provides robust protection against these diseases in 90% or more of infected individuals. In the 10% who fail to control infection and who develop clinical disease, there exists a spectrum of host immune responsiveness, more definitively described in leprosy, but also recognized in tuberculosis. Thus, clinical tuberculosis or leprosy may be associated with mycobacterium-specific Th1 immunity, albeit inadequate to prevent the emergence of disease, or with "deviant" $CD4^+$ T-cell responses, characterized by IL-10 secretion.[44–46] In both of these mycobacterial infections, primary contact is likely to be with small numbers of organisms at epithelial surfaces where antigens, including phosphoantigens and TLR-2 ligands, may encounter sentinel DCs and Vδ2 T cells. When the infectious inoculum is critically low, the importance of a Th1-amplifying mechanism, such as immediate early IFN-γ production by Vδ2 T cells, may acquire importance. Such a mechanism may have particular importance where the pathogen is a weak intrinsic stimulator of DCs, as we have found with *M. leprae*, in contrast to *M. tuberculosis* (unpublished data). Alternatively, if there is a defect in TLR signaling, our data suggest that Vδ2 T-cell activation may cause DCs to migrate to lymph nodes, where priming of nonprotective $CD4^+$ T cells can occur. Consistent with this idea, a recent study found that a loss-of-function mutation in TLR-2 is associated with the lepromatous type of leprosy,[15,47,48] a disease where uncontrolled mycobacterial proliferation is associated with IL-10–secreting $CD4^+$ T-cell responses, but where Vδ2 T cells are still efficiently activated by *M. leprae* antigens.

The data presented here, together with the reports of Leslie *et al.* and Ismaili *et al.*,[42,43] and the recent studies suggesting direct antigen-presenting activity of Vδ2 T cells,[40] suggest that pharmacologic stimulation of the latter cells with synthetic phosphoantigens, in combination with TLR ligands, may be an applicable immune adjuvant strategy to optimize vaccine-induced Th1 immunity.

ACKNOWLEDGMENTS

This work was supported by The Dana Foundation Human Immunology Research Program (P.A.J.H and J.A.I.) and by PHS grant NIH-AI-22616 (G.K.).

[*Competing interests*: The authors declare that they have no competing financial interests.]

REFERENCES

1. BEUTLER, B. *et al.* 2003. How we detect microbes and respond to them: the toll-like receptors and their transducers. J. Leukoc. Biol. **74:** 479–485.
2. OZINSKY, A. *et al.* 2000. The repertoire for pattern recognition of pathogens by the innate immune system is defined by cooperation between toll-like receptors. Proc. Natl. Acad. Sci. USA **97:** 13766–13771.
3. HAWIGER, D. *et al.* 2001. Dendritic cells induce peripheral T cell unresponsiveness under steady state conditions *in vivo*. J. Exp. Med. **194:** 769–779.
4. STEINMAN, R. M. *et al.* 2003. Dendritic cell function *in vivo* during the steady state: a role in peripheral tolerance. Ann. N.Y. Acad. Sci. **987:** 15–25.
5. MAHNKE, K. *et al.* 2003. Induction of CD4+/CD25+ regulatory T cells by targeting of antigens to immature dendritic cells. Blood **101:** 4862–4869.
6. VAN DER KLEIJ, D. *et al.* 2002. A novel host-parasite lipid cross-talk. Schistosomal lyso-phosphatidylserine activates toll-like receptor 2 and affects immune polarization. J. Biol. Chem. **277:** 48122–48129.
7. AGRAWAL, S. *et al.* 2003. Cutting edge: different toll-like receptor agonists instruct dendritic cells to induce distinct Th responses via differential modulation of extracellular signal-regulated kinase-mitogen-activated protein kinase and c-Fos. J. Immunol. **171:** 4984–4989.
8. PULENDRAN, B. *et al.* 2001. Lipopolysaccharides from distinct pathogens induce different classes of immune responses *in vivo*. J. Immunol. **167:** 5067–5076.
9. LIM, S.K. 2003. Freund adjuvant induces TLR2 but not TLR4 expression in the liver of mice. Int. Immunopharmacol. **3:** 115–118.
10. REILING, N. *et al.* 2002. Cutting edge: toll-like receptor (TLR)2- and TLR4-mediated pathogen recognition in resistance to airborne infection with *Mycobacterium tuberculosis*. J. Immunol. **169:** 3480–3484.
11. HELDWEIN, K.A. & M.J. FENTON. 2002. The role of toll-like receptors in immunity against mycobacterial infection. Microbes Infect. **4:** 937–944.
12. HERTZ, C.J. *et al.* 2001. Microbial lipopeptides stimulate dendritic cell maturation via toll-like receptor 2. J. Immunol. **166:** 2444–2450.
13. MEANS, T.K. *et al.* 1999. Human toll-like receptors mediate cellular activation by Mycobacterium tuberculosis. J. Immunol. **163:** 3920–3927.
14. SIELING, P.A. *et al.* 2003. Toll-like receptor 2 ligands as adjuvants for human Th1 responses. J. Immunol. **170:** 194–200.
15. BOCHUD, P.Y., T.R. HAWN & A. ADEREM. 2003. Cutting edge: a toll-like receptor 2 polymorphism that is associated with lepromatous leprosy is unable to mediate mycobacterial signaling. J. Immunol. **170:** 3451–3454.
16. KRUTZIK, S.R., *et al.* 2003. Activation and regulation of toll-like receptors 2 and 1 in human leprosy. Nat. Med. **9:** 525–532.
17. HAYDAY, A.C. 2000. [gamma][delta] cells: a right time and a right place for a conserved third way of protection. Annu. Rev. Immunol. **18:** 975–1026.
18. HAAS, W., P. PEREIRA & S. TONEGAWA. 1993. Gamma/delta cells. Annu. Rev. Immunol. **11:** 637–685.
19. TANAKA, Y. *et al.* 1995. Natural and synthetic non-peptide antigens recognized by human gamma delta T cells. Nature **375:** 155–158.
20. EBERL, M. *et al.* 2003. Microbial isoprenoid biosynthesis and human gammadelta T cell activation. FEBS Lett. **544:** 4–10.

21. HAVLIR, D.V. *et al.* 1991. Selective expansion of human gamma delta T cells by monocytes infected with live *Mycobacterium tuberculosis*. J. Clin. Invest. **87:** 729–733.
22. BARNES, P.F. *et al.* 1992. Gamma delta T lymphocytes in human tuberculosis. J. Infect. Dis. **165:** 506–512.
23. DIELI, F. *et al.* 2001. Granulysin-dependent killing of intracellular and extracellular *Mycobacterium tuberculosis* by Vgamma9/Vdelta2 T lymphocytes. J. Infect. Dis. **184:** 1082–1085.
24. PASSMORE, J.S. *et al.* 2001. Granule-dependent cytolysis of *Mycobacterium tuberculosis*-infected macrophages by human gammadelta+ T cells has no effect on intracellular mycobacterial viability. Clin. Exp. Immunol. **126:** 76–83.
25. WANG, L. *et al.* 2001. Antibacterial effect of human V gamma 2V delta 2 T cells *in vivo*. J. Clin. Invest. **108:** 1349–1357.
26. FERRICK, D.A. *et al.* 1995. Differential production of interferon-gamma and interleukin-4 in response to Th1- and Th2-stimulating pathogens by gamma delta T cells *in vivo*. Nature **373:** 255–257.
27. SHEN, Y. *et al.* 2002. Adaptive immune response of Vgamma2Vdelta2+ T cells during mycobacterial infections. Science **295:** 2255–2258.
28. JAMESON, J. *et al.* 2002. A role for skin gammadelta T cells in wound repair. Science **296:** 747–749.
29. WORKALEMAHU, G. *et al.* 2003. Human gamma delta-T lymphocytes express and synthesize connective tissue growth factor: effect of IL-15 and TGF-beta 1 and comparison with alpha beta-T lymphocytes. J. Immunol. **170:** 153–157.
30. HANNINEN, A. & L.C. HARRISON. 2000. Gamma delta T cells as mediators of mucosal tolerance: the autoimmune diabetes model. Immunol. Rev. **173:** 109–119.
31. HASLETT, P.A. *et al.* 1998. Thalidomide costimulates primary human T lymphocytes, preferentially inducing proliferation, cytokine production, and cytotoxic responses in the CD8+ subset. J. Exp. Med. **187:** 1885–1892.
32. AANDAHL, E.M. *et al.* 2002. Inhibition of antigen-specific T cell proliferation and cytokine production by protein kinase A type I. J. Immunol. **169:** 802–808.
33. MOKUNO, Y. *et al.* 2000. Expression of toll-like receptor 2 on gamma delta T cells bearing invariant V gamma 6/V delta 1 induced by *Escherichia coli* infection in mice. J. Immunol. **165:** 931–940.
34. BALAJI, K.N. *et al.* 1995. Alveolar macrophages as accessory cells for human gamma delta T cells activated by *Mycobacterium tuberculosis*. J. Immunol. **154:** 5959–5968.
35. KADOWAKI, N. *et al.* 2001. Subsets of human dendritic cell precursors express different toll-like receptors and respond to different microbial antigens. J. Exp. Med. **194:** 863–869.
36. RE, F. & J.L. STROMINGER. 2001. Toll-like receptor 2 (TLR2) and TLR4 differentially activate human dendritic cells. J. Biol. Chem. **276:** 37692–37699.
37. LEE, A.W. *et al.* 2002. A clinical grade cocktail of cytokines and PGE2 results in uniform maturation of human monocyte-derived dendritic cells: implications for immunotherapy. Vaccine **20:** A8–A22.
38. JONULEIT, H. *et al.* 1997. Pro-inflammatory cytokines and prostaglandins induce maturation of potent immunostimulatory dendritic cells under fetal calf serum-free conditions. Eur. J. Immunol. **27:** 3135–3142.
39. MAILLIARD, R.B. *et al.* 2002. Complementary dendritic cell-activating function of CD8+ and CD4+ T cells: helper role of CD8+ T cells in the development of T helper type 1 responses. J. Exp. Med. **195:** 473–483.
40. BRANDES, M. *et al.* 2003. Flexible migration program regulates {gamma}{delta} T-cell involvement in humoral immunity. Blood **24:** 24.
41. BRANDES, M., K. WILLIMANN & B. MOSER. 2005. Professional antigen-presentation function by human gammadelta T Cells. Science **309:** 264–268.
42. ISMAILI, J. *et al.* 2002. Human gamma delta T cells induce dendritic cell maturation. Clin. Immunol. **103:** 296–302.
43. LESLIE, D.S. *et al.* 2002. CD1-Mediated gamma/delta T cell maturation of dendritic cells. J. Exp. Med. **196:** 1575–1584.
44. DELGADO, J.C. *et al.* 2002. Antigen-specific and persistent tuberculin anergy in a cohort of pulmonary tuberculosis patients from rural Cambodia. Proc. Natl. Acad. Sci. USA **99:** 7576–7581.

45. BOUSSIOTIS, V.A. *et al.* 2000. IL-10-Producing T cells suppress immune responses in anergic tuberculosis patients. J. Clin. Invest. **105:** 1317–1325.
46. SALGAME, P. *et al.* 1991. Differing lymphokine profiles of functional subsets of human CD4 and CD8 T cell clones. Science **254:** 279–282.
47. KANG, T.J., S.B. LEE & G.T. CHAE. 2002. A polymorphism in the toll-like receptor 2 is associated with IL-12 production from monocyte in lepromatous leprosy. Cytokine **20:** 56–62.
48. KANG, T.J. & G.T. CHAE. 2001. Detection of toll-like receptor 2 (TLR2) mutation in the lepromatous leprosy patients. FEMS Immunol. Med. Microbiol. **31:** 53–58.

TLR1 and TLR6 Polymorphisms Are Associated with Susceptibility to Invasive Aspergillosis after Allogeneic Stem Cell Transplantation

SANDRA KESH,[a] NANA YAA MENSAH ,[a] PAOLO PETERLONGO,[b] DANA JAFFE,[a] KATHARINE HSU,[c] MARCEL VAN DEN BRINK,[c] RICHARD O'REILLY,[c,d] ERIC PAMER,[a] JAYA SATAGOPAN,[e] AND G.A. PAPANICOLAOU[a]

[a]*Department of Medicine, Service of Infectious Disease, Memorial Sloan-Kettering Cancer Center, New York, New York 10021, USA*

[b]*Cell Biology Program, Memorial Sloan-Kettering Cancer Center, New York, New York 10021, USA*

[c]*Department of Medicine, Service of Bone Marrow Transplantation, Memorial Sloan-Kettering Cancer Center, New York, New York 10021, USA*

[d]*Department of Pediatrics, Memorial Sloan-Kettering Cancer Center, New York, New York 10021, USA*

[e]*Department of Epidemiology and Biostatistics, Memorial Sloan-Kettering Cancer Center, New York, New York 10021, USA*

ABSTRACT: Toll-like receptors (TLRs) transmit signals in response to *Aspergillus fumigatus* conidia and hyphae. In this preliminary study, we examined the association between single nucleotide polymorphisms (SNPs) in TLR1, TLR4, and TLR6 genes and development of invasive aspergillosis (IA) in 127 allogeneic hematopoietic stem cell transplant recipients consisting of 22 patients with IA and 105 unaffected control subjects. The following SNPs and their pairwise interactions were considered in the model: TLR1 (239G > C, 743A > G, 914A > T, 1805G > T), TLR4 (896A > G, 1196C > T), and TLR6 (359T > C, 745C > T, 764C > T). No association was found between donor SNP and the risk of IA. Analysis of recipient SNP data showed that the presence of TLR1 239G > C (Arg80 > Thr) or the presence of both TLR1 743A > G (Asn248 > Ser) and TLR6 745C > T (Ser249 > Pro) is associated with IA (odds ratio = 1.30, 95% confidence interval = 1.13 to 1.50; *P* < .001). Further analyses using a prospective cohort may enable us to identify TLR polymorphisms associated with the susceptibility to IA within a defined interval among immunocompromised patients.

KEYWORDS: innate immune receptor; toll-like receptor; polymorphism; aspergillosis; fungal infection; mutation; bone marrow transplantation

Address for correspondence: Genovefa A. Papanicolaou, M.D., Department of Medicine, Infectious Diseases Service, Memorial Sloan Kettering Cancer Center, 1275 York Ave., Box 9, New York, NY 10021. Voice: 212-639-8361; fax: 646-422-2124.
papanicg@mskcc.org

**Ann. N.Y. Acad. Sci. 1062: 95–103 (2005). © 2005 New York Academy of Sciences.
doi: 10.1196/annals.1358.012**

INTRODUCTION

Invasive aspergillosis (IA) develops in 5%–15% of hematopoietic stem cell transplant (HSCT) recipients and is associated with up to 85% mortality.[1,2] Prolonged neutropenia, T cell depletion, graft-versus-host disease, and the administration of immunosuppressive agents all contribute to the high incidence of infection.[3,4] Nevertheless, only a small fraction of patients with similar degrees of immunosuppression develop infection, suggesting that other, yet to be defined factors contribute to susceptibility to IA.

Inhaled *Aspergillus fumigatus* conidia encounter alveolar epithelial cells and macrophages. Alveolar macrophages and dendritic cells play a central role in host defense against *Aspergillus* infection.[6–8] Alveolar macrophages are derived from circulating blood cells, and in the transplant recipient are usually of donor origin, whereas alveolar epithelial cells are of recipient origin. It is plausible, therefore, that *both* donor and recipient cells are involved in immunity against *Aspergillus*.

Toll-like receptors (TLRs), a family of germline-encoded transmembrane receptors, mediate recognition of specific microbial molecules by immune cells. Ten members of the TLR family have been identified to date.[9] *In vitro* studies have implicated TLR2, TLR4, and their adaptor protein MyD88 in mediating signaling responses following stimulation of macrophages or polymorphonuclear cells with *Aspergillus* conidia or hyphae.[10–13] Recognition of TLR2 ligands occurs through the heterodimeric association of TLR2 with either TLR1 or TLR6.[14,15] It is plausible, therefore, that in addition to TLR2 and TLR4, TLR1 and TLR6 also contribute in the recognition of *Aspergillus* molecules. The extent to which variation in the TLR gene complement contributes to susceptibility to IA in humans remains unknown.

In this study we looked for association between the presence of polymorphisms in TLR1, TLR2, TLR4, and TLR6 genes in the donor or recipient with development of IA post transplant. TLR2 and TLR4 have been sequenced in many individuals, and clinically relevant mutations have been identified. In contrast, TLR1 and TLR6 are less well characterized. For these reasons we elected to screen our patients only for the known clinically relevant mutations in TLR2 and TLR4 and sequence the entire coding region of TLR1 and TLR6. Single-nucleotide polymorphisms (SNPs) associated with IA were identified using stepwise logistic regression models.

MATERIALS AND METHODS

DNA Source

The study was approved by the Memorial Sloan-Kettering Institutional Review Board. A total of 127 patients were analyzed. Seventy-four patients who received allogeneic HSCTs from October 2003 through December 2004 were enrolled in a prospective protocol (IRB #03-017). After signing informed consent, 5–10 mL of peripheral blood was obtained from the patients once prior to stem cell infusion (for mutational analysis of the recipient) and once after full chimerism was documented (for mutational analysis of the donor). DNA was extracted from the peripheral blood and stored at –20°C. Buccal swabs were used for DNA extraction from the recipient if a pretransplant blood specimen was not available. Fifty-three patients with infections who received HSCT from January 1999 through October 2003 were retrospectively identified from a computerized database. DNA specimens for these patients were obtained through a waiver of authorization (WA0177-04).

Case Definition

Invasive aspergillosis was defined using standard criteria.[16] All cases met criteria for probable or definite aspergillosis within 18 months post transplant or study cutoff date of June 31, 2005, whichever occurred first.

Mutational Analysis of TLR Genes

Screening was performed in a blinded manner to the identity of the samples. The relevant regions of TLR2 and TLR4 genes containing the previously defined mutations TLR2 2096C > G (Arg677 > Trp) and 2258G > A (Arg753 > Gln), and TLR4 896A > G (Asp299 > Gly) and 1196C > T (Thr399 > Ile) were sequenced. The entire coding region, including the intron–exon boundaries and 5′ untranslated region (UTR), promoter, and 3′UTR regions of TLR1 and TLR6, was sequenced. Coding regions of TLR1 and TLR6 were subdivided each in five different polymerase chain reaction (PCR) fragments. Sequencing of a total of 20 fragments (five for TLR1 and five for TLR6 in both directions), each with an average size of 500 nucleotides, was performed. PCR amplifications were performed in a final volume of 50 μL containing 100 ng of DNA, 3 m*M* dNTPs, 15 pmol of each primer, and 1.5 U of *Taq* DNA polymerase (Mercury Products; Continental Lab Products, San Diego, CA). PCR conditions were as follows: denaturation at 94°C for 20 s, annealing at 60°C for 20 s, and extension at 72°C for 1 min for 35 cycles, using different annealing temperatures depending on the fragments amplified. Final extension was conducted at 72°C for 5 min. PCR products were purified for sequencing reaction using the Montage PCR_{96} plates (Millipore, Bedford, MA). Both strands of every fragment were sequenced. Sequencing was performed on an ABI 377 sequencer using Big Dye terminator chemistry (Applied Biosystems, Foster City, CA) according to the manufacturer's recommendations. Electropherograms were analyzed using the Phred and Phrap softwares (http://www.phrap.org).[17] As a condition for further analysis, generation of contigs covering the entire coding region was required. Reference sequences of TLR1, TLR2, TLR4, and TLR6 genes were obtained from GenBank <http://www.ncbi.nlm.nih.gov> and were NM003263, NM003264, NM138554, and NM006068, respectively. Sequence of primers used for PCR amplifications and sequencing are available upon request.

Statistical Analysis

Genotypes at various single nucleotide polymorphisms were recorded for the donor and recipient samples. SNPs were coded as binary variables, representing the presence or absence of at least one copy of the minor allele, separately for the donor and recipient for each patient. The association between *Aspergillus* infection and the SNPs was investigated separately using genotypes of donor and recipient. Individuals having missing SNP data were excluded from the analysis of the corresponding SNPs.

A SNP may confer infection risk individually and/or solely through interaction with other SNPs. A pairwise interaction term is represented as a product term and indicates the presence or absence of at least one copy of a minor allele at both the SNPs. Our analytic strategy, therefore, involved first investigating the significant main effects and pairwise interactions. If SNPs within the same gene exhibited interactions, we evaluated the risk associated with haplotypes of those SNPs. Otherwise we evaluated the role of individual effects and interactions on susceptibility to invasive asperillosis.

Because of the combination of prospective and retrospective ascertainment of patients, we used logistic regression models for our analyses. SNPs associated with IA were identified using stepwise logistic regression models[18] and logic regression.[19] Logic regression is a generalized regression approach that is applied primarily to binary covariate data such as the binary SNP genotypes in our analyses <http://bear.fhcrc.org/~ingor/logic>. This approach identifies Boolean or logical combinations of variables that are associated with the outcome of interest. We considered nine SNPs having minor allele frequency of approximately 2% or more in our analyses.

First, a stepwise logistic regression model was used to identify the main effect and pairwise interactions associated with *Aspergillus* infection. A variable was entered into the model if its odds ratio had a *P* value of .20 or less. We allowed for the possibility of an interaction term appearing in the model without the corresponding main effect terms since the interaction term represents the presence of at least one copy of a minor allele at both (interacting) loci. After the final model was identified using the stepwise approach, we conducted subset contingency table analyses of the SNPs in the resulting model and used Fisher's exact test for the relevant comparisons. Finally, we conducted a logic regression analysis using all nine SNPs. A logic regression model was built by specifying one logic tree and the number of leaves equal to the total number of SNPs identified in the final logistic regression model. All analyses were conducted using Stata version 6 (StataCorp, College Station, TX) and R <http://www.r-project.org>. Logic regression analyses were conducted using the R LogicReg library. Because of the exploratory nature of this study, we did not adjust the *P* values for multiple comparisons.

RESULTS

The 127 patients ascertained for this study consisted of 22 patients with IA and 105 unaffected control subjects. Pretransplant DNA specimens were available from all 127 patients to determine the recipient genotypes. However, post-transplant specimens were available from only 116 of these 127 patients to determine the donor genotypes. A total of 17 coding SNPs were identified by sequencing the TLR1, TLR4, and TLR6 genes. Of these, nine SNPs (four in TLR1, two in TLR4, and three in TLR6) occurred at frequencies of more than 2% and were considered in the analyses. Amino acid changes and allele frequencies of the nine SNPs analyzed in the study are shown in TABLE 1. Frequencies were calculated on the basis of 127 recipient samples. TABLE 2 shows the number of cases and control subjects having at least one copy of the minor allele at each SNP (denoted SNP frequencies), separately for recipient and donor samples.

The first statistical analyses were conducted for the genotypes obtained from the recipient samples. From the stepwise logistic regression analysis of the nine main-

TABLE 1. Allele frequencies and number of homozygous and heterozygous recipients for the common TLR1, TLR4, and TLR6 SNPs

Nucleotide	Major[a] allele (M) (allele frequency in %)	Minor[b] allele (m) (allele frequency in %)	Amino acid change	Number of observed genotype MM	Mm	mm	Missing
TLR1							
239	G (91.8)	C (8.2)	Arg80Thr	98	17	1	11
743	A (65.4	G (34.6)	Asn248Ser	54	41	19	11
914	A (97.4)	T (2.6)	His305Leu	110	4	1	12
1805	G (95.2)	T (41.8)	Ser602Ile	45	38	27	17
TLR4							
896	A (94.2)	G (5.8)	Asp299Gly	100	11	1	15
1196	C (58.2)	T (4.9)	Thr399Ile	103	9	1	14
TLR6							
359	T (94.2)	C (5.8)	Ile120Thr	100	11	1	15
745	C (67.1)	T (32.9)	Ser249Pro	50	49	12	16
764	C (98.2)	T (1.8)	Thr255Ile	110	2	1	14

[a]Major represents the reference allele in dbSNP public database.
[b]Minor allele represents the rare allele.

TABLE 2. Number (and frequencies in %) of recipient and donor SNPs in infectious aspergillosis cases and unaffected controls

SNP	Recipient samples: Aspergillosis total $N = 22$	Recipient samples: No aspergillosis total $N = 105$	Donor samples: Aspergillosis total $N = 21$	Donor samples: No aspergillosis total $N = 95$
TLR1 239G > C	5 (22.7)	13 (12.4)	2 (9.5)	10 (10.5)
TLR1 743A > G	12 (54.5)	48 (45.7)	10 (47.6)	35 (36.8)
TLR1 914A > T	2 (9.1)	3 (2.9)	0 (0)	5 (5.3)
TLR1 1805G > T	12 (54.5)	53 (50.5)	10 (47.6)	44 (46.3)
TLR4 896A > G	2 (9.1)	10 (9.5)	3 (14.3)	10 (10.5)
TLR4 1196C > T	2 (9.1)	8 (7.6)	3 (14.3)	12 (12.6)
TLR6 539T > C	2 (9.1)	10 (9.5)	0 (0)	3 (3.2)
TLR6 754C > T	10 (45.5)	51 (48.6)	11 (52.4)	40 (42.1)
TLR6 764C > T	0 (0)	3 (2.9)	1 (4.8)	6 (6.3)

effect terms and 36 (= 9 × 8/2) pairwise interaction terms, TLR1 G293 > C (Arg80 > Thr) (odds ratio = 1.22, 95% confidence interval [CI] = 1.02 to 1.48; $P = .04$) and the interaction between TLR1 743A > G (Asn248 > Ser) and TLR6 745C > T (Ser249 > Pro) (odds ratio = 1.23, 95% CI = 1.03 to 1.47, $P = .02$) were identified as being statistically significantly associated with aspergillosis (TABLE 3).

We then conducted contingency table analysis to compare the association between susceptibility to IA and the interaction term (i.e., the presence of at least one

TABLE 3. Final model following stepwise logistic regression of recipient genotypes and aspergillosis using 9 SNPs

SNP	N case	N control	Odds ratio	95% CI	*P*
TLR1 239G > C	5	11	1.22	1.01–1.48	.04
TLR1 743A > G and TLR6 745C > T	6	13	1.23	1.03–1.47	.02

NOTE: The columns N case and N control represent the number of cases and controls, respectively, having the variable indicated in the SNP column. The effective sample size for this logistic regression model is 103 patients (16 cases and 87 controls). The baseline category for the odds ratio calculations are individuals who do not have at least one copy of minor allele at TLR1 239G > C (row 2), and in both TLR1 743A > G and TLR6 745C > T (row 3).

TABLE 4. Result of logic regression analysis of recipient genotypes and aspergillosis using all 9 SNPs

Variable	N case	N control	Odds ratio	95% CI	*P* value
(TLR1 239G > C) or (TLR1 743A > G and TLR6 745C > T)	11	22	1.30	1.13–1.50	.0005

NOTE: The logic regression model was built by specifying 1 tree and 3 leaves. The choice of 3 leaves was motivated by 3 SNPs identified in the logistic regression model using the stepwise analysis (TABLE 3). The "logic variable" represents a variable taking value 1 if a patient has a SNP in TLR1 239G > C or a SNP in both TLR1 743A > G and TLR6 745C > T, and takes value 0 otherwise. The effective sample size for this logic regression analysis is 103 patients (16 cases and 87 controls). The columns N case and N control represent the number of cases and controls, respectively, who have the logic variable.

copy of the minor allele at both TLR1 743A > G and TLR6 745C > T) among the 98 patients who do not have a minor allele in TLR1 239G > C. Eleven of the 98 patients had a missing genotype at TLR1 743A > G or TLR6 745C > T, resulting in an effective sample size of 87 for this analysis. Of the 87 patients, 11 were aspergillosis cases and 76 were unaffected control subjects. Six (55%) of the 11 cases had a minor allele at both TLR1 743A > G and TLR6 745C >T, compared with 11 (14.5%) of 76 control subjects (Fisher's exact test $P = .006$). Next we conducted a contingency table analysis to compare the association between IA and the presence of at least one copy of a minor allele in TLR1 239G > C among the 84 patients who did not have a minor allele in both TLR1 743A > G and TLR6 745C > T. Ten of 84 patients had IA. Five (50%) of these IA case patients had a minor allele at TLR1 239G > C, compared with 9 (12%) of 74 non-IA control subjects (Fisher's exact test $P = .01$).

These results motivated us to consider logic regression to identify combinations of SNPs conferring IA risk. The logic regression analysis showed that patients having at least one copy of minor allele at TLR1 239G > C or at both TLR1 743A > G and TLR6 745C > T were at increased risk for aspergillosis (odds ratio = 1.30, 95% CI = 1.13 to 1.50; $P = .0005$) (TABLE 4).

When we performed the same analyses for genotypes of the donor samples, none of the nine SNPs or their interactions was associated with the development of aspergillosis post-transplant.

DISCUSSION

Patients undergoing allogeneic HSCT are highly vulnerable to IA with an incidence of ranging from 5% to 15%.[1,2] Recent evidence suggests that TLR polymorphisms are associated with susceptibility to infection in a pathogen-specific manner.[20–23] We postulated, therefore, that polymorphisms in these receptors are clinically important risk factors for aspergillosis. In this study we evaluated whether the presence of polymorphisms in the TLR1, TLR2, TLR4, and TRL6 genes of donors or recipients of allogeneic HSCTs are associated with developing aspergillosis post-transplant. Because allogeneic HSCT dramatically impairs various layers of the innate immune system, we postulated that subtle defects in immune recognition become clinically significant compared with healthy individuals, where the redundancy of the different innate immune pathways is likely to camouflage a subtle defect.

We looked specifically for SNPs in TLR1, TLR2, TLR4, and TLR6, as these members of the TLR family are more likely to mediate recognition of *Aspergillus* molecules.[10,12,13] TLR2 and TLR4 have been sequenced in many individuals, and clinically relevant mutations have been identified. TLR4 896A > G (Asp299 > Gly) has been associated with the development of gram-negative sepsis.[19] TLR2 2258G > A (Arg753 > Gln) has been associated with higher incidence of gram-positive sepsis and increased risk of developing tuberculosis.[20] TLR2 2096C > G (Arg677 > Trp), which occurs at a relatively high frequency in the Chinese population, is associated with lepromatous leprosy, whereas the wild-type allele is associated with tuberculoid leprosy.[22] As many individuals have been sequenced for TLR2 and TLR4, we elected to screen our patients only for the above-mentioned polymorphisms. In contrast, TLR1 and TLR6 are less well characterized, with only 47 individuals sequenced in the dbSNP public database <http://www.ncbi.nlm.nih.gov/SNP>. Therefore we elected to sequence the entire coding region of TLR1 and TLR6. The allelic frequencies for TLR1 and TLR6 SNPs identified in our patients were similar to the reported frequencies in the dbSNP public database. The SNPs in TLR2 were not polymorphic in our study population and hence were not considered suitable for data analyses presented here.

A SNP may confer risk of infection individually and/or solely through interaction with other SNPs. SNPs within the same gene exhibiting a significant interaction would indicate the presence of a haplotype effect. SNPs in two different genes may also exhibit a significant interaction effect, indicating the possibility of a common pathway through which the SNPs mediate infection risk. Our analytic strategy, therefore, involved first investigating the significant main effects of each SNP and pairwise interactions. We identified no SNPs within the same gene exhibiting interactions. Next, we evaluated the association of each of the SNPs and pairwise combination of SNPs present in the donor or recipient with *Aspergillus* infection.

None of the nine SNPs or 36 pairwise combinations in the donor were associated with *Aspergillus* infection based on the donor genotypes. Interestingly, our analysis of the recipient SNP data identified one SNP (TLR1, 239G > C [Arg80 > Thr]) and one combination of SNPs (TLR1 743A > G [Asn248 > Ser] and TLR6 745C > T [Ser249 > Pro]) that were associated with aspergillosis. This is the first report to our knowledge that suggests an association between SNPs in TLR genes and susceptibility to aspergillosis. That recipient but not donor SNPs were associated with aspergillosis suggests that alveolar epithelial cells play an important role in the recognition of *Aspergillus* molecules.

Previous studies using murine macrophages have shown a role for TLR2 and TLR4 in the recognition of *Aspergillus* molecules. We found no association between aspergillosis and the clinically important TLR4 polymorphisms (A896 > G or C1196 > T). Our study could not evaluate the role of TLR2 2096C > G or TLR2 2258G > A, as none of our patients had these DNA changes.

This preliminary study consists of samples ascertained prospectively and retrospectively. A larger study with a consistent prospective ascertainment will be required to confirm these findings, assess the role of clinically recognized factors for IA, and determine the association between genetic factors and time to the onset of IA among immunocompromised patients. Further, detailed analysis using logic regression in a larger prospective cohort will enable us to identify relevant combinations of SNPs associated with risk of IA, including SNPs in TLR4.

To our knowledge, this is the first report indicating that genetic analysis of innate immune genes may identify a subset of patients most vulnerable to infection post-transplant. The ability to predict susceptibility to specific infections is directly relevant to the design of strategies to protect the most vulnerable patients against infections associated with high mortality.

[*Competing interests*: The authors declare that they have no competing financial interests.]

REFERENCES

1. MARR, K.A., R.A. CARTER, M. BOECKH, *et al.* 2002. Invasive aspergillosis in allogeneic stem cell transplant recipients: changes in epidemiology and risk factors. Blood **100:** 4358–4366.
2. MARR, K.A., R.A. CARTER, F. CRIPPA, *et al.* 2002. Epidemiology and outcome of mould infections in hematopoietic stem cell transplant recipients. Clin. Infect. Dis. **34:** 909–917.
3. MAURY, S., J.Y. MARY, C. RABIAN, *et al.* 2001. Prolonged immune deficiency following allogeneic stem cell transplantation: risk factors and complications in adult patients. Br. J. Haematol. **115:** 630–641.
4. PARKMAN, R. & K.I. WEINBERG. 1997. Immunological reconstitution following bone marrow transplantation. Immunol. Rev. **157:** 73–78.
5. GERSON, S.L., G.H. TALBOT, S. HURWITZ, *et al.* 1984. Prolonged granulocytopenia: the major risk factor for invasive pulmonary aspergillosis in patients with acute leukemia. Ann. Intern. Med. **100:** 345–351.
6. GRAZZIUTTI, M.L., J.H. REX, R.E. COWART, *et al.* 1997. *Aspergillus fumigatus* conidia induce a Th1-type cytokine response. J. Infect. Dis. **176:** 1579–1583.
7. ROILIDES, E., A. HOLMES, C. BLAKE, *et al.* 1994. Antifungal activity of elutriated human monocytes against *Aspergillus fumigatus* hyphae: enhancement by granulocyte-macrophage colony-stimulating factor and interferon-gamma. J. Infect. Dis. **170:** 894–899.
8. ROILIDES, E., T. SEIN, A. HOLMES, *et al.* 1995. Effects of macrophage colony-stimulating factor on antifungal activity of mononuclear phagocytes against *Aspergillus fumigatus*. J. Infect. Dis. **172:** 1028–1034.
9. BEUTLER, B. 2004. Innate immunity: an overview. Mol. Immunol. **40:** 845–859.
10. BRAEDEL, S., M. RADSAK, H. EINSELE, *et al.* 2004. *Aspergillus fumigatus* antigens activate innate immune cells via toll-like receptors 2 and 4. Br. J. Haematol. **125:** 392–399.
11. MAMBULA, S.S., K. SAU, P. HENNEKE, *et al.* 2002. Toll-like receptor (TLR) signaling in response to *Aspergillus fumigatus*. J. Biol. Chem. **277:** 39320–39326.

12. MEIER, A., C.J. KIRSCHNING, T. NIKOLAUS, *et al.* 2003. Toll-like receptor (TLR) 2 and TLR4 are essential for *Aspergillus*-induced activation of murine macrophages. Cell. Microbiol. **5:** 561–570.
13. ROEDER, A., C.J. KIRSCHNING, R.A. RUPEC, *et al.* 2004. Toll-like receptors as key mediators in innate antifungal immunity. Med. Mycol. **42:** 485–498.
14. BULUT, Y., E. FAURE, L. THOMAS, *et al.* 2001. Cooperation of Toll-like receptor 2 and 6 for cellular activation by soluble tuberculosis factor and *Borrelia burgdorferi* outer surface protein A lipoprotein: role of Toll-interacting protein and IL-1 receptor signaling molecules in Toll-like receptor 2 signaling. J. Immunol. **167:** 987–994.
15. TAKEDA, K., O. TAKEUCHI & S. AKIRA. 2002. Recognition of lipopeptides by Toll-like receptors. J. Endotoxin Res. **8:** 459–463.
16. ASCIOGLU, S., J.H. REX, B. DE PAUW, *et al.* 2002. Defining opportunistic invasive fungal infections in immunocompromised patients with cancer and hematopoietic stem cell transplants: an international consensus. Clin. Infect. Dis. **34:** 7–14.
17. GREEN, P., B. EWING & D. GORDON. 2001. Phred, phrap and consed: University of Washington Genome Sciences Department. Available at: http://www.phrap.org.
18. HOSMER, D.W. & S. LEMESHOW. Applied Logistic Regression. John Wiley & Sons. New York.
19. RUCZINSKI, I., C. KOOPERBERG & M.L. LEBLANC. 2004. Exploring interactions in high-dimensional genomic data: an overview of logic regression with application. J. Multivariate Anal. **90:** 178–195.
20. KIECHL, S., E. LORENZ, M. REINDL, *et al.* 2002. Toll-like receptor 4 polymorphisms and atherogenesis. N. Engl. J. Med. **347:** 185–192.
21. LORENZ, E., J.P. MIRA, K.L. CORNISH, *et al.* 2000. A novel polymorphism in the toll-like receptor 2 gene and its potential association with staphylococcal infection. Infect. Immun. **68:** 6398–6401.
22. OGUS, A.C., B. YOLDAS, T. OZDEMIR, *et al.* 2004. The Arg753GLn polymorphism of the human toll-like receptor 2 gene in tuberculosis disease. Eur. Respir. J. **23:** 219–223.
23. KANG, T.J. & G.T. CHAE. 2001. Detection of Toll-like receptor 2 (TLR2) mutation in the lepromatous leprosy patients. FEMS Immunol. Med. Microbiol. **31:** 53–58.

T-Cell Immunotherapy for Adenoviral Infections of Stem-Cell Transplant Recipients

A.M. LEEN,[a,b] G.D. MYERS,[a,b] C.M. BOLLARD,[a,b,c] M.H. HULS,[a,b] U. SILI,[a,b,d] A.P. GEE,[a,b] H.E. HESLOP,[a,b] AND C.M. ROONEY[a,b,c,d]

[a]*Center for Cell and Gene Therapy,* [b]*Department of Pediatrics,* [c]*Department of Immunology, and* [d]*Department of Molecular Virology and Microbiology, Baylor College of Medicine, Houston, Texas 77030, USA*

ABSTRACT: Human adenoviruses are ubiquitous lytic DNA viruses that can be divided into 51 different serotypes, grouped from A to F on the basis of genome size, composition, homology, and organization. Adenovirus infections, although frequent, are rarely fatal in immunocompetent individuals, due to potent innate and adaptive immune responses. By contrast, adenoviruses are a significant cause of morbidity and mortality in immunosuppressed individuals, for whom there are limited treatment options. Since antiviral drugs have variable efficacy in the treatment of severe adenovirus disease, iatrogenic reconstitution with *in vitro* expanded virus-specific cytotoxic T lymphocytes (CTLs) is an attractive option for prophylaxis and treatment, particularly because the endogenous recovery of adenovirus-specific T cells has proved important in controlling infection *in vivo*. Thus, we have characterized human T-cell responses to adenovirus *in vitro* and explored the potential of adoptive T-cell immunotherapy as a prophylactic or therapeutic strategy for adenovirus infections posttransplant.

KEYWORDS: stem cell transplantation; adenoviral infections; immunotherapy; DNA viruses; T cells; cytotoxic T lympocytes (CTL)

INTRODUCTION

Therapy with cytotoxic T-cell lines has been effective for the prevention and treatment of Epstein-Barr virus (EBV) and cytomegalovirus (CMV) infections after allogeneic stem-cell transplantation.[1,2] Small numbers of EBV-specific T cells proliferate massively after infusion, home to tumor sites, and persist for up to eight years after infusion, retaining their ability to respond to antigenic challenge, both *in vitro* and *in vivo*.[2–5] However, adenovirus remains a major cause of morbidity and mortality after hematopoietic stem-cell transplantation (HSCT).[6] To date, there are no consistently effective antiviral drugs available. Current therapies include ribavirin or cidofovir, but responses are unpredictable and are associated with toxicities,

Address for correspondence: Cliona Rooney, Ph.D., Center for Cell and Gene Therapy, Department of Pediatrics–Hem/Onc, Baylor College of Medicine, 6621 Fannin St., MC3-3320 Houston, TX 77030. Voice: 832-824-4693; fax: 832-825-4732.
crooney@bcm.edu

Ann. N.Y. Acad. Sci. 1062: 104–115 (2005).
doi: 10.1196/annals.1358.013

making alternative approaches to adenovirus prophylaxis and treatment attractive.[7,8] Therefore, our goal has been to produce adenovirus-specific T-cell lines that can protect stem-cell recipients after adoptive transfer.

In a number of retrospective and prospective studies, adenovirus has been detected in 5% to 30% of patients post-HSCT, with a higher incidence in the pediatric population, in which adenovirus can be detected early in the posttransplant period (median 30 days posttransplant) compared with adults (median > 90 days posttransplant).[9–13] In a retrospective study of the incidence of adenovirus infection and disease at Texas Children's Hospital, adenovirus was detected in samples from 35 of 111 (32%) pediatric HSCT recipients, with 9 of 111 (8%) developing disease.[48] Importantly, development of adenovirus disease recently has been correlated with lack of antigen-specific T-cell recovery in the posttransplant period.[14–16] These findings highlight the potential benefits of an adoptive immunotherapy approach to this common posttransplant complication, and indicate that *in vitro* expanded adenovirus-specific CTLs should be infused early in the posttransplant period, particularly in pediatric patients.

Adenoviruses have evolved multiple mechanisms to evade the host immune response and allow infection to progress.[17] Several immune evasion genes are encoded in the early transcription unit, E3. E3-19K anchors MHC class I molecules in the endoplasmic reticulum (ER) and also inhibits tapasin 1 transport of peptides to the ER.[18] Other E3 genes protect adenovirus-infected cells from lysis by tumor necrosis factor α (TNF-α) and from Fas-mediated death.[18–22] Even E1A, the first viral gene to be expressed, inhibits interferon-induced gene expression.[23] We reasoned, therefore, that like CMV, adenovirus virion proteins that enter the cell before the expression of immune evasion genes should be processed and presented to T cells and may provide targets for CTLs.[24] We hypothesized that standard adenoviral vectors would provide an abundant source of virion proteins without introducing infectious virus, because both E1A, the prime transcriptional transactivator, and the entire immune inhibitory E3 region are deleted. In addition, adenovirus vectors have a long history in gene therapy studies, and, therefore, would be available as a clinical-grade product, an important consideration for future adenovirus immunotherapy protocols. Rather than the customary adenovirus 5 (Ad5)-based vector, we used an Ad5f35 vector, in which parts of the Ad5 fiber gene are replaced by Ad35 fiber.[25] This small alteration results in improved transduction of hematopoietic cells.[26,27]

There are 51 known human adenovirus serotypes that fall into 6 subgroups, A to F.[28,29] They are ubiquitous in all human communities and usually cause only mild localized disease, with infected tissues depending on serotype.[6] However, viruses from all subgroups can cause disease in immunosuppressed patients, and, thus, immunotherapeutic T cells must protect against all. Human immunity to adenoviruses has been understudied and little is known about protective T-cell immunity. Therefore, in order to achieve our ultimate goal of developing an adenovirus immunotherapy protocol, we decided to characterize the human T-cell immune response to adenovirus, to determine whether adenovirus-specific T cells could be reactivated and expanded in the laboratory, to identify immunodominant antigens and epitopes, and to establish whether these CTL lines would cross-react with adenoviruses from different serotypes and subgroups. Our ultimate goal was to ascertain whether adenovirus-specific T cells would protect stem-cell recipients against adenovirus-associated disease.

RESULTS

All Donors Respond to T-Cell Stimulation with the Ad5f35 Vector

To determine whether the Ad5f35 vector was immunogenic *in vitro* we isolated $CD4^+$ and $CD8^+$ T cells from a number of healthy seropositive donors and stimulated them with autologous dendritic cells (DCs) that had been transduced with a null (transgeneless) adenoviral vector.[30] We measured T-cell responses in an ELISPOT assay that measured antigen-induced interferon (IFN)-γ production from T cells. IFN-γ was produced by T cells from all donors screened, and this reactivity was found predominantly in the $CD4^+$ T-cell compartment.[31–36]

Adenovirus-Specific T Cells Can Be Expanded Ex Vivo *and Are Subgroup Cross-Reactive*

Responder T cells expanded in culture in response to weekly restimulation with Ad5f35-transduced DCs, and recognized and lysed autologous fibroblasts infected with wild-type adenoviruses from subgroups B, C, D, and E, suggesting that these CTL lines might respond to any infecting adenovirus strain.[32,36–38] This was an important milestone in the design of our adenovirus immunotherapy protocol.

Development of an Immunotherapy Protocol

Alternative Antigen-Presenting Cells

This work confirmed that virion proteins of adenovirus were viable targets for immunotherapy approaches, and that replication-incompetent vector could be used as a source of antigen. DCs were used as antigen-presenting cells (APCs), as they were transduced easily and could stimulate T cells efficiently. However, from a practical point of view DCs are problematic. They are limited in supply, particularly from unrelated donors; they do not proliferate in vivo; they are time-consuming to generate; and their production depends on the availability of a cocktail of cytokines, including granulocyte-macrophage colony-stimulating factor (GM-CSF), interleukin (IL)-4, IL-1, IL-6, TNF-α, and prostaglandin E2, not all of which are available as GMP-grade reagents. We considered alternative sources of APCs, such as EBV-transformed B lymphoblastoid cells lines (LCL), and means of nonspecific expansion of DC-activated T cells, including artificial APCs and beads. However, LCLs, while in plentiful supply, express a variety of lytic and latent EBV antigens, which compete with adenoviral antigens available in the vector, and preliminary experiments confirmed that Ad5f35-transduced LCLs could induce preferential expansion of EBV-specific T cells. Nonspecific expansion protocols are useful for the expansion of T-cell clones, but when applied to polyclonal T-cell lines produce significant losses in specificity.[39]

We therefore examined peripheral blood monocytes, which after activation by simple adherence without exogenous cytokines, attain a mature DC-like phenotype signified by the upregulation of a number of activation and costimulatory molecules, including CD80 and CD83[40,41](Leen *et al.*, manuscript in preparation; FIG. 1). Because autologous monocytes are (1) easily isolated, either by adherence or using magnetic beads coupled to the monocyte marker CD14, (2) efficiently transduced by

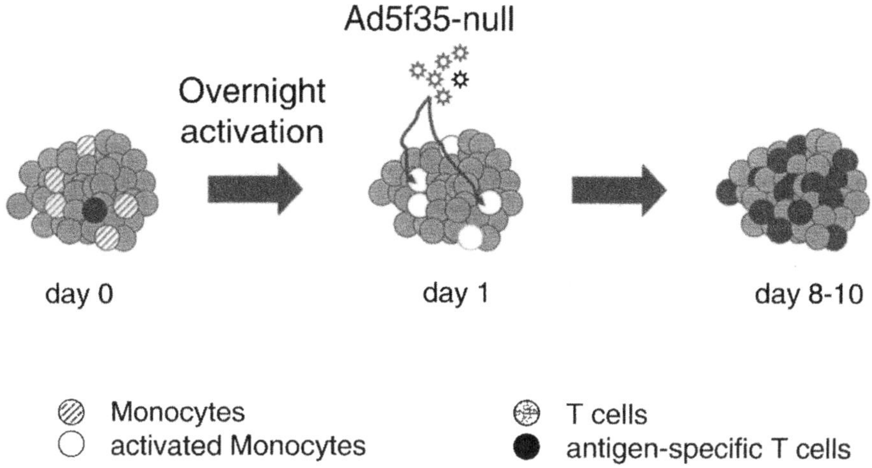

FIGURE 1. Activation of adenovirus-specific T cells. Peripheral blood monocytes can be activated by adherence to plastic overnight, attain an activated DC-like phenotype signified by the upregulation of a number of activation and co-stimulatory molecules, including CD80 and CD83. These activated monocytes are capable or reactivating adenovirus-specific T cells following transduction with the Ad5f35-null vector.

the Ad5f35 vector,[32] and (3) capable of activating T cells,[32,37–42] we investigated their ability to activate adenovirus-specific T cells *in vitro*. We hypothesized that after activation, reactive T cells could be expanded further using autologous Ad5f35-transduced LCLs, with only minor competition from the EBV antigens expressed in the LCLs. To test this hypothesis, T-cell lines from several healthy donors were stimulated with Ad5f35-transduced monocytes, and then expanded with Ad5f35-transduced LCLs.[32] All the lines retained adenovirus specificity, but most contained, in addition, an EBV-specific T-cell component (FIG. 2). Because allogeneic SCT recipients are at risk for both adenovirus and EBV infection, we reasoned that the infusion of a CTL line specific for both viruses would be a bonus.

Characterization of Adenovirus Vector-Specific T Cells

Optimal evaluation of the persistence and function of infused T cells requires detailed knowledge of the specificity of the infused T cells, so that peptide ELISPOT and tetramer assays can be performed on patient blood pre- and postinfusion. Therefore, we analyzed the antigen and epitope specificity of the T cells reactivated with Ad5f35-null. The adenovirus virion contains 11 proteins that are potential targets for T cells. We focused our preliminary studies on the three most abundant antigens, hexon, penton, and fiber, that have been shown by Hamel and colleagues to be immunogenic.[43] T-Cell clones were isolated from the polyclonal lines by magnetic isolation and were cloned by limiting dilution into microwells containing allogeneic feeder cells and autologous Ad5f35-transduced APCs in the presence of high-dose

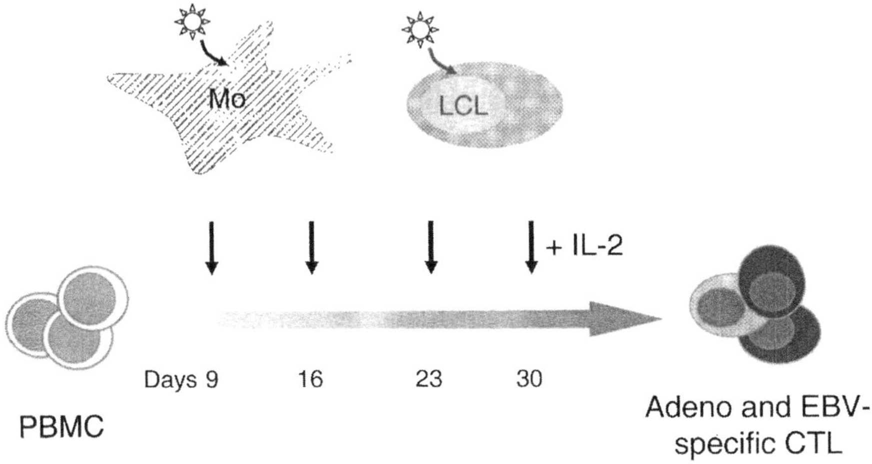

FIGURE 2. CTL activation protocol. T-Cell lines for infusion can be activated with Ad5f35-transduced monocytes, and then expanded with Ad5f35-transduced LCLs. The resultant lines are both adenovirus and EBV-specific.

IL-2. We initially focused on the $CD8^+$ response, as $CD8^+$ T-cell epitopes are only 8 to 11 amino acids long, and presented in the context of a single class I allele, each with characteristic amino acids at anchor positions so that epitopes can be predicted using computer algorithms.

Adenovirus specificity was confirmed by exposing each $CD8^+$ clone to Ad5f35-null–transduced autologous APCs in IFN-γ ELISPOT assays. Then their ability to kill fibroblasts transduced with retroviral vectors expressing hexon or penton constructs was assessed using a standard chromium release assay. Fiber proved toxic to cells, and we were unable to produce the vector. However, all the adenovirus-specific $CD8^+$ T-cell clones killed target cells expressing hexon, with no recognition of penton. This was confirmed using clones generated from a number of different donors with different HLA backgrounds, indicating that hexon may be an immunodominant T-cell target.[37]

We next addressed whether these $CD8^+$ T-cell clones recognized adenoviruses from other subgroups. All clones recognized viruses from at least two, and in most cases up to four, different subgroups, indicating that the immunodominant T-cell epitopes were conserved between different viral serotypes. Thus, identification of the individual HLA-restricting molecules could be narrowed down to regions of the hexon molecule that were conserved among different serotypes. Finally, the epitope prediction algorithms BIMAS and SYFPEITHI were used to define the minimal epitopes recognized. Using this technique, we identified five novel $CD8^+$ T-cell epitopes presented in the context of HLA-A1 (TDLGQNLLY), A2 (TFYLNHT-FKKV), A24 (TYFSLNNKF), and B7 (MPNRPNYIAFR and KPYSGTAYNSL), which will be useful tools, both as tetramers and in ELISPOT assays, for characterizing adenovirus-specific CTL lines and for rational immunological monitoring of patients pre- and post–T-cell infusion.[37]

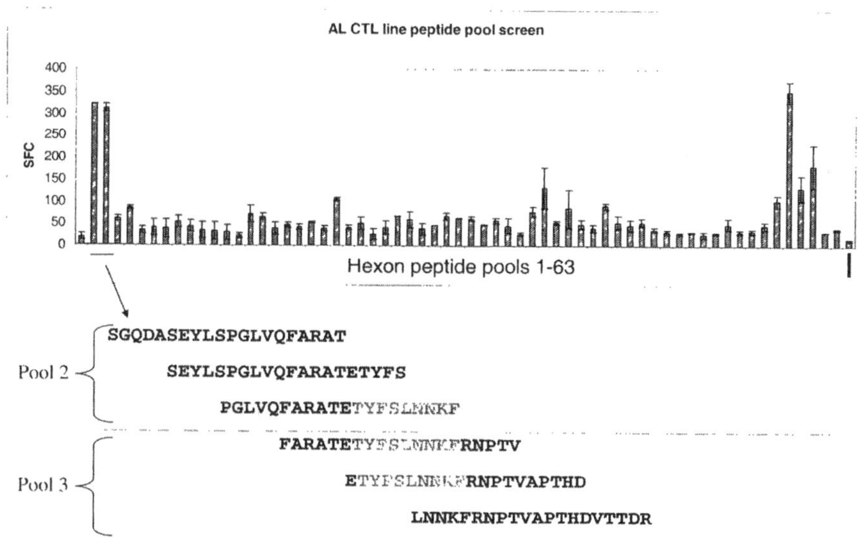

FIGURE 3. Hexon epitope screening. Using a dodecamer peptide library overlapping by 15 amino acids (aa) and spanning the 952 aa sequence of this hexon serotype 5 protein, we were able to ientify known CD8+ T-cell epitopes, as well as novel CD4+ and CD8+ T-cell epitopes.

Because hexon appeared to be the immunodominant T-cell target of adenoviral vector-specific T cells, we produced a dodecamer peptide library overlapping by 15 amino acids (aa) and spanning the 952 aa sequence of the hexon serotype 5 protein. This library was designed to identify both class I and class II epitopes. Adenovirus-specific T-cell lines and clones were screened against 63 pools of three peptides, an approach that has proved successful for the identification of both $CD4^+$ and $CD8^+$ T-cell epitopes in other viral systems.[44,45] Using CTL lines from five healthy seropositive donors, we identified previously published $CD8^+$ T-cell epitopes (FIG. 3), as well as ten additional $CD8^+$ and six $CD4^+$ T cell-epitopes (Leen *et al.*, unpublished data). It should be noted that 21 of 22 epitopes map to conserved regions of hexon (FIG. 4). Work is ongoing to identify the restricting HLA alleles, and to examine the frequency of these responses in other donors who share the restricting HLA type.

Clinical Trial to Determine the Protective Capacity of Adenoviral Vector-Specific CTLs for the Prevention and Treatment of Adenovirus Infections in HSCT Recipients

A clinical protocol for the infusion of adenovirus-specific CTLs into allogeneic SCT recipients has been approved by the Baylor College of Medicine Institutional Review Board (IRB), the Recombinant DNA Advisory Committee (RAC), and the Food and Drug Administration (FDA).

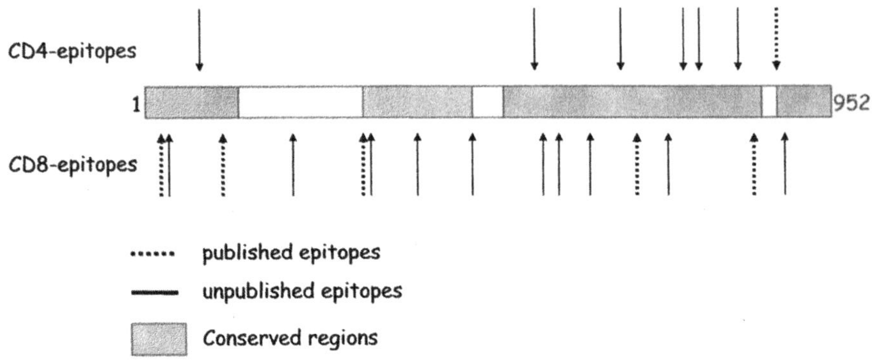

FIGURE 4. Epitope locations. Both CD4+ and CD8+ T-cell epitopes map to the conserved regions of the hexon molecule.

The trial is designed as a standard phase I dose-escalation study, with donor-derived CTLs infused at four different dose levels:

$$\text{Level } 1 = 5 \times 10^6 \text{ CTL/m}^2$$

$$\text{Level } 2 = 1.5 \times 10^7 \text{ CTL/m}^2$$

$$\text{Level } 3 = 4.5 \times 10^7 \text{ CTL/m}^2$$

$$\text{Level } 4 = 1.35 \times 10^8 \text{ CTL/m}^2$$

Two to six patients will be enrolled at each dose level, and, providing there is no toxicity, we will move to the next level. The patient eligibility criteria are as follows:

(1) Recipients of allogeneic (i.e., HLA matched or mismatched related or unrelated);
(2) No evidence of GVHD > Grade II at time of enrollment;
(3) Life expectancy > 30 days;
(4) No severe intercurrent infections;
(5) Lansky/Karnofsky scores ≥ 60;
(6) Absence of severe renal disease (Creatinine > × 3 normal for age);
(7) Absence of severe hepatic disease (direct bilirubin > 3 mg/dL or SGOT > 500);
(8) Patient must be at least 30 days posttransplant to be eligible to receive CTL;
(9) Not receiving Cidofovir;
(10) Patient has not received other viral-specific CTL prophylactically within 4 weeks of receiving Adv-CTL;
(11) Patient/guardian able to give informed consent.

Both children and adults will be enrolled, but we anticipate that the majority of patients in the study will be children, as they are at a higher risk of developing infection and disease post-HSCT. Because CTL lines will take six to eight weeks to manufacture, patients will be enrolled and CTLs produced regardless of adenovirus infection status, and cells will be given to patients both as prophylaxis and as treatment for active infection. Although there may be too few patients in this study to determine antiviral efficacy, we will be able to monitor T-cell survival postinfusion. For this reason, we will preferentially enroll patients with informative HLA types, that is, for which we have identified epitopes. This will allow us to characterize the adenovirus-specific T-cell product, evaluate patient adenovirus-specific immunity preinfusion, and track infused T cells to evaluate their ability to expand, reconstitute immunity to adenovirus and persist *in vivo*. Samples for immune monitoring will be collected immediately preinfusion, then 24 h, 1, 2, 4, and 6 weeks postinfusion, and then at 3, 6, 9, and 12 months. In addition to tetramer analysis, IFN-γ ELISPOT assays will be performed using the overlapping hexon library to cover patients from whom epitopes may not have been identified and to evaluate T-cell function.

Extensive virological monitoring of patients for the presence of EBV and adenovirus pre- and postinfusion will also be performed. EBV will be monitored using real-time quantitative reverse transcription polymerase chain reaction (RT-PCR) of peripheral blood mononuclear cell (PBMC) DNA, and adenovirus will be monitored by RT-PCR analysis of blood, urine, and stool samples. Initially, a generic primer–probe combination that detects all adenovirus serotypes will be used. However, if an infection is detected, the infecting subgroup(s) will be identified using a primer–probe combination that is particular to each subgroup. This virological monitoring will be carried out pretreatment, then weekly for 60 days postinfusion, and then as per standard of care for each patient.

DISCUSSION

Adenovirus infections and disease remain a major cause of morbidity and mortality, particularly in patients who receive an allogeneic HSCT. In pediatric transplant recipients, the high incidence of infection has been correlated with a lack of T-cell recovery. Thus, in the absence of effective antiviral therapies, adoptive T-cell therapy is an attractive option. To date, however, there have been no immunotherapy trials, mainly because of a lack of information on cellular immune responses to adenoviral antigens. However, a number of laboratories are now addressing this deficiency. We have identified the virion hexon protein as an immunodominant target of the adenovirus-specific immune response. Within hexon, we have identified multiple CD4 and CD8 epitopes that will allow us to track the fate of adoptively transferred cells. Our group has developed a protocol for the generation and infusion of adenovirus-specific CTLs; patients will be enrolled in the upcoming months. The safety and efficacy data from infused patients should allow us to establish a link between virus-specific T cells and protection against adenovirus infection.

The major question that we hope to address is whether hexon-specific T cells can provide protection against adenovirus infection and disease. However, the primary endpoint of a phase I trial is safety and we may enroll an insufficient number of patients to determine efficacy in this trial. Another interesting question is whether antigen is required for the optimal expansion and persistence of infused T cells. Although CMV and EBV-specific T cells expand after infusion, most patients are chronically infected with these viruses, so it is not clear whether expansion is driven by homeostatic mechanisms or by antigen. By contrast, only a fraction (5–32%) of our patients may have an active adenovirus infection. Therefore, it will be interesting to determine whether T-cell expansion is largely homeostatic or is driven by infection.

Although adoptive T-cell transfer is a promising therapeutic approach to viral infections in the immunocompromised patient, there are few centers worldwide that have the facilities to produce clinical-grade CTLs for infusion. While many facilities perform short-term processing of primary tissues for stem-cell infusions, few can maintain long-term cultures using good manufacturing practices (GMP). Therefore, adoptive immunotherapy currently is beyond the reach of most institutions. However, there is increasing interest in T-cell therapies for cancer, and so adenovirus-specific T cells, if effective, may be adopted more widely until a safe and effective antiadenoviral drug is developed. Unfortunately, to date there are no approved antiviral agents with proven efficacy in the treatment of severe adenoviral disease, nor are there any prospective randomized, controlled trials of potentially useful anti-adenoviral therapies.

Future studies will be aimed at shortening the time required for CTL generation. A major reduction could be made if LCLs, which require about six weeks to generate, could be eliminated for the expansion phase. If adenovirus-specific T cells expand effectively after infusion, this could reduce the dose infused, so that a single activation cycle may suffice to produce sufficient cells for infusion. However, a shortened activation period would require a selection step to eliminate alloreactive T cells. A reverse strategy has been adopted by a number of groups who, instead of selecting viral antigen-specific T cells, deplete alloreactive T cells. Recipient-derived APCs are used to activate allospecific T cells, which are then eliminated based on their activation markers. The remaining cells, containing T cells specific for all the pathogens to which the donor has been exposed, can then be infused.[46,47] Either strategy would simplify and greatly shorten the time for T-cell production, ultimately making adoptive immunotherapy a more attractive therapy option.

ACKNOWLEDGMENTS

This work was supported by the DANA Foundation (C.M.R.), the Methodist Foundation (A.M.L.), the GCRC at Baylor College of Medicine (RR00188). H.E. Heslop was supported by a Doris Duke Distinguished Clinical Scientist Award, and C.M. Bollard by an Amy Stelzer Manasevit Scholar Award.

[*Competing interests*: The authors declare that they have no competing financial interests.]

REFERENCES

1. WALTER, E.A., P.D. GREENBERG, M.J. GILBERT, *et al.* 1995. Reconstitution of cellular immunity against cytomegalovirus in recipients of allogeneic bone marrow by transfer of T-cell clones from the donor. N. Engl. J. Med. **333:** 1038–1044.

2. Rooney, C.M., C.A. Smith, C. Ng, *et al.* 1995. Use of gene-modified virus-specific T lymphocytes to control Epstein-Barr virus-related lymphoproliferation. Lancet **345:** 9–13.
3. Heslop, H.E., C.Y.C. Ng, C. Li, *et al.* 1996. Long-term restoration of immunity against Epstein-Barr virus infection by adoptive transfer of gene-modified virus-specific T lymphocytes. Nat. Med. **2:** 551–555.
4. Peggs, K.S. & S. MacKinnon. 2004. Augmentation of virus-specific immunity after hematopoietic stem cell transplantation by adoptive T-cell therapy. Hum. Immunol. **65:** 550–557.
5. Rooney, C.M., C.A. Smith, C.Y. Ng, *et al.* 1998. Infusion of cytotoxic T cells for the prevention and treatment of Epstein-Barr virus-induced lymphoma in allogeneic transplant recipients. Blood **92:** 1549–1555.
6. Kojaoghlanian, T., P. Flomenberg & M.S. Horwitz. 2003. The impact of adenovirus infection on the immunocompromised host. Rev. Med. Virol. **13:** 155–171.
7. Gavin, P.J. & B.Z. Katz. 2002. Intravenous ribavirin treatment for severe adenovirus disease in immunocompromised children. Pediatrics **110:** e9.
8. Hoffman, J.A., A.J. Shah, L.A. Ross & N. Kapoor. 2001. Adenoviral infections and a prospective trial of cidofovir in pediatric hematopoietic stem cell transplantation. Biol. Blood Marrow Transplant. **7:** 388–394.
9. Flomenberg, P., J. Babbitt, W.R. Drobyski, *et al.* 1994. Increasing incidence of adenovirus disease in bone marrow transplant recipients. J. Infect. Dis. **169:** 775–781.
10. Hale, G.A., H.E. Heslop, R.A. Krance, *et al.* 1999. Adenovirus infection after pediatric bone marrow transplantation. Bone Marrow Transplant. **23:** 277–282.
11. Lion, T., R. Baumgartinger, F. Watzinger, *et al.* 2003. Molecular monitoring of adenovirus in peripheral blood after allogeneic bone marrow transplantation permits early diagnosis of disseminated disease. Blood **102:** 1114–1120.
12. Chakrabarti, S., V. Mautner, H. Osman, *et al.* 2002. Adenovirus infections following allogeneic stem cell transplantation: incidence and outcome in relation to graft manipulation, immunosuppression, and immune recovery. Blood **100:** 1619–1627.
13. Avivi, I., S. Chakrabarti, D.W. Milligan, *et al.* 2004. Incidence and outcome of adenovirus disease in transplant recipients after reduced-intensity conditioning with alemtuzumab. Biol. Blood Marrow Transplant. **10:** 186–194.
14. Van Tol, M.J., A.C. Kroes, J. Schinkel, *et al.* 2005. Adenovirus infection in paediatric stem cell transplant recipients: increased risk in young children with a delayed immune recovery. Bone Marrow Transplant. **36:** 39–50.
15. Heemskerk, B., A.C. Lankester, T. van Vreeswijk, *et al.* 2005. Immune reconstitution and clearance of human adenovirus viremia in pediatric stem-cell recipients. J. Infect. Dis. **191:** 520–530.
16. Feuchtinger, T., J. Lucke, K. Hamprecht, *et al.* 2005. Detection of adenovirus-specific T cells in children with adenovirus infection after allogeneic stem cell transplantation. Br. J. Haematol. **128:** 503–509.
17. Burgert, H.G., Z. Ruzsics, S. Obermeier, *et al.* 2002. Subversion of host defense mechanisms by adenoviruses. Curr. Top. Microbiol. Immunol. **269:** 273–318.
18. Elsing, A. & H.G. Burgert. 1998. The adenovirus E3/10.4K-14.5K proteins down-modulate the apoptosis receptor Fas/Apo-1 by inducing its internalization. Proc. Natl. Acad. Sci. USA **95:** 10072–10077.
19. Burgert, H.G. & S. Kvist. 1987. The E3/19K protein of adenovirus type 2 binds to the domains of histocompatibility antigens required for CTL recognition. EMBO J. **6:** 2019–2026.
20. Wold, W.S., K. Doronin, K. Toth, *et al.* 1999. Immune responses to adenoviruses: viral evasion mechanisms and their implications for the clinic. Curr. Opin. Immunol. **11:** 380–386.
21. Wold, W.S. & L.R. Gooding. 1991. Region E3 of adenovirus: a cassette of genes involved in host immunosurveillance and virus-cell interactions. Virology **184:** 1–8.
22. Wold, W.S. & L.R. Gooding. 1989. Adenovirus region E3 proteins that prevent cytolysis by cytotoxic T cells and tumor necrosis factor. Mol. Biol. Med. **6:** 433–452.
23. Anderson, K.P. & E.H. Fennie. 1987. Adenovirus early region 1A modulation of interferon antiviral activity. J. Virol. **61:** 787–795.

24. GILBERT, M.J., S.R. RIDDELL, B. PLACHTER & P.D. GREENBERG. 1996. Cytomegalovirus selectively blocks antigen processing and presentation of its intermediate-early gene product. Nature **383:** 720–722.
25. SHAYAKHMETOV, D.M. & A. LIEBER. 2000. Dependence of adenovirus infectivity on length of the fiber shaft domain. J. Virol. **74:** 10274–10286.
26. SHAYAKHMETOV, D.M., T. PAPAYANNOPOULOU, G. STAMATOYANNOPOULOS & A. LIEBER. 2000. Efficient gene transfer into human CD34(+) cells by a retargeted adenovirus vector. J. Virol. **74:** 2567–2583.
27. YOTNDA, P., H. ONISHI, H.E. HESLOP, *et al.* 2001. Efficient infection of primitive hematopoietic stem cells by modified adenovirus. Gene Ther. **8:** 930–937.
28. HORWITZ, M.S. 2001. Adenoviruses. *In* Fields Virology, 4th ed. D.M. Knipe, P.M. Howley, D.E. Griffin, Eds.: 2301–2326. Lippincott, Williams & Wilkins. Philadelphia.
29. SHENK, T.E. 2002. Adenoviridae: The Viruses and Their Replication. *In* Fields Virology, 4th ed. D.M. Knipe, P.M. Howley, D.E. Griffin, Eds.: 2265–2300. Lippincott, Williams & Wilkins. Philadelphia.
30. SMITH, C.A., L.S. WOODRUFF, G.R. KITCHINGMAN & C.M. ROONEY. 1996. Adenovirus-pulsed dendritic cells stimulate human virus-specific T-cell responses in vitro. J. Virol. **70:** 6733–6740.
31. FLOMENBERG, P., V. PIASKOWSKI, R.L. TRUITT & J.T. CASPER. 1995. Characterization of human proliferative T cell responses to adenovirus. J. Infect. Dis. **171:** 1090–1096.
32. LEEN, A.M., U. SILI, B. SAVOLDO, *et al.* 2004. Fiber-modified adenoviruses generate subgroup cross-reactive, adenovirus-specific cytotoxic T lymphocytes for therapeutic applications. Blood **103:** 1011–1019.
33. OLIVE, M., L.C. EISENLOHR & P. FLOMENBERG. 2001. Quantitative analysis of adenovirus-specific CD4+ T-cell responses from healthy adults. Viral Immunol. **14:** 403–413.
34. OLIVE, M., L. EISENLOHR, N. FLOMENBERG, *et al.* 2002. The adenovirus capsid protein hexon contains a highly conserved human CD4+ T-cell epitope. Hum. Gene Ther. **13:** 1167–1178.
35. TANG, J., M. OLIVE, K. CHAMPAGNE, *et al.* 2004. Adenovirus hexon T-cell epitope is recognized by most adults and is restricted by HLA DP4, the most common class II allele. Gene Ther. **11:** 1408–1415.
36. HEEMSKERK, B., L.A. VELTROP-DUITS, T. VAN VREESWIJK, *et al.* 2003. Extensive cross-reactivity of CD4+ adenovirus-specific T cells: implications for immunotherapy and gene therapy. J. Virol. **77:** 6562–6566.
37. LEEN, A.M., U. SILI, E.F. VANIN, *et al.* 2004. Conserved CTL epitopes on the adenovirus hexon protein expand subgroup cross-reactive and subgroup-specific CD8+ T cells. Blood **104:** 2432–2440.
38. SMITH, C.A., L.S. WOODRUFF, C. ROONEY & G.R. KITCHINGMAN. 1998. Extensive cross-reactivity of adenovirus-specific cytotoxic T cells. Hum. Gene Ther. **9:** 1419–1427.
39. SILI, U., M.H. HULS, A.R. DAVIS, *et al.* 2003. Large-scale expansion of dendritic cell-primed polyclonal human cytotoxic T-lymphocytes using lymphoblastoid cell lines for adoptive immunotherapy. J. Immunother. **26:** 241–256.
40. EIERMAN, D.F., C.E. JOHNSON & J.S. HASKILL. 1989. Human monocyte inflammatory mediator gene expression is selectively regulated by adherence substrates. J. Immunol. **142:** 1970–1976.
41. HASKILL, S., C. JOHNSON, D. EIERMAN, *et al.* 1988. Adherence induces selective mRNA expression of monocyte mediators and proto-oncogenes. J. Immunol. **140:** 1690–1694.
42. OSUGI, Y., S. VUCKOVIC & D.N. HART. 2002. Myeloid blood CD11c(+) dendritic cells and monocyte-derived dendritic cells differ in their ability to stimulate T lymphocytes. Blood **100:** 2858–2866.
43. HAMEL, Y., N. BLAKE, S. GABRIELSSON, *et al.* 2002. Adenovirally transduced dendritic cells induce bispecific cytotoxic T lymphocyte responses against adenovirus and cytomegalovirus pp65 or against adenovirus and Epstein-Barr virus EBNA3C protein: a novel approach for immunotherapy. Hum. Gene Ther. **13:** 855–866.
44. LEEN, A., P. MEIJ, I. REDCHENKO, *et al.* 2001. Differential immunogenicity of Epstein-Barr virus latent-cycle proteins for human CD4(+) T-helper 1 responses. J. Virol. **75:** 8649–8659.

45. MEIJ, P., A. LEEN, A.B. RICKINSON, *et al.* 2002. Identification and prevalence of CD8(+) T-cell responses directed against Epstein-Barr virus-encoded latent membrane protein 1 and latent membrane protein 2. Int. J. Cancer **99:** 93–99.
46. AMROLIA, P.J., G. MUCIOLI-CASADEI, H. HULS, *et al.* 2005. Add-back of allodepleted donor T cells to improve immune reconstitution after haplo-identical stem cell transplantation. Cytotherapy **7:** 116–125.
47. MONTAGNA, D., E. YVON, V. CALCATERRA, *et al.* 1999. Depletion of alloreactive T cells by a specific anti-interleukin-2 receptor p55 chain immunotoxin does not impair *in vitro* antileukemia and antiviral activity. Blood **93:** 3550–3557.
48. MYERS, G.D., R.A. KRANCE, H. WEISS, *et al.* 2005. Adenovirus infection rates in pediatric recipients of alternate donor allogeneic bone marrow transplants receiving either antithymocyte globulin (ATG) or alemtuzumab (Campath). Bone Marrow Transplant. In press.

Human B Cell Tolerance and Its Failure in Rheumatoid Arthritis

JONATHAN SAMUELS,[a] YEN-SHING NG,[a] CLAIRE COUPILLAUD,[a] DANIEL PAGET,[a] AND ERIC MEFFRE[a,b]

[a]*Laboratory of Biochemistry and Molecular Immunology, Hospital for Special Surgery, New York, New York 10021, USA*

[b]*Weill Medical College of Cornell University, New York, New York 10021, USA*

ABSTRACT: Random V(D)J gene assembly generates many autoreactive B cell receptors (BCRs). In healthy donors, most autoreactive developing B cells are removed either in the bone marrow or in the periphery, revealing two B cell tolerance checkpoints. The regulation and the mechanisms that ensure this human B cell tolerance are poorly characterized, but they require proper BCR signaling. Indeed, patients with X-linked agammaglobulinemia who carry mutations in the *BTK* gene, which encodes an essential BCR signaling component, fail to establish proper central B cell tolerance, as demonstrated by the release of self-reactive B cells in the periphery. In autoimmune diseases such as rheumatoid arthritis (RA), B cell tolerance is broken and autoantibodies are secreted. Our recent results show that RA patients suffer from defective central and peripheral B cell tolerance checkpoints, which may favor the development of autoimmunity. Also, about half of our RA patients display unusual immunoglobulin light chain repertoires showing impaired secondary recombination regulation, which indicates that receptor editing, one of the mechanisms that normally ensures B cell tolerance, may often be defective in RA.

KEYWORDS: rheumatoid arthritis; B lymphocyte; X-linked agammaglobulinemia; receptor editing; autoantibody

INTRODUCTION

Rheumatoid arthritis (RA) is a chronic inflammatory disease that affects about 1% of the population. RA has been extensively investigated, yet its etiology and pathogenesis remain elusive.[1] An important characteristic that distinguishes RA from the other inflammatory and degenerative joint diseases such as psoriatic arthritis or osteoarthritis is the production of autoantibodies directed against self-antigens, including antibody Fc regions (rheumatoid factors), type II collagen, and cyclic citrullinated peptides (CCPs).[2–5] Autoantibodies can be found as soluble immune complexes (ICs) in RA synovium fluid and as insoluble ICs in synovial tissue and cartilage. The involvement of ICs in the pathogenesis of RA has long been an accepted mechanism, and extensive analysis of ICs, particularly those containing rheuma-

Address for correspondence: Eric Meffre, Hospital for Special Surgery, Research Department, 535 E. 70th St., New York, NY 10021. Voice: 212-774-2347; fax: 212-717-1192. meffree@hss.edu

Ann. N.Y. Acad. Sci. 1062: 116–126 (2005). © 2005 New York Academy of Sciences. doi: 10.1196/annals.1358.014

toid factor, showed the presence of immunoglobulin G (IgG) as well as IgM antibodies in RA.[6,7] In experimental models of inflammatory and destructive arthritis, passive transfer of serum from animals with collagen-induced arthritis or transfer of anticollagen antibodies induced an arthritis similar to RA.[8,9] Despite these strong indications of a pathogenic role for B cells in RA, research focus had shifted toward the discovery that cytokines were essential effectors in driving and maintaining inflammation and cartilage damage, and investigation of B cells and their autoantibodies in disease pathogenesis fell out of favor.[1]

The emergence in the mid-1990s of a new arthritis mouse model described by D. Mathis, C. Benoist, *et al.* further demonstrated a major role for B cells and self-reactive antibodies in the development of inflammatory arthritis.[10,11] Recently, an important role for B cells in RA has been supported by successful treatment of RA patients with anti-CD20 monoclonal antibodies that eliminate B cells.[12,13]

The underlying mechanisms that account for autoreactive B cells and autoantibody production in RA have not been defined. Alterations in the counterselection of autoreactive B cells generated during early B cell development may allow the accumulation of self-reactive mature naïve B cells in the periphery, and stimulations by self- or xenoantigens may favor the emergence of autoreactive antibody specificities. Extrinsic signals from T cells, cytokines, or other factors may also drive B cells normally present in the repertoire to generate pathogenic isotypes and high-affinity self-reactive antibodies. Here we summarize our recent findings on the establishment and the regulation of B cell tolerance in humans and its dysregulation in RA patients.

ESTABLISHMENT OF HUMAN B CELL TOLERANCE

Engineered models using transgenic and knock-in mice have revealed that developing B cells expressing self-reactive receptors are normally silenced by receptor editing, deletion, or anergy.[14–17] However, the frequency of self-reactive antibodies that arise during unmanipulated B cell development could not be assessed using these mice, nor could it be determined when such antibodies were actually removed from the repertoire under physiologic circumstances. To determine the proportion of autoreactive B cells that were removed from the nascent repertoire and how central B cell tolerance was established in humans, we examined the antibody specificity of developing B cell precursors in the bone marrow and the blood of healthy donors.[18]

Immunoglobulin heavy (IgH) and light chain-kappa (Igκ) or -lambda (Igλ) transcripts were amplified from single developing B cells by two rounds of reverse transcription–polymerase chain reaction (PCR). The second PCR used primers with restriction sites compatible with cloning vectors that contained IgH or light chain constant regions. Antibody heavy and light chain expression vectors were cotransfected into A293 cells, and 1 week later the supernatants that contained secreted antibodies were harvested and their concentrations determined by enzyme-linked immunosorbent assay (ELISA). Recombinant antibodies from 29 single pre-B cells (CD34–CD19+CD10+IgM–) and 72 immature B cells (CD34–CD19+CD10+IgM+) purified from the bone marrow, and 54 newly emigrated B cells (CD19+CD10+IgM+CD27–) and 93 mature naive B cells (CD19+CD10–IgM+CD27–) from the blood of three healthy donors were tested for reactivity by ELISA against HEp-2 cell lysates and a panel of defined antigens including double-

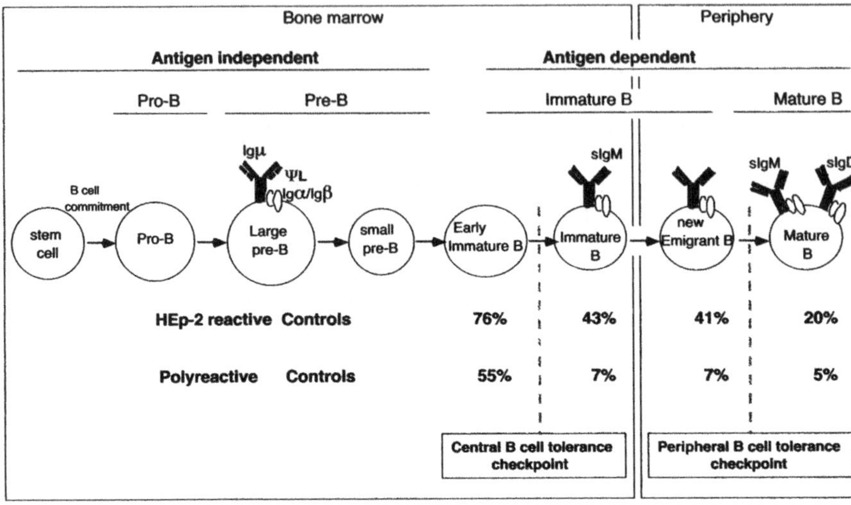

FIGURE 1. Two early B cell tolerance checkpoints in healthy donors. Developmental stages of B cell lymphopoiesis and cell surface expression of pre–B (Igμ, ψL [surrogate light chains] and Igα–Igβ) or B- (Igμ, Igκ, or Igλ and Igα–Igβ) cell receptors are shown. The frequency of B cells expressing HEp-2–reactive and polyreactive antibodies is indicated under each fraction analyzed. A central B cell tolerance checkpoint removes some HEp-2–reactive and most polyreactive antibodies between the early immature and immature B cell stage in the bone marrow. A peripheral B cell tolerance checkpoint eliminates further HEp-2–reactive B cells between new emigrant and mature naïve B cell stage.

stranded DNA, single-stranded DNA, insulin, and lipopolysaccharide.[19–24] Antibodies that bound to more than one of these antigens were considered polyreactive. We found that during normal B cell development, random V(D)J joining generated many HEp-2–reactive and polyreactive B cells. About 75% of early immature B cells expressed HEp-2–reactive antibodies that often recognized nuclear antigens, and 55% of those cells expressed polyreactive antibodies (FIG. 1). The analysis of the frequency of developing B cells expressing HEp-2–reactive and/or polyreactive antibodies revealed that autoreactive B cell clones were removed at two discrete checkpoints. First, a central checkpoint in the bone marrow between early immature and immature B cells removed most B cells expressing polyreactive and antinuclear antibodies. A peripheral checkpoint at the transition between new emigrant and mature naïve B cells further counterselected some HEp-2–reactive B cells that may encounter peripheral autoantigens probably not expressed in the bone marrow environment. Nonetheless, we found that 20% of mature naïve B cells still expressed HEp-2–reactive antibodies mostly recognizing cytoplasmic structures (FIG. 1). It is unclear whether those cells escape B cell tolerance or are ignored by the organism, but some of these B cells expressed antibodies with low levels of polyreactivity and may produce natural antibodies. Thus, two checkpoints allow the counterselection of autoreactive B cells first in the bone marrow, then in the periphery, thereby ensuring early B cell tolerance in humans.

BCR SIGNALING IS ESSENTIAL TO ESTABLISHING CENTRAL B CELL TOLERANCE

The next challenge in studying B cell tolerance in humans consists of identifying pathways and molecules involved in the regulation of these checkpoints. Two complementary approaches can be used to characterize mechanisms and molecules controlling B cell tolerance. The first approach consists of generating and analyzing engineered mouse models. They revealed that the regulation and induction of tolerance mechanisms involve antigen binding to self-reactive B cell receptors (BCRs), and BCR signaling thresholds are therefore essential to mediate B cell tolerance.[14] Alterations in the expression levels of BCR co-receptors such as CD19 or CD22 and PD-1 and their associated signaling molecules Lyn and SHIP all affect B cell tolerance.[25–28] A second strategy involves the study of patients suffering from primary immunodeficiencies. To investigate the role of BCR signaling in the regulation of B cell tolerance in humans, we analyzed the reactivity of antibodies from X-linked agammaglobulinemia (XLA) B cells. These patients carry mutations in the *BTK* gene that encodes an essential BCR signaling component.[29,30] B cell differentiation in XLA patients is severely affected at the pro-B–to–pre-B cell transition, but a few B cell precursors develop into new emigrant B cells.[31–33] We found that in the absence of Btk, the new emigrant B cells showed a distinct antibody repertoire consistent with extensive secondary light chain gene recombination, suggesting that receptor editing at the pre-B–immature B cell stage requires appropriate BCR signaling to be downregulated.[34] Nevertheless, XLA new emigrant B cells were enriched with autoreactive and polyreactive clones, which demonstrate that Btk is essential in regulating the central B cell tolerance checkpoint in humans.

DEFECTIVE B CELL TOLERANCE CHECKPOINTS IN RA

Autoantibody production is a characteristic of most autoimmune diseases, including RA. The role of these autoantibodies in the pathogenesis of RA remains elusive, but they appear in the serum many years before the onset of clinical disease, suggesting an early break in B cell tolerance.[35] We aimed to determine the stage of B cell development at which B cell tolerance is broken in RA. Two nonexclusive scenarios can be considered: B cell tolerance may be broken during early B cell development and may result in the accumulation of autoreactive B cell clones in the periphery; alternatively, early B cell tolerance checkpoints may be functional and B cells present in a normal repertoire may receive signals from T cells, cytokines, or other factors to develop into clones secreting high-affinity self-reactive antibodies. Focusing on the first scenario, we amplified, cloned, and expressed *in vitro* 176 and 177 antibodies from single new emigrant and mature naive RA B cells, respectively, isolated from six untreated active RA patients.[36] The reactivity of recombinant antibodies was tested by ELISA on HEp-2 lysates and a panel of classic antigens as well as specific RA antigens such as IgG and CCPs.[36] Despite the broad age range (28–64 years) and duration of disease (1–13 years), all six patients showed elevated percentages of polyreactive B cells in both new emigrant (24% versus 7% in control

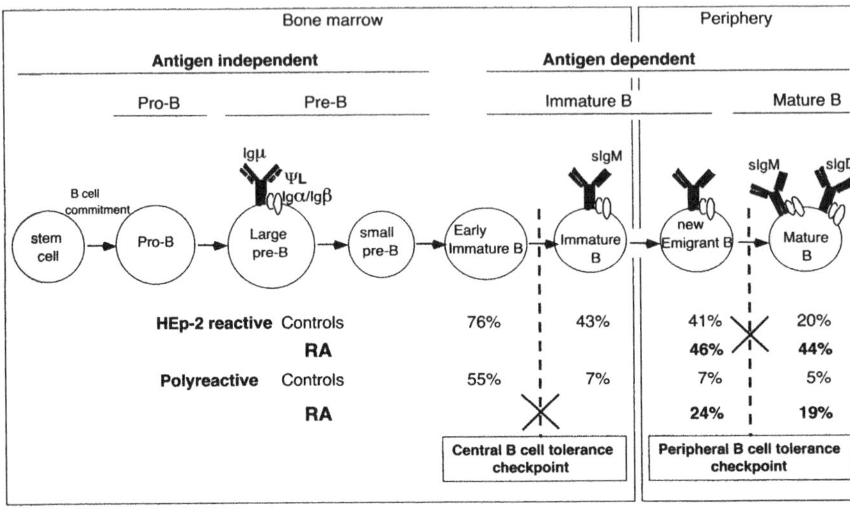

FIGURE 2. Defective central and peripheral B cell tolerance checkpoints in RA. The frequency of B cells expressing HEp-2–reactive and polyreactive antibodies in control subjects and RA patients is indicated. Only peripheral B cell fractions were analyzed in RA patients. The higher percentage of polyreactive B cells in RA versus control new emigrant B cells reveals a defective central B cell tolerance checkpoint in RA, whereas the increased frequency of HEp-2–reactive B cells in RA versus control mature naïve B cells demonstrates a defective peripheral B cell tolerance checkpoint in those patients.

subjects) and mature naïve (19% versus 5% in control subjects) B cell compartments and therefore differ from the six adult control donors[18,36–38] (FIG. 2). Some of those polyreactive B cells expressed antibodies that could recognize RA-specific antigens IgG and CCP with low affinity. Since most polyreactive B cells from healthy donors are removed in the bone marrow, the elevated frequency of polyreactive B cells in RA patients reveals a defective central B cell tolerance checkpoint in these patients. To determine the efficiency of the peripheral B cell tolerance checkpoint in removing autoreactive B cells in RA patients, we analyzed the reactivity of RA recombinant antibodies against HEp-2 cell lysates. The proportion of HEp-2–reactive antibodies in RA new emigrant B cells was not significantly different from that of control new emigrant antibodies previously reported (46% in RA patients versus 41% in healthy control subjects).[18,36,38] In contrast, all six RA patients revealed an increase of HEp-2–reactive mature naïve B cells (44% in RA patients versus 20% in healthy control subjects)[36] (FIG. 2). Thus, the inability to remove autoreactive B cells between new emigrant and mature naïve B cells reveals a defective peripheral B cell tolerance checkpoint in RA patients. In conclusion, RA patients showed defective central and peripheral B cell tolerance checkpoints that result in the accumulation of autoreactive and polyreactive B cells in the periphery.[36]

IMPAIRED TOLERANCE MECHANISMS IN RA

Defects in secondary recombination, the mechanism that allows receptor editing, have been reported in systemic lupus erythematosus (SLE) by several groups.[39–41] Igκ gene editing occurs through secondary recombination in which incoming Vκ genes delete preexisting VκJκ genes by recombining with downstream Jκs.[42] Therefore, light chain editing results in increased usage of upstream Vκs and downstream Jκs. In humans, there are five Jκs, and Jκ1 is the most upstream Jκ gene segment found in about a third of VκJκ rearrangements in new emigrant B cells from healthy donors. In contrast, Jκ gene segment usage in RA patients revealed abnormal secondary recombination regulation in four of nine patients analyzed.[36] Some RA patients showed increased usage of Jκ1 that could be identified in more than 50% of κ chains. Also, upstream Vκ gene usage was decreased in these patients. Abundant VκJκ1 rearrangements combined with a dearth in upstream Vκ genes in new emigrant B cells suggests a premature termination of secondary recombination and therefore impaired receptor editing in these RA patients' B cells.[36] Moreover, RA new emigrant B cells can display the opposite pattern characterized by an increase in downstream Jκ3-4-5 and upstream Vκ gene usage. Here RA B cells suffered extensive secondary recombination that may fail to be downregulated.[36] As with RA, both an increase and decrease in secondary recombination have been reported in other rheumatic diseases such as SLE and suggest that defects in receptor editing can be a common feature shared by different rheumatic diseases.[39–41]

What defective pathways may result in an inability to regulate secondary recombination? One clue came from the analysis of XLA new emigrant B cells that showed extensive secondary recombination events and expressed autoreactive BCRs.[38] In mice, BCR signaling has been shown to control receptor editing by regulating recombination activating genes.[43–45] Defects in BCR signaling may therefore result in a failure either to induce or to downregulate secondary recombination and receptor editing. Little is known about BCR signaling defects in RA B cells, but abnormal BCR signaling has been reported in SLE B cells that also suffer from defective B cell tolerance.[46,47] On line with this hypothesis, a missense polymorphism in the protein tyrosine phosphatase *PTPN22* gene has been recently shown to segregate with RA and SLE patients.[48,49] This missense polymorphism replaces one amino acid in PTPN22 that disrupts its interaction with Csk tyrosine kinase and may therefore affect the BCR signaling threshold.[48]

About half of the analyzed RA patients showed no significant evidence of defective secondary recombination. However, new emigrant B cells from those patients expressed unusually long Igκ chains that contained 11 or more amino acids in their CDR3.[36,50,51] The production of 11-amino-acid-long CDR3 Igκ chains mostly requires the addition of nontemplate nucleotides to V–J junctions by the terminal deoxynucleotidyl transferase (TdT). Since TdT expression is downregulated by pre-BCR expression at the pre–B cell stage, abnormal pre-BCR signaling may fail to downregulate TdT expression and may result in the generation of 11-amino-acid-long CDR3 Igκ chains found in these RA patients.[52,53]

In conclusion, defects in BCR signaling may explain the different unusual Igκ repertoires observed in RA B cells and may therefore be a common feature to all RA patients.

DISCUSSION

RA patients suffer from defective B cell tolerance checkpoints that result in the accumulation of many autoreactive mature naïve B cells in their blood.[36] Some of those autoreactive B cells express polyreactive antibodies and recognize classical RA autoantigens with low affinity. SLE patients suffer from similar defective B cell tolerance checkpoints in that they also show an increase in autoreactive and polyreactive mature naïve B cells in the periphery.[47] Impaired B cell tolerance checkpoints may therefore be a common feature to rheumatic diseases. Breaks in early B cell tolerance probably occur early in the pathogenesis of rheumatic diseases because serum autoantibodies can be detected in RA and SLE patients many years before the clinical onset of those diseases.[35,54]

How could RA and SLE B cells expressing autoreactive/polyreactive antibodies with apparent poor specificity develop into clones that produce high-affinity antibodies to autoantigens specific for each disease? Genetic predispositions may play an important role in mounting immune reactions toward autoantigens specific to each disease. For instance, defects in clearing apoptotic cells favor the persistence of cellular debris and nuclear autoantigens in SLE patients.[55,56] B cells expressing polyreactive antibodies may bind to nucleosomal DNA that can simultaneously trigger BCR and toll-like receptor (TLR) signaling pathways, leading to further B cell maturation and autoantibody production.[57–60] Polyreactive antibodies expressed by naïve SLE B cells may not be pathogenic, but they may become so by acquiring higher affinity through somatic hypermutation and by switching to downstream isotypes once B cells are activated.[61–64] In contrast to SLE, RA patients are not known to suffer from antigen clearance defects and rarely produce antinuclear antibodies. Autoantibodies in RA are rather directed toward IgG and CCP. Polyreactive RA B cells with low rheumatoid factor reactivity may bind IgG–chromatin immune complexes in the joints of RA patients. Dual engagement of BCR and TLRs such as TLR9 may activate such B cells and induce their development into specific anti-IgG–producing B cells.[59,60] Anti-CCP B cells may originate from clones that can present citrullinated peptides bound to RA-associated HLA-DRB1*0401 major histocompatibility class II molecules and activate specific autoreactive T cells.[65] In return, those T cells may further activate CCP-reactive B cells and induce the formation of ectopic germinal centers, causing the production of specific high-affinity anti-CCP autoantibodies.[62,66]

The efficiency of anti–B cell treatments is currently not understood. However, T cell–driven inflammation in the synovial membrane has been shown to be B cell–dependent and cannot be supported by macrophages and dendritic cells.[67] We postulate that the accumulation of autoreactive B cells in the mature compartment of RA patients may favor the development of the disease as a pool of autoantigen-presenting cells that eventually get recruited and activated in the joints of those patients. The nature of the events that allow such recruitment and the antigens recognized *in situ* by RA autoreactive B cells remain to be characterized.

ACKNOWLEDGMENTS

We thank Dr. S. Rudchenko for help with the single-cell sorter and Drs. S. Paget and M. Crow for comments and discussions.

This work was supported by the Arthritis Foundation (New York Chapter) Fellowship Award (to J.S.) and by grants from the Dana Foundation, the Gosden-Robinson Early Arthritis Center, and the Florence Gould Foundation (to E.M.).

[*Competing interests*: The authors declare that they have no competing financial interests.]

REFERENCES

1. FELDMANN, M., F.M. BRENNAN & R.N. MAINI. 1996. Rheumatoid arthritis. Cell **85:** 307–310.
2. LESLIE, D., P. LIPSKY & A.L. NOTKINS. 2001. Autoantibodies as predictors of disease. J. Clin. Invest. **108**: 1417–1422.
3. SMOLEN, J.S. & G. STEINER. 2001. Rheumatoid arthritis is more than cytokines: autoimmunity and rheumatoid arthritis. Arthritis Rheum. **44:** 2218–2220.
4. SEBBAG, M., M. SIMON, C. VINCENT, *et al.* 1995. The anti-perinuclear factor and the so-called anti-keratin antibodies are the same rheumatoid arthritis-specific autoantibodies. J. Clin. Invest. **95:** 2672–2679.
5. SCHELLEKENS, G.A., B.A.W. DE JONG, F.H.J. VAN DEN HOOGEN, *et al.* 1998. Citrulline is an essential constituent of antigenic determinants recognized by rheumatoid arthritis-specific autoantibodies. J. Clin. Invest. **101:** 273–281.
6. ZVAIFLER, N.J. 1973. The immunopathology of joint inflammation in rheumatoid arthritis. Adv. Immunol. **16:** 265–336.
7. POPE, R.M., D.C. TELLER & M. MANNIK. 1975. Intermediate complexes formed by self-association of IgG-rheumatoid factors. Ann. N.Y. Acad. Sci. **256:** 82–87.
8. STUART, J. M., M.A. CREMER, A.S. TOWNES, *et al.* 1982. Type II collagen-induced arthritis in rats. Passive transfer with serum and evidence that IgG anticollagen antibodies can cause arthritis. J. Exp. Med. **155:** 1–16.
9. STUART, J.M. & F.J. DIXON. 1983. Serum transfer of collagen-induced arthritis in mice. J. Exp. Med. **158:** 378–392.
10. KOUSKOFF, V., A.S. KORGANOW, V. DUCHATELLE, *et al.* 1996. Organ-specific disease provoked by systemic autoimmunity. Cell **87:** 811–822.
11. KORGANOW, A.S., H. JI, S. MANGIALAIO, *et al.* 1999. From systemic T cell self-reactivity to organ-specific autoimmune disease via immunoglobulins. Immunity **10:** 451–461.
12. SILVERMAN, G.J. & S. WEISMAN. 2003. Rituximab therapy and autoimmune disorders: prospects for anti-B cell therapy. Arthritis Rheum. **48:** 1484–1492.
13. EDWARDS, J.C.W., L. SZCZEPANSKI, J. SZECHINSKI, *et al.* 2004. Efficacy of B cell-targeted therapy with Rituximab in patients with rheumatoid arthritis. N. Engl. J. Med. **350:** 2572–2581.
14. GOODNOW, C.C. 1996. Balancing immunity and tolerance: deleting and tuning lymphocyte repertoires. Proc. Natl. Acad. Sci. USA **93:** 2264–2271.
15. NEMAZEE, D. 1995. Does immunological tolerance explain the waste in the B-lymphocyte immune system? Experiment and theory. Ann. N.Y. Acad. Sci. **764:** 397–401.
16. RADIC, M.Z. & M. WEIGERT. 1995. Origins of anti-DNA antibodies and their implications for B-cell tolerance. Ann. N.Y. Acad. Sci. **764:** 384–396.
17. HALVERSON, R., R.M. TORRES & R. PELANDA. 2004. Receptor editing is the main mechanism of B cell tolerance toward membrane antigens. Nat. Immunol. **6:** 645–650.
18. WARDEMANN, H., S. YURASOV, A. SCHAEFER, *et al.* 2003. Predominant autoantibody production by early human B cell precursors. Science **301:** 1374–1377.
19. UCKUN, F.M., S. HAISSIG, J.A. LEDBETTER, *et al.* 1992. Developmental hierarchy during early human B-cell ontogeny after autologous bone marrow transplantation using autografts depleted of CD19+ B-cell precursors by an anti-CD19 pan-B-cell immunotoxin containing pokeweed antiviral protein. Blood **79:** 3369–3379.
20. MEFFRE, E., E. DAVIS, C. SCHIFF, *et al.* 2000. Circulating human B cells that express surrogate light chains and edited receptors. Nat. Immunol. **1:** 207–213.

21. BILLIPS, L.G., K. LASSOUED, C. NUNEZ, *et al.* 1995. Human B-cell development. Ann. N.Y. Acad. Sci. **764:** 1–8.
22. KLEIN, U., K. RAJEWSKY & R. KUPPERS. 1998. Human immunoglobulin (Ig)M+IgD+ peripheral blood B cells expressing the CD27 cell surface antigen carry somatically mutated variable region genes: CD27 as a general marker for somatically mutated (memory) B cells. J. Exp. Med. **188:** 1679–1689.
23. TANGYE, S.G., Y.J. LIU, G. AVERSA, *et al.* 1998. Identification of functional human splenic memory B cells by expression of CD148 and CD27. J. Exp. Med. **188:** 1691–1703.
24. SIMS, G.P., R. ETTINGER, Y. SHIROTA, *et al.* 2005. Identification and characterization of circulating human transitional B cells. Blood **105:** 4390–4398.
25. TEDDER, T.F., M. INAOKI & S. SATO. 1997. The CD19-CD21 complex regulates signal transduction thresholds governing humoral immunity and autoimmunity. Immunity. **6:** 107–118.
26. CORNALL, R.J., J.G. CYSTER, M.L. HIBBS, *et al.* 1998. Polygenic autoimmune traits: Lyn, CD22, and SHP-1 are limiting elements of a biochemical pathway regulating BCR signaling and selection. Immunity **8:** 497–508.
27. NISHIMURA, H., M. NOSE, H. HIAI, *et al.* 1999. Development of lupus-like autoimmune diseases by disruption of the PD-1 gene encoding an ITIM motif-carrying immunoreceptor. Immunity **11:** 141–151.
28. OKAZAKI, T., A. MAEDA, H. NISHIMURA, *et al.* 2001. PD-1 immunoreceptor inhibits B cell receptor-mediated signaling by recruiting src homology 2-domain-containing tyrosine phosphatase 2 to phosphotyrosine. Proc. Natl. Acad. Sci. USA **98:** 13866–13871.
29. DE WEERS, M., G.S. BROUNS, S. HINSHELWOOD, *et al.* 1994. B-cell antigen receptor stimulation activates the human Bruton's tyrosine kinase, which is deficient in X-linked agammaglobulinemia. J. Biol. Chem. **269:** 23857–60.
30. KUROSAKI, T. & S. TSUKADA. 2000. BLNK: connecting Syk and Btk to calcium signals. Immunity **12:** 1–5.
31. CONLEY, M.E. 1985. B cells in patients with X-linked agammaglobulinemia. J. Immunol. **134:** 3070–3074.
32. CAMPANA, D., J. FARRANT, N. INAMDAR, *et al.* 1990. Phenotypic features and proliferative activity of B cell progenitors in X-linked agammaglobulinemia. J. Immunol. **145:** 1675–1680.
33. MEFFRE, E., F. LEDEIST, G. DE SAINT-BASILE, *et al.* 1997. A non-XLA primary deficiency causes the earliest known defect of B cell differentiation in humans: a comparison with an XLA case. Immunol. Lett. **57:** 93–99.
34. MEFFRE, E., M. MILILI, C. BLANCO-BETANCOURT, *et al.* 2001. Immunoglobulin heavy chain expression shapes the B cell receptor repertoire in human B cell development. J. Clin. Invest. **108:** 879–886.
35. RANTAPAA-DAHLQVIST, S., B.A.W. DE JONG, E. BERGLIN, *et al.* 2003. Antibodies against cyclic citrullinated peptide and IgA rheumatoid factor predict the development of rheumatoid arthritis. Arthritis Rheum. **48:** 2741–2749.
36. SAMUELS, J., Y.-S. NG, C. COUPILLAUD, *et al.* 2005. Impaired early B cell tolerance in patients with rheumatoid arthritis. J. Exp. Med. **201:** 1659–1667.
37. MEFFRE, E., A. SCHAEFER, H. WARDEMANN, *et al.* 2004. Surrogate Light Chain Expressing Human Peripheral B Cells Produce Self-Reactive Antibodies. J. Exp. Med. **199:** 145–150.
38. NG, Y.-S., H. WARDEMANN, J. CHELNIS, *et al.* 2004. Bruton's tyrosine kinase (Btk) is essential for human B cell tolerance. J. Exp. Med. **200:** 927–934.
39. BENSIMON, C., P. CHASTAGNER & M. ZOUALI. 1994. Human lupus anti-DNA autoantibodies undergo essentially primary V kappa gene rearrangements. EMBO J. **13:** 2951–2962.
40. SUZUKI, N., T. HARADA, S. MIHARA, *et al.* 1996. Characterization of a germline Vk gene encoding cationic anti-DNA antibody and role of receptor editing for development of the autoantibody in patients with systemic lupus erythematosus. J. Clin. Invest. **98:** 1843–1850.
41. DORNER, T., S.J. FOSTER, N.L. FARNER, *et al.* 1998. Immunoglobulin kappa chain receptor editing in systemic lupus erythematosus. J. Clin. Invest. **102:** 688–94.

42. PRAK, E.L. & M. WEIGERT. 1995. Light chain replacement: a new model for antibody gene rearrangement. J. Exp. Med. **182:** 541–548.
43. MELAMED, D. & D. NEMAZEE. 1997. Self-antigen does not accelerate immature B cell apoptosis, but stimulates receptor editing as a consequence of developmental arrest. Proc. Natl. Acad. Sci. USA **94:** 9267–9272.
44. HERTZ, M. & D. NEMAZEE. 1997. BCR ligation induces receptor editing in IgM+IgD- bone marrow B cells in vitro. Immunity **6:** 429–436.
45. TZE, L.E., K.L. HIPPEN & T.W. BEHRENS. 2003. Late immature B cells (IgM(high)IgD(neg)) undergo a light chain receptor editing response to soluble self-antigen. J. Immunol. **171:** 678–682.
46. LIOSSIS, S.N., B. KOVACS, G. DENNIS, *et al.* 1996. B cells from patients with systemic lupus erythematosus display abnormal antigen receptor-mediated early signal transduction events. J. Clin. Invest. **98:** 2549–2557.
47. YURASOV, S., H. WARDEMANN, J. HAMMERSEN, *et al.* 2005. Defective B cell tolerance checkpoints in systemic lupus erythematosus. J. Exp. Med. **201:** 703–711.
48. BEGOVICH, A.B., V.E.H. CARLTON, L.A. HONIGBERG, *et al.* 2004. A missense single-nucleotide polymorphism in a gene encoding a protein tyrosine phosphatase (PTPN22) is associated with rheumatoid arthritis. Am. J. Hum. Genet. **75:** 330–337.
49. KYOGOKU, C., C.D. LANGFELD, W.A. ORTMANN, *et al.* 2004. Genetic association of the R620W polymorphism of protein tyrosine phosphatase PTPN22 with human SLE. Am. J. Hum. Genet. **75:** 504–507.
50. VICTOR, K.D., I. RANDEN, K. THOMPSON, *et al.* 1991. Rheumatoid factors isolated from patients with autoimmune disorders are derived from germline genes distinct from those encoding the Wa, Po, and Bla cross-reactive idiotypes. J. Clin. Invest. **87:** 1603–1613.
51. BRIDGES, S.L., JR., S.K. LEE, M.L. JOHNSON, *et al.* 1995. Somatic mutation and CDR3 lengths of immunoglobulin kappa light chains expressed in patients with rheumatoid arthritis and in normal individuals. J. Clin. Invest. **96:** 831–841.
52. WASSERMAN, R., Y.S. LI & R.R. HARDY. 1997. Down-regulation of terminal deoxynucleotidyl transferase by Ig heavy chain in B lineage cells. J. Immunol. **158:** 1133–1138.
53. GHIA, P., E. TEN BOEKEL, E. SANZ, *et al.* 1996. Ordering of human bone marrow B lymphocyte precursors by single-cell polymerase chain reaction analyses of the rearrangement status of the immunoglobulin H and L chain loci. J. Exp. Med. **184:** 2217–2229.
54. ARBUCKLE, M.R., M.T. MCCLAIN, M.V. RUBERTONE, *et al.* 2003. Development of autoantibodies before the clinical onset of systemic lupus erythematosus. N. Engl. J. Med. **349:** 1526–1533.
55. CARROLL, M. 2001. Innate immunity in the etiopathology of autoimmunity. Nat. Immunol. **2:** 1089–1090.
56. MANDERSON, A.P., M. BOTTO & M.J. WALPORT. 2004. The role of complement in the development of systemic lupus erythematosus. Annu. Rev. Immunol. **22:** 431–456.
57. CASCIOLA-ROSEN, L.A., G. ANHALT & A. ROSEN. 1994. Autoantigens targeted in systemic lupus erythematosus are clustered in two populations of surface structures on apoptotic keratinocytes. J. Exp. Med. **179:** 1317–1330.
58. KIM, S.J., D. GERSHOV, X. MA, *et al.* 2002. I-PLA(2) activation during apoptosis promotes the exposure of membrane lysophosphatidylcholine leading to binding by natural immunoglobulin M antibodies and complement activation. J. Exp. Med. **196:** 655–665.
59. LEADBETTER, E.A., I.R. RIFKIN, A.M. HOHLBAUM, *et al.* 2002. Chromatin-IgG complexes activate B cells by dual engagement of IgM and Toll-like receptors. Nature **416:** 603–607.
60. VIGLIANTI, G.A., C.M. LAU, T.M. HANLEY, *et al.* 2003. Activation of autoreactive B cells by CpG dsDNA. Immunity **19:** 837–847.
61. SHLOMCHIK, M.J., A.H. AUCOIN, D.S. PISETSKY, *et al.* 1987. Structure and function of anti-DNA autoantibodies derived from a single autoimmune mouse. Proc. Natl. Acad. Sci. USA **84:** 9150–9154.
62. SHLOMCHIK, M.J., A. MARSHAK-ROTHSTEIN, C.B. WOLFOWICZ, *et al.* 1987. The role of clonal selection and somatic mutation in autoimmunity. Nature **328:** 805–811.

63. RADIC, M.Z., J. MACKLE, J. ERIKSON, *et al.* 1993. Residues that mediate DNA binding of autoimmune antibodies. J. Immunol. **150:** 4966–4977.
64. LI, H., Y. JIANG, H. CAO, *et al.* 2003. Regulation of anti-phosphatidylserine antibodies. Immunity **18:** 185–192.
65. HILL, J.A., S. SOUTHWOOD, A. SETTE, *et al.* 2003. Cutting edge: The conversion of arginine to citrulline allows for a high-affinity peptide interaction with the rheumatoid arthritis-associated HLA-DBRB1*0401 MHC class II molecule. J. Immunol. **171:** 538–541.
66. WEYAND, C.M. & J.J. GORONZY. 2003. Ectopic germinal center formation in rheumatoid synovitis. Ann. N.Y. Acad. Sci. **987:** 140–149.
67. TAKEMURA, S., P.A. KLIMIUK, A. BRAUN, *et al.* 2001. T cell activation in rheumatoid synovium is B cell dependent. J. Immunol. **167:** 4710–4718.

Autoantigens

The Critical Partner in Initiating and Propagating Systemic Autoimmunity

WEI D. DUAN-PORTER, LIVIA CASCIOLA-ROSEN, AND ANTONY ROSEN

Division of Rhematology, Johns Hopkins University, Baltimore, Maryland 21224, USA

ABSTRACT: The increasing recognition that cancer is frequently associated with an autoantibody response, and observations that systemic autoimmunity is sometimes associated with the diagnosis of a variety of malignancies (many detected near the onset of autoimmune disease), strongly underscore a potential mechanistic connection between cancer immunity and systemic autoimmunity. Accumulating data suggest that autoantigens are critical partners in driving the autoimmune response. Futhermore, unique changes in antigen expression and conformation in the immunizing tumor and the target tissue may play a role in antigen selection and ongoing damage. This construct has important implications for disgnosis, monitoring, and treatment of autoimmunity and, potentially, cancer immunotherapy.

KEYWORDS: autoimmunity; autoantigens; cancer; nucleophosmin; myositis; B23

INTRODUCTION

Systemic autoimmune diseases are complex phenomena in which the immune system recognizes and destroys the body's own tissues. The causes and mechanisms of systemic autoimmune diseases remain unclear. These disorders deserve attention not only because they are often devastating clinically but also because of their immense potential to teach us about the fundamentals of immunologic perception. In this review, we focus on autoantigens in systemic autoimmunity and the powerful insights they can provide into disease initiation and propagation, particularly when studied in the relevant target tissues.

AUTOANTIBODIES

Historically, studies of disease mechanism in systemic autoimmunity have focused on characterization of autoantibodies and identification of their antigenic targets.[1] Although the pathogenic role of autoantibodies remains unclear except in a

Address for correspondence: Antony Rosen, M.D., Director, Division of Rheumatology, Johns Hopkins University, Mason F. Lord Building, Central Tower, Suite 4100, Room 411, Baltimore, MD. Voice: 410-550-1894; fax: 410-550-2072.
arosen@jhmi.edu

**Ann. N.Y. Acad. Sci. 1062: 127–136 (2005). © 2005 New York Academy of Sciences.
doi: 10.1196/annals.1358.015**

few rare cases,[2] this body of work has revealed a profound conundrum in human autoimmunity—while many autoantigens can be widely expressed, autoantibodies recognizing specific molecules correlate strongly with certain clinical patterns of organ-specific damage.[3,4] For example, antibodies to topoisomerase I are found exclusively in patients with the diffuse form of scleroderma, where they are frequently associated with interstitial lung disease.[5–7] Similarly, antibodies recognizing several aminoacyl tRNA synthetases are found in autoimmune myositis, where they are associated with a distinct phenotype called the synthetase syndrome.[8–11] Antibodies to the Sm ribonucleoprotein (part of the mRNA splicing complex) are specific for systemic lupus erythematosus (SLE).[12,13] Interestingly, in some cases, similar targets of autoantibodies are found in a systemic autoimmune disease as well as in cancer. For example, B23/nucleophosmin (B23/NPM) is recognized by antibodies in scleroderma patients with pulmonary hypertension,[14] as well as in patients with hepatocellular[15] or breast[16] cancer. In hepatocellular cancer, autoantibodies seem to appear first around the time of diagnosis.[17] The mechanisms underlying this striking association of specific immune response and phenotype remain unclear.

There are at least three components that interact to produce systemic autoimmune disease: (i) The T-cell and B-cell repertoires capable of immunological specificity and memory, (ii) the physiological context (e.g., infection, Toll-like receptor ligation) integrated by antigen-presenting cells, and (iii) the antigen that initiates and drives the ongoing autoimmune response. Autoantibodies and antigen-specific T cells provide invaluable information about which antigens (or antigenic complexes) are relevant to autoimmune disease. However, they are but enigmatic clues to the complex chronology of autoimmunity.

Most investigations into human autoimmune disease deal with a more mature phase of autoimmunity, when autoimmune processes have generated observable clinical phenotypes. Thus, the specific patterns of autoantibodies and self-reactive T cells seen at these moments result from immunologic integration and filtering of critical events that have already occurred, some of which may have been recent but many of which were probably distant in time.[18] Recent investigations indicate that studying autoantigens in the affected tissue itself will constitute an additional, critically important resource in the analysis of autoimmune initiation and propagation.

Antigen Structure and Conformation Affect Processing and Epitope Selection: Implications for Proteolysis of Autoantigens during Apoptosis

Significant data have demonstrated that antigen-specific T cells are central orchestrators of autoimmunity, making it particularly vital to understand the mechanisms by which T cells become activated and respond to self-antigens. One theory of immunologic perception is especially powerful in explaining how potentially self-reactive T cells may escape central and peripheral tolerance (reviewed in Ref. 19). In the Sercarz construct of immunodominance, T lymphocytes are exposed to a limited number of all the possible peptide fragments that could be derived from protein antigens. Those peptides that can stimulate T cells, having been effectively loaded into the groove of major histocompatibility complex (MHC) molecules during normal pathways of antigen processing, are termed dominant. Those peptides that fail to compete effectively for MHC loading are termed cryptic. The structure of the antigen itself, the presence of interacting proteins, and the nature of processing and presentation pathways all determine which peptides are efficiently presented and therefore seen by T cells. Any given set of circumstances consistently produces a certain small set of such dominant epitopes in the steady state. T cells undergoing negative selection in the thymus or periphery will be deleted only if they recognize dominant epitopes of autoantigens, namely those peptides that are preferentially generated and presented in that particular microenvironment. Therefore, the T-cell repertoire retains reactivity to cryptic autoantigen epitopes that are not usually presented (or presented only at subthreshold levels) *in vivo*. If changes occur in antigen structure and/or the processing and presentation pathways, cryptic epitopes may be revealed in suprathreshold amounts. Under proinflammatory circumstances, an immune response may ensue and spread to other epitopes of the same molecule.[20–22]

The hierarchy of processing and the critical role of certain proteases in the selection of epitopes have been shown experimentally in several model systems. Colin Watts' group demonstrated that an asparaginyl endopeptidase (AEP) activity was required in B cells to process tetanus toxin and reveal the dominant epitopes recognized by reactive T cells.[23,24] The cleavage site for this protease was distant in primary sequence from the T-cell epitopes generated, occurring instead in a hinge region between two domains of the antigen. Thus, an early proteolytic event can determine the accessibility of certain regions to subsequent processing and presentation, thereby influencing the final antigenic image perceived by the immune system. For other antigens, proteases may also cleave and destroy certain epitopes, rendering these sequences cryptic.[25,26]

Additionally, posttranslational modifications of antigens can affect proteolytic processing, epitope selection, and epitope structure itself. Manoury *et al.*[24] found that *N*-glycosylation of the cleavage site asparagine inhibited AEP activity, suggesting that epitopes generated downstream of AEP would be sensitive to this modification. In a mouse model of autoimmunity, Mamula *et al.*[27] showed that a minor posttranslational change in protein structure can break tolerance. The conversion of one aspartate to an isoaspartyl linkage in a 25-amino-acid cytochrome *c* peptide produced a potent immunogen, generating robust T-cell responses in their mouse model. T lymphocytes isolated from mice immunized with the isoaspartyl peptide responded only to this form of the antigen in *ex vivo* proliferation assays and not to the aspartyl form of the peptide. Interestingly, autoantibodies from similarly immunized mice recognized both the aspartyl and the isoaspartyl cytochrome *c* peptides by enzyme-linked immunosorbent assay.

Collectively, the above studies demonstrate that the generation and selection of epitopes for presentation to T cells, although generally operating by predictable rules for a specific antigen–APC pair, may be profoundly affected by even subtle modifications of the antigen itself. As noted previously, there is a paucity of data examining autoantigen structural changes in disease-relevant tissues and the role such alterations may play in autoimmune pathogenesis.

Autoantigen Structure Is Modified during Cell Death

In an initial series of studies examining autoantigen structure in a variety of physiological states, we observed that a striking, near-unifying feature of autoantigens is their susceptibility to undergo proteolytic modification during cell death.[28–31] Of particular relevance in this regard is the cytotoxic T lymphocyte (CTL)–mediated destruction of virally infected or cancerous cells, in which unique autoantigen fragments are generated by granzyme B.[30] Granzyme B, a serine protease found in CTL granules, is essential for initiation of apoptosis in target cells.[32,33] Also, granzyme B displays great specificity in substrate and site selection, with clear primary sequence requirements surrounding the cleavage site of its substrate,[34–36] as well as probable macromolecular preferences.[37] The autoantigen fragments produced by granzyme B were not generated during other forms of cell death and were especially prominent when caspase activity was inhibited during granule-mediated death.[30] There is currently little information available about the function of the CTL granule pathway and its effects on autoantigens in the actual tissues targeted by autoimmune processes during human disease.

To understand autoimmune initiation and propagation, the expression, structure, and cleavage of autoantigens in the most biologically and immunologically relevant microenvironments must be defined. Clinically affected tissues and organs offer appropriate sites in which to examine the forms of autoantigens that propagate autoimmune diseases. In contrast, we know much less about the circumstances of disease initiation, making studies of the status of specific autoantigens in the immunizing tissue difficult. Recent work indicates that a variety of autoimmunity-associated cancers may be appropriate in this regard.

Autoimmunity and Cancer

Previous groups have noted a striking association between various autoimmune disorders (e.g., myositis, scleroderma, SLE, vasculitis) and cancer, with cancer diagnosis and autoimmune detection frequently clustering in time.[38–40] The association of distinct autoantibodies with unique phenotypes in systemic autoimmune disease is reminiscent of a variety of paraneoplastic autoimmune syndromes where autoantibody and T-cell responses target a set of autoantigens expressed only in the inciting tumor and the tissue under immune attack.[41–43] For example, expression of neurooncological ventral antigen (NOVA) proteins is increased in tumor tissue from patients with the clinically distinct paraneoplastic opsoclonus–myoclonus ataxia,[44] and expression of NOVA in healthy adults is restricted to neuronal tissue.[45,46] Similarly, a high-titer autoantibody response to the Hu antigen is observed in patients with paraneoplastic encephalomyelitis and sensory neuropathy, and elevated levels of Hu antigens are present in small-cell lung cancers and various neuronal tissues.[47–49] These studies indicate that cancerous tissues may present an altered and proimmune microenvironment where self-proteins with abnormal expression and/or structure are first registered by the immune system. The autoimmune responses originally directed against tumor antigens then spreads to nontumor tissues with shared antigen profiles, leading to tissue destruction manifesting as a paraneoplastic syndrome.

The above findings have focused our attention on whether analogous connections exist in systemic autoimmune diseases, namely that cancer tissues associated with certain syndromes are the appropriate sites of autoimmune initiation in those disorders. We have therefore examined autoantigen expression and structure in relevant tumor tissues to determine if immunogenic properties may be altered in these biological settings. Furthermore, we have investigated the possible pathogenic role of a cross-reactive antitumor response by studying autoantigen expression in the specific tissues targeted in a particular human disease, as well as in the corresponding tumors.

Hepatocellular Carcinoma Antigen B23/NPM Has a Unique Conformation in Liver Tumor Tissues

The initial model chosen for study was that of hepatocellular carcinoma (HCC), in which patient autoantibodies recognize a variety of nucleolar antigens including B23/NPM. B23/NPM is an abundant and ubiquitously expressed nucleolar protein targeted by autoantibodies in scleroderma[14] and HCC.[15,17] Imai *et al.*[17] found that several patients with chronic hepatitis or cirrhosis showed increases in antinucleolar antibody titers before diagnoses of liver cancer, indicating that the immune response to nucleolar antigens may reflect changes in the structure and function of these molecules.

When B23/NPM expression levels in HCC liver or nontumor liver were analyzed by immunoblotting, liver cancer expressed increased amounts of B23/NPM compared with nontumor liver. Furthermore, HCC B23/NPM ran slightly faster by sodium dodecyl sulfate–polyacrylamide gel electrophoresis (SDS–PAGE) when compared with nontumor liver, both from healthy individuals and from the surrounding cirrhotic tissue of HCC patients. We also examined the susceptibility of B23/NPM to cleavage by granzyme B in these different lysates: whereas B23/NPM in nontumor liver was extremely resistant to proteolysis by granzyme B, the form in HCC samples was efficiently cleaved. This enhanced susceptibility to cleavage, along with the formation of an SDS-stable oligomeric complex not seen in normal and cirrhotic samples, indicated that B23/NPM had an altered conformation distinct from that of normal liver protein.

We defined the granzyme B cleavage sites in B23/NPM and generated an antibody specific for the amino-terminal fragment resulting from proteolysis at aspartate 161. Using this antibody for immunohistochemistry, we found a robust signal in tumor tissue alone, although we could not detect granzyme B fragments by immunoblot analysis of tumor lysates. These data strongly suggested that HCC B23/NPM displays a novel structure, thus exposing a normally hidden granzyme B cleavage site. A mutant protein lacking only the first six amino acids had similar biochemical properties to HCC B23/NPM, as well as an increased susceptibility to granzyme B cleavage. Hence, truncation (or other posttranslational modifications) at the amino terminus may be responsible for the conformational differences seen in tumor samples.

That small changes in the amino terminus of B23/NPM may significantly affect its three-dimensional structure has interesting implications for the role of altered B23/NPM function in liver tumorigenesis. B23/NPM was found to interact with critical tumor suppressors[50–54] $p14^{ARF}$ and p53 and is overexpressed in several cancer tissues and cell lines.[55–57] Several groups have also described phosphorylation of B23/NPM by various cell cycle–regulated kinases, including CDK2/cyclin E,[58] casein kinase II,[59] and Polo-like kinase 1 (Plk1).[60] Of particular note, Plk1, which has critical functions in proper spindle maturation and chromosomal segregation during mitosis,[61] phosphorylates B23/NPM on serine 4.[60] Thus, reversible modification of the amino terminus likely occurs during normal physiological processes, with subsequent changes in B23/NPM activity and structure. A tantalizing model is that a more permanent change in the amino terminus is favored and propagated in cancer tissues because of some growth advantage conferred by altered B23/NPM function, and the resulting conformational changes then reveal key cryptic epitopes for autoimmune initiation.

More studies are required to confirm the proposed changes in HCC B23/NPM and to demonstrate structural consequences. Furthermore, alterations in processing and presentation of the tumor form of B23/NPM need to be investigated. Defining the T-cell response to B23/NPM in HCC will be invaluable in these efforts.

Autoantigens in the Target Tissue in Systemic Autoimmunity: Insights from Autoimmune Inflammatory Myopathies

Although B23/NPM provided an excellent view into autoantigen expression and structure in tumors, there was not a natural extension to an associated autoimmune syndrome that had corresponding autoantibodies to B23/NPM. We therefore proceeded to study autoimmune myositis, since a correlation between autoimmune myositis and cancer has been demonstrated repeatedly.[39,62,63] Interestingly, the most frequent cancers associated with both dermatomyositis (DM) and polymyositis (PM) are adenocarcinomas, being approximately 80% of cancers in patients with cancer and DM and 70% of patients with cancer and PM.[39] Also, the muscle tissue targeted in these diseases is readily available for biochemical and histological analysis of antigen expression.

When we examined skeletal muscle tissues from patients with myositis, we observed several striking features of myositis-specific autoantigen expression: (i) myositis autoantigens were expressed at low levels in control muscle but at high levels in myositis muscle and (ii) increased autoantigen expression correlated with differentiation state, such that myositis autoantigens were particularly abundant in cells demonstrating features of muscle cell regeneration. For example, histidyl tRNA synthetase (HRS) is a myositis autoantigen with 10%–20% of patients showing this autoantibody specificity.[11] Myositis muscle lysates contained at least fourfold the amount of HRS found in normal control samples. We also detected abundant signal for HRS by immunocytochemistry in diseased muscle sections, whereas few cells showed positive staining in normal tissues. Analysis of serial sections for markers of muscle regeneration, such as neural cell adhesion molecule (NCAM) or neonatal myosin heavy chain, revealed that regions expressing HRS contained differentiating muscle cells. Furthermore, HRS and several other myositis autoantigens were plentifully expressed early on during *ex vivo* differentiation of cultured myoblasts but decreased substantially in myotubes. Finally, we found increased autoantigen expression in several cancers associated with autoimmune myositis, but not in the related normal tissues, demonstrating that tumor cells and undifferentiated myoblasts are antigenically similar.

These data strongly implicate regenerating muscle cells rather than mature myotubes as (i) targets of cytolytic attack in autoimmune myositis and (ii) the source of ongoing antigen supply in this disease. Taking into consideration the additional resemblance of differentiating myoblasts to cancer cells in autoantigen profile, we proposed that cancerous tissue is the relevant microenvironment for disease initiation in autoimmune myositis. A variety of inducers of change (e.g., trauma, exercise, infection) could stimulate muscle cells to regenerate and express suprathreshold levels of autoantigens recognized by the antitumor response. This would then enable a feed-forward loop with further cycles of damage and regeneration in muscle tissues. Our model provides a plausible explanation for the self-sustaining nature of the autoimmune response and the exacerbations that are general features of autoimmune diseases.

CONCLUSION

Human autoimmune rheumatic diseases are highly complex processes, exhibiting marked genetic, environmental, and kinetic diversity. Despite this, there is a striking correlation between the targets of the immune response in each disease and the clinical phenotype manifested, indicating that the specificity of the autoimmune response marks a centrally important pathogenic principle. The increasing recognition that cancer is frequently associated with an autoantibody response, and observations that systemic autoimmunity is sometimes associated with the diagnosis of a variety of malignancies (many detected near the onset of autoimmune disease), strongly underscore a potential mechanistic connection between cancer immunity and systemic autoimmunity. Accumulating data suggest that autoantigens are critical partners in driving the autoimmune response. Furthermore, unique changes in antigen expression and conformation in the immunizing tumor and the target tissue may play a role in antigen selection and ongoing damage. This construct has important implications for diagnosis, monitoring, and treatment of autoimmunity and, potentially, cancer immunotherapy.

[*Competing interests*: The authors declare that they have no competing financial interests.]

REFERENCES

1. TAN, E.M. 1991. Autoantibodies in pathology and cell biology. Cell **67:** 841–842.
2. NAPARSTEK, Y. & P.H. PLOTZ. 1993. The role of autoantibodies in autoimmune disease. Annu. Rev. Immunol. **11:** 79–104.
3. VON MUHLEN, C.A. & E.M. TAN. 1995. Autoantibodies in the diagnosis of systemic rheumatic diseases. Semin. Arthritis Rheum. **24:** 323–358.
4. PLOTZ, P.H. 2003. The autoantibody repertoire: searching for order. Nat. Rev. Immunol. **3:** 73–78.
5. WEINER, E.S., W.C. EARNSHAW, J.L. SENECAL, *et al.* 1988. Clinical associations of anticentromere antibodies and antibodies to topoisomerase I. A study of 355 patients. Arthritis Rheum. **31:** 378–385.
6. ROTHFIELD, N.F. 1992. Autoantibodies in scleroderma. Rheum. Dis. Clin. North Am. **18:** 483–498.
7. GREIDINGER, E.L., K.T. FLAHERTY, B. WHITE, *et al.* 1998. African-American race and antibodies to topoisomerase I are associated with increased severity of scleroderma lung disease. Chest **114:** 801–807.
8. ARNETT, F.C., T.J. HIRSCH, W.B. BIAS, *et al.* 1981. The Jo-1 antibody system in myositis: relationships to clinical features and HLA. J. Rheumatol. **8:** 925–930.
9. LOVE, L.A., R.L. LEFF, D.D. FRASER, *et al.* 1991. A new approach to the classification of idiopathic inflammatory myopathy: myositis-specific autoantibodies define useful homogeneous patient groups. Medicine (Baltimore). **70:** 360–374.
10. TARGOFF, I.N. 1992. Autoantibodies in polymyositis. Rheum. Dis. Clin. North Am. **18:** 455–482.

11. Levine, S.M., A. Rosen & L.A. Casciola-Rosen. 2003. Anti-aminoacyl tRNA synthetase immune responses: insights into the pathogenesis of the idiopathic inflammatory myopathies. Curr. Opin. Rheumatol. **15:** 708–713.
12. Koffler, D., R. Carr, V. Agnello, *et al.* 1971. Antibodies to polynucleotides in human sera: antigenic specificity and relation to disease. J. Exp. Med. **134:** 294–312.
13. Hughes, G.R. 1973. The diagnosis of systemic lupus erythematosus. Br. J. Haematol. **25:** 409–413.
14. Ulanet, D.B., F.M. Wigley, A.C. Gelber & A. Rosen. 2003. Autoantibodies against B23, a nucleolar phosphoprotein, occur in scleroderma and are associated with pulmonary hypertension. Arthritis Rheum. **49:** 85–92.
15. Imai, H., K. Kiyosawa, E.K. Chan & E.M. Tan. 1993. Autoantibodies in viral hepatitis-related hepatocellular carcinoma. Intervirology **35:** 73–85.
16. Brankin, B., T.C. Skaar, M. Brotzman, *et al.* 1998. Autoantibodies to the nuclear phosphoprotein nucleophosmin in breast cancer patients. Cancer Epidemiol. Biomarkers Prev. **7:** 1109–1115.
17. Imai, H., Y. Nakano, K. Kiyosawa & E.M. Tan. 1993. Increasing titers and changing specificities of antinuclear antibodies in patients with chronic liver disease who develop hepatocellular carcinoma. Cancer **71:** 26–35.
18. Arbuckle, M.R., M.T. McClain, M.V. Rubertone, *et al.* 2003. Development of autoantibodies before the clinical onset of systemic lupus erythematosus. N. Engl. J. Med. **349:** 1526–1533.
19. Sercarz, E.E., P.V. Lehmann, A. Ametani, *et al.* 1993. Dominance and crypticity of T cell antigenic determinants. Annu. Rev. Immunol. **11:** 729–766.
20. Bockenstedt, L.K., R.J. Gee & M.J. Mamula. 1995. Self-peptides in the initiation of lupus autoimmunity. J. Immunol. **154:** 3516–3524.
21. Lehmann, P.V., T. Forsthuber, A. Miller & E.E. Sercarz. 1992. Spreading of T-cell autoimmunity to cryptic determinants of an autoantigen. Nature **358:** 155–157.
22. Lanzavecchia, A. 1995. How can cryptic epitopes trigger autoimmunity? J. Exp. Med. **181:** 1945–1948.
23. Antoniou, A.N., S.L. Blackwood, D. Mazzeo & C. Watts. 2000. Control of antigen presentation by a single protease cleavage site. Immunity **12:** 391–398.
24. Manoury, B., E.W. Hewitt, N. Morrice, *et al.* 1998. An asparaginyl endopeptidase processes a microbial antigen for class II MHC presentation. Nature **396:** 695–699.
25. Manoury, B., D. Mazzeo, L. Fugger, *et al.* 2002. Destructive processing by asparagine endopeptidase limits presentation of a dominant T cell epitope in MBP. Nat. unol. **3:** 169–174.
26. Burster, T., A. Beck, E. Tolosa, *et al.* 2004. Cathepsin G, and not the asparagine-specific endoprotease, controls the processing of myelin basic protein in lysosomes from human B lymphocytes. J. Immunol. **172:** 5495–5503.
27. Mamula, M.J., R.J. Gee, J.I. Elliott, *et al.* 1999. Isoaspartyl post-translational modification triggers autoimmune responses to self-proteins. J. Biol. Chem. **274:** 22321–22327.
28. Casciola-Rosen, L., G.J. Anhalt & A. Rosen. 1995. DNA-dependent protein kinase is one of a subset of autoantigens specifically cleaved early during apoptosis. J. Exp. Med. **182:** 1625–1634.
29. Casciola-Rosen, L., D.K. Miller, G.J. Anhalt & A. Rosen. 1994. Specific cleavage of the 70kDa protein component of the U1 snRNP is a characteristic biochemical feature of apoptotic cell death. J. Biol. Chem. **269:** 30757–30760.
30. Casciola-Rosen, L., F. Andrade, D. Ulanet, *et al.* 1999. Cleavage by granzyme B is strongly predictive of autoantigen status: implications for initiation of autoimmunity. J. Exp. Med. **190:** 815–825.
31. Hall, J.C., L. Casciola-Rosen & A. Rosen. 2004. Altered structure of autoantigens during apoptosis. Rheum. Dis. Clin. North Am. **30:** 455–71, vii.
32. Heusel, J.W., R.L. Wesselschmidt, S. Shresta, *et al.* 1994. Cytotoxic lymphocytes require granzyme B for the rapid induction of DNA fragmentation and apoptosis in allogeneic target cells. Cell **76:** 977–987.
33. Shresta, S., D.M. MacIvor, J.W. Heusel, *et al.* 1995. Natural killer and lymphokine-activated killer cells require granzyme B for the rapid induction of apoptosis in susceptible target cells. Proc. Natl. Acad. Sci. USA **92:** 5679–5683.

34. HARRIS, J.L., E.P. PETERSON, D. HUDIG, *et al.* 1998. Definition and redesign of the extended substrate specificity of granzyme B. J. Biol. Chem. **273:** 27364–27373.
35. WAUGH, S.M., J.L. HARRIS, R. FLETTERICK & C.S. CRAIK. 2000. The structure of the pro-apoptotic protease granzyme B reveals the molecular determinants of its specificity. Nat. Struct. Biol. **7:** 762–765.
36. ESTEBANEZ-PERPINA, E., P. FUENTES-PRIOR, D. BELORGEY, *et al.* 2000. Crystal structure of the caspase activator human granzyme B, a proteinase highly specific for an Asp-P1 residue. Biol. Chem. **381:** 1203–1214.
37. ANDRADE, F., L.A. CASCIOLA-ROSEN & A. ROSEN. 2003. A novel domain in adenovirus L4-100K is required for stable binding and efficient inhibition of human granzyme B: possible interaction with a species-specific exosite. Mol. Cell. Biol. **23:** 6315–6326.
38. SILMAN, A.J. 1997. Scleroderma—demographics and survival. J. Rheumatol. **24:** 58–61.
39. HILL, C.L., Y. ZHANG, B. SIGURGEIRSSON, *et al.* 2001. Frequency of specific cancer types in dermatomyositis and polymyositis: a population-based study. Lancet **357:** 96–100.
40. BERNATSKY, S., J.F. BOIVIN, L. JOSEPH, *et al.* 2005. An international cohort study of cancer in systemic lupus erythematosus. Arthritis Rheum. **52:** 1481–1490.
41. ALBERT, M.L. & R.B. DARNELL. 2004. Paraneoplastic neurological degenerations: keys to tumour immunity. Nat. Rev. Cancer **4:** 36–44.
42. DARNELL, R.B. 2004. Paraneoplastic neurologic disorders: windows into neuronal function and tumor immunity. Arch. Neurol. **61:** 30–32.
43. ROBERTS, W.K. & R.B. DARNELL. 2004. Neuroimmunology of the paraneoplastic neurological degenerations. Curr. Opin. Immunol. **16:** 616–622.
44. LUQUE, F.A., H.M. FURNEAUX, R. FERZIGER, *et al.* 1991. Anti-Ri: an antibody associated with paraneoplastic opsoclonus and breast cancer. Ann. Neurol. **29:** 241–251.
45. GRAUS, F., G. ROWE, J. FUEYO, *et al.* 1993. The neuronal nuclear antigen recognized by the human anti-Ri autoantibody is expressed in central but not peripheral nervous system neurons. Neurosci. Lett. **150:** 212–214.
46. BUCKANOVICH, R.J., Y.Y. YANG & R.B. DARNELL. 1996. The onconeural antigen Nova-1 is a neuron-specific RNA-binding protein, the activity of which is inhibited by paraneoplastic antibodies. J. Neurosci. **16:** 1114–1122.
47. DALMAU, J., H.M. FURNEAUX, M.K. ROSENBLUM, *et al.* 1991. Detection of the anti-Hu antibody in specific regions of the nervous system and tumor from patients with paraneoplastic encephalomyelitis/sensory neuronopathy. Neurology **41:** 1757–1764.
48. MANLEY, G.T., P.S. SMITT, J. DALMAU & J.B. POSNER. 1995. Hu antigens: reactivity with Hu antibodies, tumor expression, and major immunogenic sites. Ann. Neurol. **38:** 102–110.
49. GRAUS, F., J. DALMOU, R. RENE, *et al.* 1997. Anti-Hu antibodies in patients with small-cell lung cancer: association with complete response to therapy and improved survival. J. Clin. Oncol. **15:** 2866–2872.
50. ITAHANA, K., K.P. BHAT, A. JIN, *et al.* 2003. Tumor suppressor ARF degrades B23, a nucleolar protein involved in ribosome biogenesis and cell proliferation. Mol. Cell **12:** 1151–1164.
51. BERTWISTLE, D., M. SUGIMOTO & C.J. SHERR. 2004. Physical and functional interactions of the Arf tumor suppressor protein with nucleophosmin/B23. Mol. Cell. Biol. **24:** 985–996.
52. KUO, M.L., W. DEN BESTEN, D. BERTWISTLE, *et al.* 2004. N-terminal polyubiquitination and degradation of the Arf tumor suppressor. Genes Dev. **18:** 1862–1874.
53. COLOMBO, E., J.C. MARINE, D. DANOVI, *et al.* 2002. Nucleophosmin regulates the stability and transcriptional activity of p53. Nat. Cell Biol. **4:** 529–533.
54. KURKI, S., K. PELTONEN, L. LATONEN, *et al.* 2004. Nucleolar protein NPM interacts with HDM2 and protects tumor suppressor protein p53 from HDM2-mediated degradation. Cancer Cell **5:** 465–475.
55. CHAN, W.Y., Q.R. LIU, J. BORJIGIN, *et al.* 1989. Characterization of the cDNA encoding human nucleophosmin and studies of its role in normal and abnormal growth. Biochemistry **28:** 1033–1039.

56. WANG, D., H. UMEKAWA & M.O. OLSON. 1993. Expression and subcellular locations of two forms of nucleolar protein B23 in rat tissues and cells. Cell. Mol. Biol. Res. **39:** 33–42.
57. SKAAR, T.C., S.C. PRASAD, S. SHARAREH, *et al.* 1998. Two-dimensional gel electrophoresis analyses identify nucleophosmin as an estrogen regulated protein associated with acquired estrogen–independence in human breast cancer cells. J. Steroid Biochem. Mol. Biol. **67:** 391–402.
58. OKUDA, M., H.F. HORN, P. TARAPORE, *et al.* 2000. Nucleophosmin/B23 is a target of CDK2/cyclin E in centrosome duplication. Cell **103:** 127–140.
59. JIANG, P.S., J.H. CHANG & B.Y. YUNG. 2000. Different kinases phosphorylate nucleophosmin/B23 at different sites during G(2) and M phases of the cell cycle. Cancer Lett. **153:** 151–160.
60. ZHANG, H., X. SHI, H. PADDON, *et al.* 2004. B23/nucleophosmin serine 4 phosphorylation mediates mitotic functions of polo-like kinase 1. J. Biol. Chem. **279:** 35726–35734.
61. GLOVER, D.M., I.M. HAGAN & A.A. TAVARES. 1998. Polo-like kinases: a team that plays throughout mitosis. Genes Dev. **12:** 3777–3787.
62. SIGURGEIRSSON, B., B. LINDELOF, O. EDHAG & E. ALLANDER. 1992. Risk of cancer in patients with dermatomyositis or polymyositis. N. Engl. J. Med. **326:** 363–367.
63. BUCHBINDER, R., A. FORBES, S. HALL, *et al.* 2001. Incidence of malignant disease in biopsy-proven inflammatory myopathy. A population-based cohort study. Ann. Intern. Med. **134:** 1087–1095.

Evaluation of Topoisomerase-1–Specific CD8$^+$ T-Cell Response in Systemic Sclerosis

FRANCESCO BOIN,[a] FREDRICK M. WIGLEY,[a] JONATHAN P. SCHNECK,[b] MATHIAS OELKE,[b] AND ANTONY ROSEN[a]

[a]*Division of Rheumatology, Department of Medicine, Johns Hopkins School of Medicine, Baltimore, Maryland 21224, USA*

[b]*Department of Pathology, Johns Hopkins School of Medicine, Baltimore, Maryland 21224, USA*

ABSTRACT: Measurement of disease activity in systemic autoimmune disorders is often unreliable, and immunosuppressive therapy is often titrated to crude clinical response and/or onset of complications. Systemic sclerosis (SSc) presents a distinct clinical phenotype associated with specific autoantibodies. Anti–topoisomerase-1 (SCL-70) is selectively detected in 30–60% of subjects with diffuse skin and interstitial lung involvement. Such patients offer an ideal clinical model to characterize and quantify the autoantigen-specific T-cell response and its correlation with disease phenotype and activity. Human leukocyte antigen A2 (HLA-A2)–restricted topo-1 peptides were selected based on an epitope prediction algorithm. For initial studies, the best binder topo-1$_{262–270}$ KMLDHEYTT (#262) was used alone or loaded onto an artificial antigen-presenting platform generated by coupling a dimeric major histocompatibility complex–immunoglobulin G fusion protein (HLA-A2–Ig) and anti-CD28 antibodies onto magnetic beads (artificial antigen-presenting cells). Blood samples (100 µL) from HLA-A2$^+$ SSc patients and cytomegalovirus (CMV) seropositive healthy control subjects were tested in an intracellular cytokine staining assay. Gamma interferon production by CD8$^+$ T cells was measured after stimulation with peptide #262, CMVpp65, or MART-1 (irrelevant peptide). In two of five SCL-70$^+$ patients, peptide #262–loaded aAPCs induced a specific CD8$^+$ T-cell response (0.45% ± 0.23% of total CD8$^+$ cells). This response was not observed in the seven SCL-70$^-$ (five SSc and two CMV$^+$) control subjects studied (0.03% ± 0.02%). Interestingly, bronchoalveolar lavage fluid obtained from one topo-1–responsive SSc patient who had worsening respiratory function and active alveolitis showed striking enrichment of topo-1–specific CD8$^+$ T cells (3.94%). This small-volume *ex vivo* assay may prove to be a sensitive and specific tool to assess disease activity and to monitor response to therapy in patients with scleroderma.

KEYWORDS: systemic sclerosis; topoisomerase-1; autoantigen; CD8$^+$ T cells

Address for correspondence: Francesco Boin, M.D., Division of Rheumatology, The Johns Hopkins University School of Medicine, 5200 Eastern Ave., Mason F. Lord Bldg., Center Tower, Ste. 4100, Baltimore, MD 21224. Voice: 410-550-7715; fax: 410-550-2072.
fboin1@jhmi.edu

**Ann. N.Y. Acad. Sci. 1062: 137–145 (2005). © 2005 New York Academy of Sciences.
doi: 10.1196/annals.1358.016**

INTRODUCTION

Scleroderma, or systemic sclerosis (SSc), is a connective tissue disorder characterized by proliferative and occlusive vasculopathy of small blood vessels, associated with excessive extracellular matrix deposition and fibrosis in a variety of target tissues. Although the skin represents a prominent target, many internal organs can be affected as well (e.g., lung, heart, gastrointestinal tract, and kidneys).[1] Autoimmunity against a limited set of ubiquitously expressed autoantigens is an early feature of the disease and appears to represent an antigen-driven, T-cell–dependent process.[2] The mechanisms responsible for initiation of autoimmunity in scleroderma, and the role of immune effector pathways in generating the characteristic phenotype, remain uncertain.

One of the striking features of the disease is the remarkable association between clinical phenotype and specific autoantibodies.[3] For example, anti–topoisomerase-1 (topo-1 or SCL-70) is selectively detected in 30–60% of subjects with diffuse skin and interstitial lung involvement, where autoantibody titers have been shown to correlate broadly with disease activity.[4] Similarly, autoantibodies against nucleolar autoantigens B23 and fibrillarin are associated with isolated pulmonary hypertension, whereas autoantibodies against centromere proteins are associated with limited skin disease and ischemic digital loss.[3] Whether autoantigen-specific T cells are amplified in individuals with active disease and participate in generating these distinct phenotypes is unknown. This question has been difficult to investigate due to the inaccessibility of target tissues for study. Furthermore, *ex vivo* detection and quantification of autoantigen-specific T cells constitutes a significant technical challenge due to low circulating precursor frequency (usually $\ll 1\%$), particularly in patients receiving immunosuppressive therapy.[5,6]

The lung in scleroderma provides an excellent opportunity to study these questions, as alveolar contents are routinely sampled during clinical care, and pulmonary manifestations as well as functional impairment can easily be quantified. The degree of involvement and progression throughout the disease is readily and precisely definable by structural high-resolution computed tomography (CT) and studies with the functional forced vital capacity (FVC) carbon monoxide–diffusing capacity (DLCO) 6-minutes walking test. Furthermore, local disease activity and immune system activation can be explored by bronchoscopy and bronchoalveolar lavage (BAL) studies. Evidence for active lung inflammation is determined in SSc patients when BAL differential cell count shows increased percentages of neutrophils and/or eosinophils (>3% or >2% of total cells, respectively).[7]

This study focused on establishing the necessary methods and infrastructure to begin to detect and quantify topoisomerase-1–specific $CD8^+$ T cells in well-characterized patients with scleroderma and to gather preliminary data on any correlation with clinical phenotype and/or disease activity. Autoreactive T cells are identified directly *ex vivo* using small volumes of peripheral blood or BAL and without prior *in vitro* amplification.

METHODS

Case Patients and Control Subjects

Samples were collected from selected SSc patients evaluated at the Johns Hopkins University Scleroderma Center. All of them met American College of Rheumatology classification criteria for diffuse scleroderma.[8] Anti–topoisomerase-1 antibody status was routinely determined as part of their assessment through the Central Laboratory of Johns Hopkins Hospital. Two healthy cytomegalovirus (CMV)-seropositive volunteers were also recruited through public posting. All donors gave written informed consent before enrolling in the study, as required by the institutional review board. Healthy volunteers and SSc patients were confirmed to be human leukocyte antigen (HLA)–A2.1$^+$ by flow cytometry.

Bronchoalveolar Lavage

The SSc patients presenting with a clinical history (worsening respiratory symptoms) and recent investigations (declining FVC and DLCO, new detection of ground-glass opacities on high-resolution chest CT) suspicious of active lung disease were referred for bronchoscopy and BAL to guide the decision whether to start immunosuppressive treatment. The procedure was performed as described elsewhere.[9] BAL cell differential counts were performed on cytocentrifuged slides stained with modified Giemsa. Lung inflammation (alveolitis) was defined by neutrophils more than 3% and/or eosinophils more than 2% (three standard deviations above the mean of controls in the testing laboratory) of total cells. BAL fluid and cells remaining after diagnostic studies were then used for the antigen-specific stimulation assay described in the following subsections.

Antigenic Peptides

We adopted a candidate peptide approach. Using an Internet-based epitope prediction algorithm, we identified multiple topo-1 HLA-A2–restricted nonamers.[10] For our preliminary experiments, we selected and synthesized the best binder topoisomerase-$1_{262–270}$ KMLDHEYTT (#262) at the Johns Hopkins University Peptide core facility. We used CMV-$pp65_{495–503}$ NLVPMVATV peptide (CMVpp65) for stimulation on blood from CMV$^+$ donors (setup experiments) and as a positive control on study patients. We used MART-1 as negative control (irrelevant peptide). We confirmed peptide binding to HLA-A2 by means of a T2 cell stabilization assay, as previously described.[11]

Antigen-Presenting Platform

We generated artificial antigen-presenting cells (aAPCs) by coupling HLA-IgG– and CD28-specific antibodies onto microbeads (Dynal, Lake Success, NY), as previously described.[11,12] In brief, beads were washed twice in sterile 0.1 *M* borate buffer. Then they were incubated with a 1:1 mixture of HLA-A2–Ig and the CD-28–specific monoclonal antibody 9.3 in borate buffer for 24 h at 4°C on a rotator, washed twice with bead-wash buffer, incubated again for 24 h at 4°C in bead-wash buffer, and placed in fresh buffer. For peptide loading, HLA-Ig–coated aAPCs were washed twice with phosphate-buffered saline and adjusted to 10^7 beads/mL in final peptide concentration of 30 μg/mL.

Tetramer Staining

After separation from heparinized whole blood by Ficoll–Paque PLUS density gradient centrifugation (Amersham Pharmacia, Uppsala, Sweden), peripheral blood mononuclear cells (PBMCs) were washed twice in phosphate-buffered saline. Staining was then performed at 4°C for 25 minutes with fluorescein isothiocyanate–conjugated CD8-specific monoclonal antibody (Sigma-Aldrich, St. Louis, MO) and phycoerythrin-conjugated HLA A*02 CMV-pp65 tetramers (NLVPMVATV) (Beckman Coulter Immunomics, San Diego, CA).[14] Major histocompatibility complex tetramers (phycoerythrin conjugated) loaded with irrelevant peptide MART-1 (Beckman Coulter Immunomics) were used for control staining. Gating was set on lymphocytes for acquisition by flow cytometry (FACSCalibur; BD BioSciences, San Jose, CA), and analysis was performed using CellQuest software (BD BioSciences).

Intracellular Cytokine Staining

Intracellular cytokine staining (ICS) for gamma interferon (IFN-γ) was performed as described in the manufacturer's protocol (BD Pharmingen). The only modification was that 100 μL of heparinized whole blood was stimulated for 6 h at 37°C and 5% CO_2 with 2×10^5 peptide-loaded aAPCs or 20 μg/mL of peptide alone. Data were acquired by flow cytometry (FACScalibur; BD BioSciences) and analyzed using CellQuest software (BD BioSciences).

RESULTS

Defining the number and phenotype of autoantigen-specific lymphocytes in systemic autoimmune disorders has the potential to provide important insights into the pathogenesis of these diseases, and particularly to provide a method for monitoring the specific response to therapy. The low precursor frequency in peripheral blood and the inability to easily access lymphoid or relevant target tissues make detecting and characterizing these relatively rare T cells difficult. Studies using actual samples from the lung and blood of patients with SSc provide an outstanding opportunity with which to optimize such assays.

MHC Tetramer Staining and ICS Assay Detect Similar Levels of Antigen-Specific T Cell Reactive to CMVpp65

To establish an intracellular cytokine assay on small blood volumes and define its sensitivity, CMV-$pp65_{495-503}$–specific $CD8^+$ T-cell responses in healthy CMV-seropositive donors were evaluated and compared by using a tetramer assay. Different volumes of blood (50–200 μL) were tested. One hundred microliters was found to be equivalent to larger volumes for detection of CMV $CD8^+$ T-cell responses and was therefore used in later experiments. In one individual (FIG. 1), CMVpp65–HLA-A2 tetramer staining estimated a precursor frequency of 7.3% of total $CD8^+$ T cells. In this subject, the ICS assay detected approximately 68% of the CMV-specific

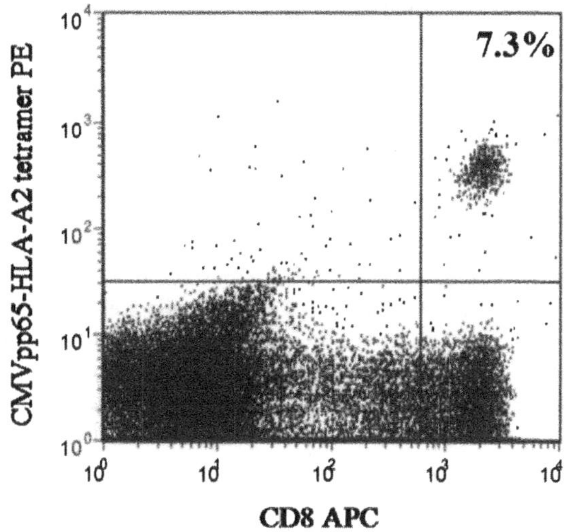

FIGURE 1. CMV-pp65$_{495-503}$–HLA-A2 tetramer staining of PBMCs from a CMV-seropositive donor. Gating was set on live lymphocytes and the estimated precursor frequency was 7.3% of total CD8⁺ T cells.

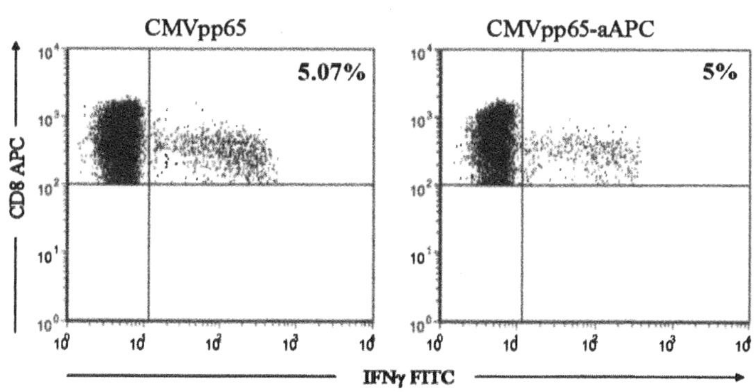

FIGURE 2. CMVpp65-loaded aAPCs and peptide alone were equally effective in inducing a CMVpp65-specific $CD8^+$ T-cell (INF-γ) response expressed as percentage of total $CD8^+$ T cells. Data are representative of $n = 6$ experiments with 100 μL of whole blood. Gating was set on live lymphocytes and $CD8^+$ cells.

CD8+ T cells detected by tetramer staining. CMVpp65 peptide and peptide-loaded aAPCs induced IFN-γ responses of 4.63% ± 0.4% and 4.85% ± 0.22%, respectively (FIG. 2).

Detection of Topoisomerase-1–Specific CD8+ T-Cell Responses in Peripheral Blood and BAL of SSc Patients

The ICS assay measuring IFN-γ production optimized as described earlier was applied to patients with diffuse SSc. Although peptide alone did not induce IFN-γ production, peptide #262–loaded aAPCs were successful in inducing antigen-specific responses (FIG. 3). Topo-1 (#262)–specific CD8+ T cells were detected in two of five topo-1–positive subjects (0.45% ± 0.23% of total CD8+ T cells), but in none of the seven topo-1–negative subjects tested (0.03% ± 0.02%). Interestingly, we could simultaneously obtain and analyze the BAL fluid from one patient who showed a positive topo-1 CD8+ T-cell response in the peripheral blood. This subject was referred

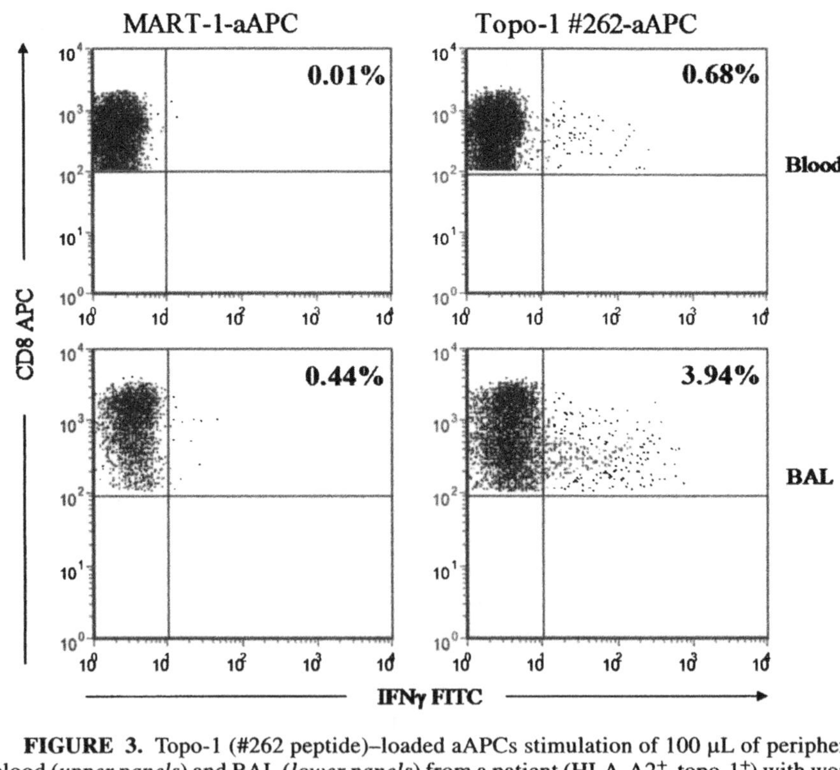

FIGURE 3. Topo-1 (#262 peptide)–loaded aAPCs stimulation of 100 μL of peripheral blood (*upper panels*) and BAL (*lower panels*) from a patient (HLA-A2+, topo-1+) with worsening respiratory symptoms, new onset of ground-glass infiltrates on high-resolution CT, and declining FVC and DLCO. INF-γ topo-1–specific response is shown as percentage of total CD8+ T cells. Gating was set on live lymphocytes and CD8+ cells. MART-1 is used as negative control (irrelevant peptide).

to bronchoscopy and BAL fluid study based on the clinical suspicion for active pulmonary involvement (worsening respiratory symptoms, declining FVC and DLCO, new onset of ground-glass infiltrates on high-resolution CT). Upon separation, BAL mononuclear cells were stimulated with #262 topo-1 peptide followed by ICS. Compared with the peripheral blood, #262-specific $CD8^+$ T-cell response was significantly enriched (3.94%) (FIG. 3). BAL cell-count analysis in the same sample revealed the presence of cells consistent with very active alveolitis (neutrophils, 13.2% and eosinophils, 4.5% of total cells).

The possibility that an antigen-specific assay offers a more accurate and dependable tool for identification and monitoring of patients with active lung disease is appealing. In fact, in scleroderma lung disease, the distinction between disease-related interstitial lung inflammation and other pulmonary or extrapulmonary processes that cause clinical and laboratory manifestations is often unclear. Such distinction is important so that prompt immunosuppressive therapy is instituted only when appropriate. However, the standard BAL criteria for alveolitis are based on surrogate markers like alveolar neutrophilia and/or eosinophilia, which are not considered to be responsible for the initial immune-mediated lung insult.[15] Furthermore, different clinical studies have shown that some patients develop progressive lung disease despite negative BAL eosinophilia and neutrophilia, whereas others maintain a stable clinical course and testing parameters despite the presence of alveolitis on BAL.

DISCUSSION

Detection, quantification, and characterization of autoantigen-specific T cells represent important steps to refine the approach to diagnosis, monitoring, and treatment of systemic autoimmune diseases. The development of a highly sensitive and specific assay able to detect the low frequency of circulating autoreactive T cells in patients with autoimmune disorders is a major priority.

Topoisomerase-1 and scleroderma lung involvement are selectively associated and represent a prototypical model of autoantigen–disease phenotype correlation. Taken together with the fact that the lungs are extremely accessible to functional, structural, and immunological studies, clinical samples from patients with scleroderma lung disease offer an excellent opportunity to investigate autoantigen-specific immune responses and their relationship with disease activity, clinical phenotype, and outcome.

In this study, a small-volume, *ex vivo* assay for antigen-specific $CD8^+$ T-cell detection was developed using 100 μL of whole blood and without prior *in vitro* expansion, and applied to topo-1–positive and –negative patients. This approach is appealing since it allows a direct and relatively rapid analysis of antigen-specific T-cell responses on small amounts of peripheral blood, minimizing the inconvenience of large blood draws in patients with difficult venous access and often with low cellular counts because of therapy. Moreover, the application of this technique was extended to specimens, like BAL, obtained from the tissues (lungs) selectively targeted by the autoimmune response.

Autoantigen-specific (topo-1 #262 nonamer) $CD8^+$ T cells were detected and quantified in the peripheral blood (100 μL) of topo-1–positive patients. Although topoisomerase-specific T cells were present at frequencies of less than 1%, this response was highly specific. No response against an irrelevant peptide was observed, and neither topo-1–negative patients nor control subjects showed any circulating topo-1–reactive T lymphocytes.

There was a striking enrichment of topo-1 (#262)–specific $CD8^+$ T cells in the BAL fluid from a patient with declining respiratory function, ground-glass opacities on high-resolution chest CT, and a BAL differential cell count significant for active alveolitis. If such findings are representative of other patients with alveolitis, a correlation with disease activity in the lung might be possible. This observation is of significant interest, since previous investigations have found no relationship between total BAL lymphocyte count and active lung disease.[7] Furthermore, the prognostic value of neutrophilia and/or eosinophilia in BAL fluid is limited.[16] Thus, a substantial number of patients (15–30%) with normal BAL findings evolve toward progressive pulmonary fibrosis. Conversely, others with active lung inflammation by BAL cell counts may have a stable disease course for many years. It is therefore plausible that the identification of specific autoreactive T cells in peripheral blood and more importantly in the context of target tissues (i.e., lungs) carries a stronger predictive power and has a more specific prognostic value.

Important future steps need to be undertaken to confirm and expand these preliminary findings: (1) performing studies with a large population of scleroderma patients who are monitored to determine clinical outcomes; (2) quantitation of topo-1–specific $CD8^+$ T-cell response in the peripheral blood as well as in the BAL (target tissue) of subjects, and correlation with disease activity; (3) phenotyping of detected topo-1–specific T cells and characterization of their functional status, particularly in terms of cytokine secretion profiles; (4) switching from a predictive to an overlapping peptide approach to screen the entire topoisomerase-1 molecule for immunorelevant epitopes; and (5) extending the investigation to autoantigen-specific $CD4^+$ and regulatory T cells.

The availability of accurate and sensitive tools for studying antigen-specific immune responses in human subjects is essential to understanding the mechanisms of ongoing tissue injury in systemic autoimmune diseases. Currently we do not have ideal biomarkers that predict and follow the course of autoimmune diseases. Measuring antigen-specific cellular responses will potentially provide a significant tool for quantifying disease activity and response to therapy. We hope that earlier and more selective treatment strategies focused on the elimination of autoreactive cells or the induction of antigen-specific regulatory function will substantially decrease the morbidity and mortality commonly associated with immunosuppressive treatments.

ACKNOWLEDGMENTS

This work was supported by Irvington Institute/Dana Foundation Human Immunology Fellowship (awarded to F.B.) and NIH Grant DE 12354 (A.R.).

[*Competing interests*: The authors declare that they have no competing financial interests.]

REFERENCES

1. WIGLEY, F.M. & L.K. HUMMERS. 2003. Clinical features of systemic sclerosis. *In* Rheumatology, 3rd ed. Marc C. Hochberg et al., Eds.: 1463–1480. Mosby. St. Louis, MO.
2. SAKKAS, L.I. & C.D. PATSOUCAS. 2004. Is systemic sclerosis an antigen-driven T cell disease? Arthritis Rheum. **50:** 1721–1733.
3. HARRIS, M.L. & A. ROSEN. 2003. Autoimmunity in scleroderma: the origin, pathogenetic role, and clinical significance of autoantibodies. Curr. Opin. Rheumatol. **15:** 778–784.
4. HU, P.Q., N. FERTIG, T.A. MEDSGER, JR. & T.M. WRIGHT. 2003. Correlation of serum anti-DNA topoisomerase I antibody levels with disease severity and activity in systemic sclerosis. Arthritis Rheum. **48:** 1363–1373.
5. WINEK, J., A. MUELLER, E. CSERNOK, *et al.* 2004. Frequency of proteinase 3 (PR3)-specific autoreactive T cells determined by cytokine flow cytometry in Wegener's granulomatosis. J. Autoimmun. **22:** 79–85.
6. NAIK, R.G., C. BECKERS, R. WENTWOORD, *et al.* 2004. Precursor frequencies of T-cells reactive to insulin in recent onset type 1 diabetes mellitus. J. Autoimmun. **23:** 55–61.
7. SILVER, R.M., K.S. MILLER, M.B. KINSELLA, *et al.* 1990. Evaluation and management of scleroderma lung disease using bronchoalveolar lavage. Am. J. Med. **88:** 470–476.
8. SUBCOMMITTEE FOR SCLERODERMA CRITERIA OF THE AMERICAN RHEUMATISM ASSOCIATION DIAGNOSTIC AND THERAPEUTIC CRITERIA COMMITTEE. 1980. Preliminary criteria for the classification of systemic sclerosis (scleroderma). Arthritis Rheum. **23:** 581–590.
9. ATAMAS, S.P. 1999. Production of type 2 cytokines by CD8+ lung cells is associated with greater decline in pulmonary function in patients with systemic sclerosis. Arthritis Rheum. **42:** 1168–1178.
10. SINGH, H. & G.P. RAGHAVA. 2003. ProPred1: prediction of promiscuous MHC Class-I binding sites. Bioinformatics **19:** 1009–1014.
11. CERUNDOLO, V., J. ALEXANDER, K. ANDERSON, *et al.* 1990. Presentation of viral antigen controlled by a gene in the major histocompatibility complex. Nature **345:** 449–452.
12. SCHNECK, J.P. 2000. Monitoring antigen-specific T cells using MHC-Ig dimers. Immunol. Invest. **29:** 163–169.
13. OELKE, M., M.V. MAUS, D. DIDIANO, *et al.* 2003. *Ex vivo* induction and expansion of antigen-specific cytotoxic T cells by HLA-Ig-coated artificial antigen-presenting cells. Nat. Med. **9:** 619–624.
14. GRETEN, T.F., J.E. SLANSKY, R. KUBOTA, *et al.* 1998. Direct visualization of antigen-specific T cells: HTLV-1 Tax11-19- specific CD8(+) T cells are activated in peripheral blood and accumulate in cerebrospinal fluid from HAM/TSP patients. Proc. Natl. Acad. Sci. USA **95:** 7568–7573.
15. LATSI, P.I. & A.U. WELLS. 2003. Evaluation and management of alveolitis and interstitial lung disease in scleroderma. Curr. Opin. Rheumatol. **15:** 748–755.
16. WHITE, B., W.C. MOORE, F.M. WIGLEY, *et al.* 2000. Cyclophosphamide is associated with pulmonary function and survival benefit in patients with scleroderma and alveolitis. Ann. Intern. Med. **132:** 947–954.

Analysis of Significance Patterns Identifies Ubiquitous and Disease-Specific Gene-Expression Signatures in Patient Peripheral Blood Leukocytes

DAMIEN CHAUSSABEL,[a] WINDY ALLMAN,[a] ASUNCION MEJIAS,[b] WENDY CHUNG,[b] LYNDA BENNETT,[a] OCTAVIO RAMILO,[b] VIRGINIA PASCUAL,[a] A. KAROLINA PALUCKA,[a] AND JACQUES BANCHEREAU[a]

[a]*The Baylor NIAID Cooperative Center for Translational Research on Human Immunology and Biodefense and Baylor Institute for Immunology Research, Dallas, Texas 75204, USA*

[b]*Division of Pediatric Infectious Diseases, UT Southwestern Medical Center and Children's Medical Center Dallas, Dallas, Texas, USA*

ABSTRACT: The utilization of gene-expression microarrays in patient-based research creates new prospects for the discovery of diagnostic biomarkers and the identification of genes or pathways linked to pathogenesis. Gene-expression signatures in peripheral blood mononuclear cells isolated from over one hundred patients with conditions presenting a strong immunological component (patient with autoimmune, graft versus host and infectious diseases, as well as immunosuppressed transplant recipients) were generated. This dataset provides the opportunity to carry out comparative analyses and define disease signatures in a broader context. Transcriptional changes of 22,283 probe sets were evaluated through statistical group comparison performed systematically for seven diseases versus their respective healthy control group. Patterns of significance were generated by hierarchical clustering of *P*-values. This approach led to the identification of a SLE-specific "diagnostic signature," formed by genes that did not change compared to healthy subjects in the other six diseases. Conversely, a "sentinel signature" that was common to all seven diseases was characterized. These findings bring new perspectives for the application of blood leukocyte expression signatures for diagnosis and early disease detection.

KEYWORDS: systemic lupus erythematosus; influenze A; gene expression; pathogenesis; immunology; leukocyte

Address for correspondence: Damien Chaussabel, Baylor Institute for Immunology Research, 3434 Live Oak Street, Suite 205, Dallas, TX 75204. Voice: 214-820-4818; fax: 214-820-4813. damienc@baylorhealth.edu

Ann. N.Y. Acad. Sci. 1062: 146–154 (2005). © 2005 New York Academy of Sciences. doi: 10.1196/annals.1358.017

INTRODUCTION

Blood is a reservoir and migration compartment for immune cells exposed to infectious agents, allergens, tumors, transplants, or autoimmune reactions. Leukocytes isolated from the peripheral blood of patients constitute an accessible source of clinically relevant information, and a comprehensive molecular phenotype of these cells can be obtained by microarray analysis. Gene expression microarrays have been extensively used in cancer research,[1,2] and proof of principle studies analyzing peripheral blood mononuclear cell (PBMC) samples isolated from patients with systemic lupus erythematosus (SLE) lead to a better understanding of mechanisms of disease onset and responses to treatment.[3,4] Two main applications have been found for gene-expression microarrays in the context of patient-based research: (1) the discovery of biomarkers and the establishment of diagnosis/prognosis signatures (e.g., prediction of survival of breast cancer patients[5]); (2) the identification of genes/pathways involved in pathogenesis, leading, for instance, to the discovery of the role of interleukin-1 in the pathogenesis of systemic onset juvenile idiopathic arthritis.[6] However, the analysis of microarray data still constitutes a considerable challenge. The ability to simultaneously acquire data for tens of thousands of features in a single test is one of the most appealing characteristics of microarrays, but it can also be a major shortcoming.[7] This "curse of dimensionality" is compounded by the fact that the numbers of samples analyzed is usually small. The imbalance between the numbers of genes and conditions analyzed considerably weakens data-interpretation capabilities. We are creating a microarray gene-expression database constituted of samples obtained from patients with diseases that possess a strong immune component. We present preliminary results obtained using a meta-analysis strategy that led to the identification of ubiquitous as well as disease-specific signatures.

METHODS

Processing of Blood Samples

Blood samples were collected by venipuncture and immediately delivered at room temperature to the Baylor Institute for Immunology Research, Dallas, TX, for processing. Peripheral blood mononuclear cells (PBMCs) from 3-4 mL of blood were isolated via Ficoll gradient and immediately lysed in RLT reagent (Qiagen, Valencia, CA) with beta-mercaptoethanol (BME) and stored at −80°C prior to the RNA extraction step.

Microarray Analysis

Total RNA was isolated using the RNeasy kit (Qiagen, Valencia, CA) according to the manufacturer's instructions, and RNA integrity was assessed by using an Agilent 2100 Bioanalyzer (Agilent, Palo Alto, CA). Target labeling was performed according to the manufacturer's standard protocol (Affymetrix Inc., Santa Clara, CA). Biotinylated cRNA targets were purified and subsequently hybridized to Affymetrix HG-U133A GeneChips (22,283 probe sets). Arrays were scanned using an Affymetrix confocal laser scanner. Microarray Suite, Version 5.0 (MAS 5.0; Affymetrix) software was used to assess fluorescent hybridization signals, to normalize signals, and to evaluate signal-detection calls. Normalization of signal values per chip was achieved using the MAS 5.0 global method of scaling to the target intensity value of 500 per GeneChip. A gene-expression analysis software program, GeneSpring, Version 7.1 (Agilent), was used to perform statistical analysis, hierarchical clustering, and classification of samples.

Analysis of Significance Patterns

Gene-expression data were generated for PBMCs obtained from patients and healthy volunteers using Affymetrix HG-U133A GeneChips that were run on the same Affymetrix system, using standard operating procedures. *P*-Values were obtained by comparing seven groups of patients to their respective healthy control groups (Mann-Whitney rank test). The groups were composed of pediatric patients with: (1) systemic lupus erythomatosus [(SLE), 16 samples], (2) influenza A (16 samples), (3) *Staphylococcus aureus* (16 samples), (4) *Escherichia coli* (16 samples), and (5) *Streptococcus pneumoniae* (14 samples); as well as adult transplant recipients: (6) liver transplant patients that have accepted the graft under immunosuppressive therapy (16 samples), and (7) bone marrow transplant recipients undergoing graft versus host disease [(GVHD), 12 samples]. Control groups were also formed taking into account age, sex, and project (10 samples in each group). Genes significantly changed ($P < .01$) in the "study group" (influenza A and/or SLE) were divided in two sets: overexpressed versus control and underexpressed versus control. *P*-Values of the genes forming the overexpressed set were obtained for the "reference groups" (infections with *E. coli*, *S. aureus*, *S. penumoniae*, liver transplant recipients, and graft versus host disease). *P*-Values of the reference groups were set to 1 when genes were underexpressed. The same procedure was used in the set of genes underexpressed in the study group, only this time *P*-values of the reference group were set to 1 when genes were overexpressed. *P*-Value data were processed with a gene expression analysis software program, GeneSpring, Version 7.1 (Agilent), that was used to perform hierarchical clustering and group genes based on significance patterns.

RESULTS AND DISCUSSION

Identification of blood leukocytes transcriptional signatures associated with acute influenza A infection and SLE

Microarray gene-expression data obtained from pediatric patients with either SLE or acute influenza A infections were used to identify transcriptional signatures characteristic of these two diseases (FIG. 1). Statistical comparison of a similar number of patients (18 samples) to their respective control group (10 samples) identified (1) 1826 differentially expressed genes that formed the Influenza signature [of those, 703 were overexpressed (red) relative to controls, and 1123 were underexpressed (blue); see FIG. 1(a)]; (2) 3382 differentially expressed genes formed the SLE signature [of those 1019 were overexpressed relative to controls and 2363 were underexpressed, see FIG. 1(b)].

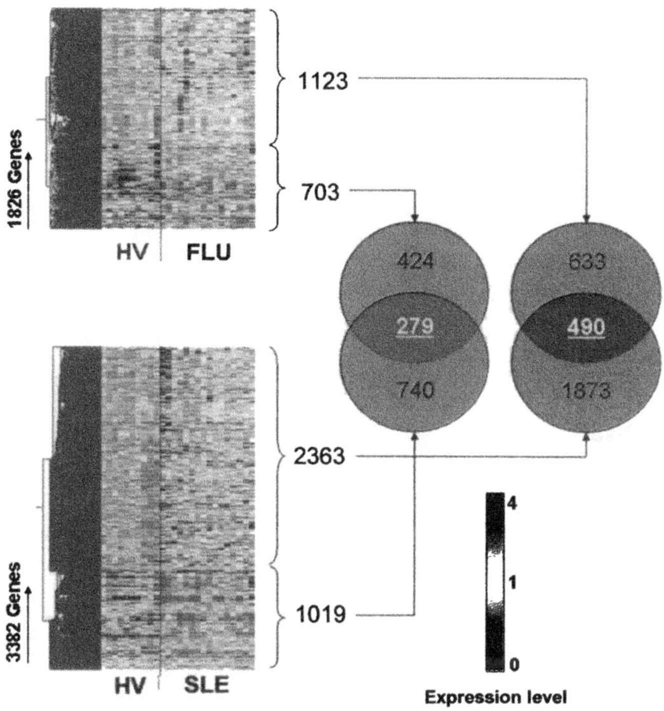

FIGURE 1. Statistical group comparison between patients and their respective controls. (**a**) Microarray expression obtained for PBMC isolated from 16 children with acute influenza A infection (FLU) and 10 healthy volunteers (HV) were compared (Mann-Whitney rank test, $P < .01$). Out of 1826 differentially expressed genes, 703 were overexpressed and 1123 underexpressed in patients. (**b**) An equivalent number of children with systemic lupus erythomatosus (SLE) were compared to their respective set of 10 healthy volunteers (HV) (Mann-Whitney rank test, $P < .01$). Out of 3382 differentially expressed genes, 1019 were overexpressed and 2363 underexpressed in patients. (**c**) Comparison of overexpressed and underexpressed gene lists obtained for SLE and FLU samples relative to their respective control groups (healthy volunteers). Transformed expression levels are indicated by color scale, with red representing relatively high expression and blue indicating relatively low expression compared to the median expression for each gene across all donors.

Analysis of Significance Patterns

Next, we determined the specificity of these signatures for each disease. We found substantial overlap between the sets of genes that were differentially expressed in FLU and SLE [FIG. 1(c)], with 279 overexpressed and 490 underexpressed genes common to both diseases (19% and 16% of similarities, respectively). This observation prompted us to ask whether a specific disease signature could be obtained in the context of a broader set of diseases.

In order to address this question, we extended the analysis to PBMC transcriptional datasets obtained for patients with acute infections caused by bacteria (*E. coli*, *S. aureus*, and *S. pneumoniae*), as well as transplant recipients (liver recipients who

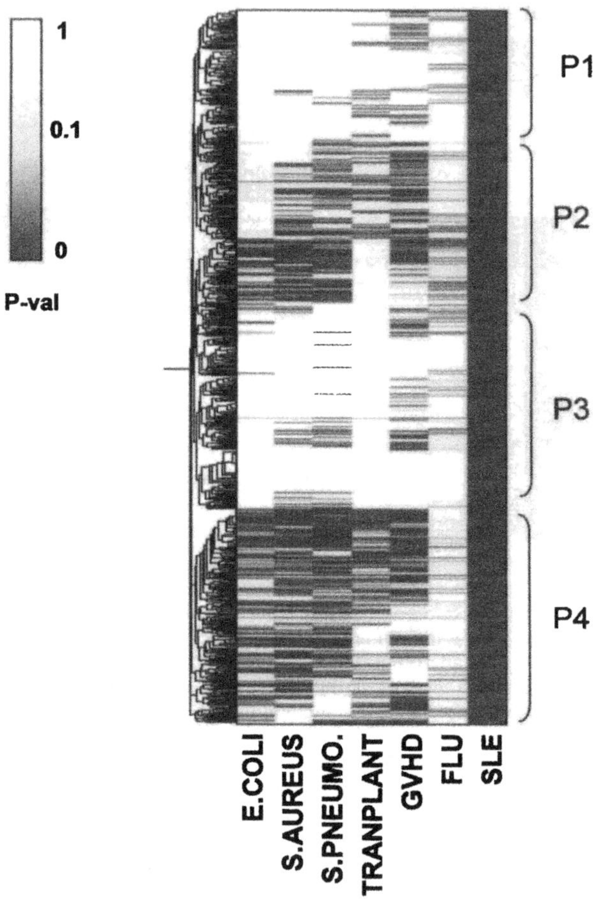

FIGURE 2. Analysis of significance patterns for genes overexpressed in SLE patients, but not in patients with acute influenza A infection. The genes used for this analysis were significantly overexpressed in patients with SLE compared to their respective control group (Mann-Whitney $P < .05$) and not in patients with acute influenza A infection were selected for this analysis (740 genes). *P*-Values were obtained for five additional groups of patients: *E. coli*, *S. aureus*, *S. pneumoniae*, liver transplant recipients, and patients with graft versus host disease. The values were imported into a microarray data-analysis software package (see METHODS for details). Four patterns were identified: SLE-1 to -4. Significance levels are indicated by color scale, with darker green representing lower *P*-values and white indicating a *P*-value of 1.

have accepted the allograft under pharmacological immunosuppressive therapy and bone marrow recipients with graft versus host disease). We analyzed patterns of significance for genes that were specifically overexpressed in SLE compared to influenza (FIG. 1, 740 genes). This approach permits visualization of the significance of changes in levels of gene expression for each disease compared to its respective control group (age- and sex-matched healthy volunteers). Genes were arranged according to significance patterns by hierarchical clustering (see METHODS for details).

Of the four patterns identified, two were found to be largely specific to SLE (FIG. 2: P1—98 genes, and P3—193 genes). In conclusion, we were able to identify sets of genes, particularly among P3, that displayed a high degree of specificity for SLE when compared to six other diseases.

Identification of a Common Disease Signature

We observed that an important proportion of genes from FIGURE 2 were induced ubiquitously (P2—222 genes, and P4—225 genes). This finding suggests that these different diseases may share common transcriptional components in the blood, constituting a "sickness" signature. In order to investigate this possibility, we analyzed sets of genes that were shared between influenza and SLE signatures [FIG. 1(c): 279 genes overexpressed, and 490 underexpressed].

Patterns of significance were generated for these genes across all seven diseases, as previously described. Three subsets were identified among the genes that were overexpressed in patients with influenza A infection and SLE: one changing in most diseases, another presenting significant differences in all diseases, while the third was more specific to influenza and SLE [FIG. 3(a), respectively P1, P2, and P3]. Equivalent patterns can be found upon analysis of a set of underexpressed genes common to influenza and SLE [FIG. 3(b), P4-7]. Interestingly, the group of patient with significance patterns that were the most similar to Influenza and SLE had GVHD. The parallelism was particularly striking for the set of underexpressed genes [FIG. 3(b)].

Functional Analysis of Significance Patterns

Finally, we extracted functional annotations associated to the patterns identified in FIGURE 3. Genes associated with "defense response" were preferentially found in two patterns (P2-3 in FIGS. 3 and 4; Fisher's test for overrepresentation of this functional category: $P < .0005$). These genes were expressed at higher levels compared to healthy. The list includes Defensin alpha 3, Azurocidin 1, Stabilin 1 (P2); the tumor necrosis factor family member TRAIL, and Galectin 3 binding protein (P3). Conversely underexpressed genes belonging to patterns P4–P6 were preferentially associated with "structural constituent of ribosome" (Fisher's test for overrepresentation of this functional category in P4–P6: $P < .0001$). These genes include multiple ribosomal protein family members (e.g., RPS10, RPL37, and RPL13). Genes belonging to the set of overexpressed genes, the most specific to influenza and SLE (P3) were preferentially associated to "interferon response" ($P < .0001$, e.g., myxovirus resistance 1, interferon alpha–inducible protein 16, double-stranded RNA inducible protein kinase), while genes in P1 were uniquely associated to "heavy metal binding" ($P < .0001$, reflecting an overabundance of members of the metallothionein family).

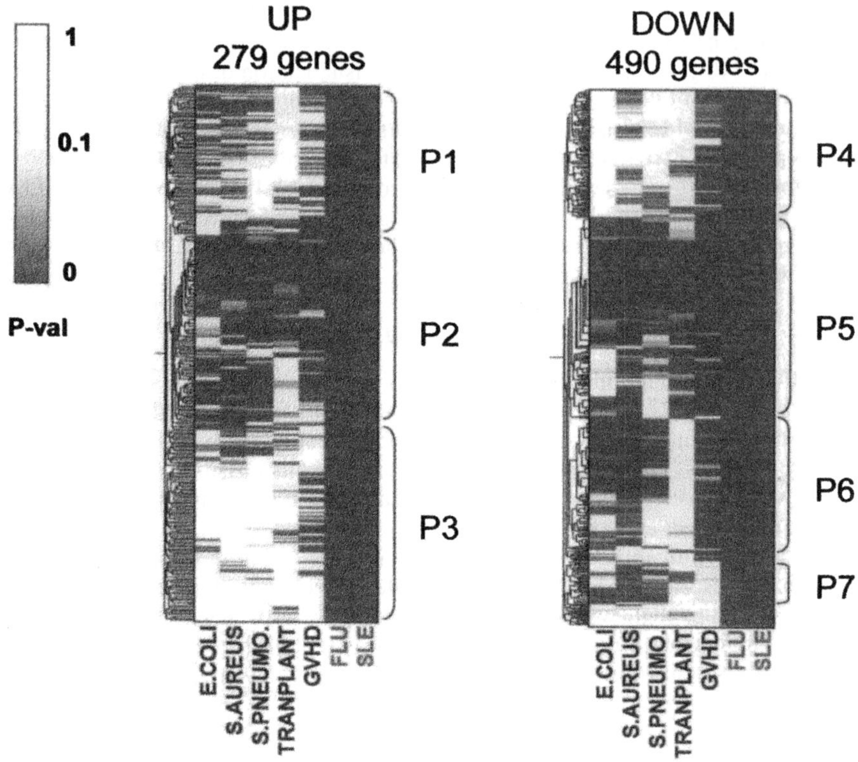

FIGURE 3. Patterns of significance for genes common to influenza A and SLE. Genes overexpressed (**a**) and underexpressed (**b**) in both patients with influenza A (FLU) and SLE were examined in the context of other diseases: acute infections with *E. coli*, *S. aureus*, *S. pneumoniae*, liver transplant recipients (transplant), and bone marrow recipients with graft versus host disease (GVHD). Significance levels are indicated by color scale, with dark green representing lower *P*-values and white indicating a *P*-value of 1.

CONCLUSIONS

The comparative analysis of PBMC transcriptional patterns identified disease-specific as well as ubiquitous expression signatures. We distinguished different degrees of disease specificity among the genes found to be common between the transcriptional profiles of PBMCs obtained from patients with influenza infection and SLE. Differences in significance patterns were translated into distinct functional associations. Indeed, the genes that were most specific to influenza and SLE relative to five other diseases were the most strongly associated to biological themes such as: "Interferon induction" (overexpressed genes; FIGS. 3 and 4: P3) or "structural constituent of ribosome" (underexpressed genes; FIGS. 3 and 4: P4). These observations permit validation of the relevance of this approach. This analysis facilitates the in-

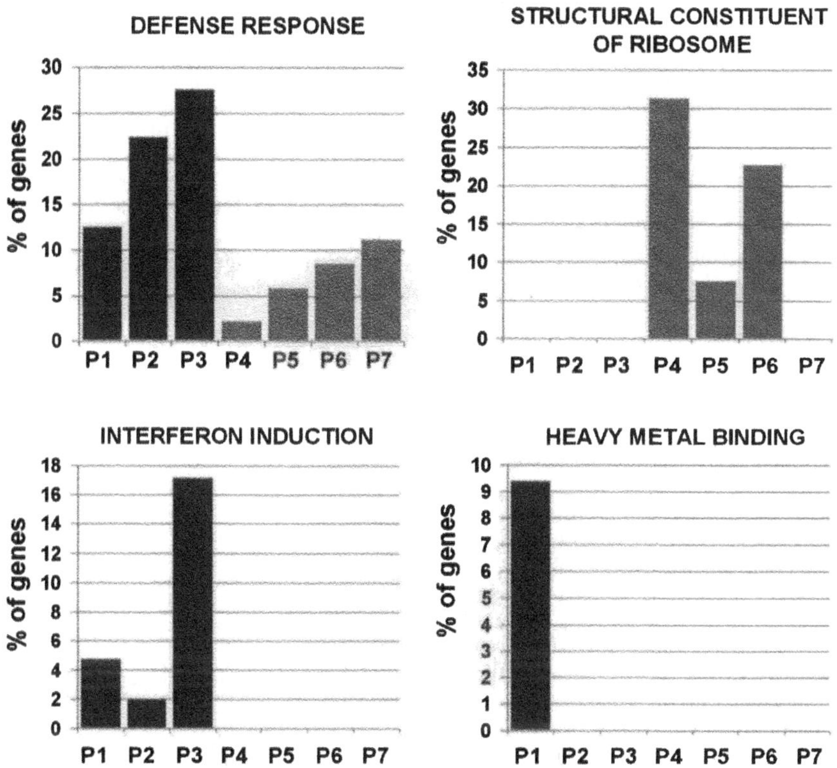

FIGURE 4. Functional analysis of genes shared by patients with influenza infection and lupus grouped according to significance patterns. Sets of genes forming the different patterns indicated on FIGURE 3 (P1–P7) were subjected to functional analyses. The histograms indicate the percentage of genes associated to a given annotation for each of the sets. Overexpressed genes = red, underexpressed = blue. P1, $n = 71$ genes; P2, $n = 118$; P3, $n = 85$; P4, $n = 117$; P5, $n = 184$; P6, $n = 120$; P7, $n = 46$.

terpretation of microarray data by placing disease signatures in a much broader context.

In addition to contributing to a better understanding of disease processes, the meta-analysis of PBMC transcriptional datasets has important implications for clinical diagnostic with (1) the identification of discriminatory disease-specific signatures; as the screening of tens of thousands of potential markers will in most cases permit to pinpoint a limited number of transcripts that uniquely characterize a disease, and (2) the identification of a sentinel signature; as sets of genes for which expression changes in a wide range of health disorders could potentially be used in a screening assay for early disease detection.

ACKNOWLEDGMENTS

One of the authors (A.K.P.) was supported by the Baylor Health Care Systems Foundation, the Children's Medical Center, the Dallas Foundation, and the DANA Foundation; another of the authors (J.B.) was supported by the Defense Advanced Research Planning Agency, and the National Institutes of Health (Grants U19 AIO57234-02 and CA78846. J.B. is the recipient of the W.W. Caruth Chair in Organ Transplantation Immunology. A.K.P. is the recipient of the Michael A. Ramsay Chair for Cancer Immunology Research.

We thank our patients and their parents/guardians for agreeing to participate in the study. We thank Dr. Michael Ramsay for continuous support.

[*Competing interests*: The authors declare that they have no competing financial interests.]

REFERENCES

1. ALIZADEH, A.A. *et al.* 2000. Distinct types of diffuse large B-cell lymphoma identified by gene expression profiling. Nature **403:** 503–511.
2. GOLUB, T.R. *et al.* 1999. Molecular classification of cancer: class discovery and class prediction by gene expression monitoring. Science **286:** 531–537.
3. BAECHLER, E.C. *et al.* 2003. Interferon-inducible gene expression signature in peripheral blood cells of patients with severe lupus. Proc. Natl. Acad. Sci. USA **100:** 2610–2615.
4. BENNETT, L. *et al.* 2003. Interferon and granulopoiesis signatures in systemic lupus erythematosus blood. J. Exp. Med. **197:** 711–723.
5. VAN DE VIJVER, M.J. *et al.* 2002. A gene-expression signature as a predictor of survival in breast cancer. N. Engl. J. Med. **347:** 1999–2009.
6. PASCUAL, V. *et al.* 2005. Role of interleukin-1 (IL-1) in the pathogenesis of systemic onset juvenile idiopathic arthritis and clinical response to IL-1 blockade. J. Exp. Med. **201:** 1479–1486.
7. SOMORJAI, R.L., B. DOLENKO & R. BAUMGARTNER. 2003. Class prediction and discovery using gene microarray and proteomics mass spectroscopy data: curses, caveats, cautions. Bioinformatics **19:** 1484–1491.
8. HOSACK, D.A. *et al.* 2003. Identifying biological themes within lists of genes with EASE. Genome Biol. **4:** R70.

Appreciating the Heterogeneity in Autoimmune Disease

Multiparameter Assessment of Intracellular Signaling Mechanisms

OMAR D. PEREZ

The Baxter Laboratory for Genetic Pharmacology, Department of Microbiology and Immunology, Stanford University School of Medicine, Stanford, California 94305, USA

ABSTRACT: Autoimmune disease pathologies are multifactorial with complex interactive networks of cells and chemical messengers that initiate cascades of aberrant cellular activity. Rheumatoid arthritis (RA) is a chronic inflammatory disease that is characterized by systemic inflammation, destruction of the joints, and production of autoantibodies recognizing dozens of putative autoantigens. The presence of autoreactive T cells in individuals leads to pathological autoimmunity by activating additional cellular constituents to mediate inflammation and joint destruction. The etiology of RA is unknown, and knowledge is lacking of the molecular mechanisms underlying the production and subsequent regulation of autoreactive T cells and predicting patient responses to treatments. Biochemical investigations into mechanisms of the disease have relied on animal models that are helpful in dissecting elements of the disease but that are not necessarily reflective of human RA development. The study of multiple activated signaling pathways in complex populations of cells, such as peripheral blood, at the single-cell level has not previously been possible. This article describes how intracellular phosphoepitope staining methodology in conjunction with surface-cell immunophenotyping can be used to deconvolute cellular subsets and allow functional characterization of patient-derived material. Multiparameter flow cytometric analysis allows for small subpopulations—representing different cellular subsets and differentiation or activation states—to be discerned and simultaneously assessed for intracellular biochemical activities. This article also describes how single-cell signal network analysis can be used to stratify patients and may be useful for understanding mechanisms of disease progression, treatment resistance, and development of diagnostic indicators.

KEYWORDS: flow cytometry; phosphoproteomics; kinase; signal transduction; patient stratification

Address for correspondence: Omar D. Perez, The Baxter Laboratory for Genetic Pharmacology, Department of Microbiology & Immunology, Stanford University, 269 Campus Dr., CCSR 4225, Stanford, CA 94305. Voice: 650-724-4847; fax: 650-725-6193.
email: operez@stanford.edu

Ann. N.Y. Acad. Sci. 1062: 155–164 (2005).
doi: 10.1196/annals.1358.018

INTRODUCTION

Rheumatoid arthritis (RA) is a systemic and chronic inflammatory autoimmune disease that targets synovial joints. Disease pathogenesis is multifactorial and extends beyond T-cell–mediated destruction of cartilage. Production of proinflammatory cytokines such as tumor necrosis factor α (TNF-α) and interleukin 1 (IL-1) by activated monocytes and macrophages contributes to tissue destruction by activation of chondrocytes and fibroblasts, which release metalloproteinases and collagenases into the synovial cavity.[1,2] Cartilage loss and bone erosion are physical manifestations of disease progression. Additional blood-borne compartments, such as B cells, contribute to production of autoantibodies and rheumatoid factor and have been regarded as playing an important role.[3] Both T- and B-cell lymphocyte deregulation and the involvement of chondrocytes and fibroblasts suggest that a dynamic interaction of cell-to-cell communications contributes to the pathogenesis of RA (FIG. 1).

The nature of the intracellular pathways activated with most primary immune-cell interactions is not well understood *in vivo* and less clear in disease states. Often it is understood using only derived cell lines, *in vitro*, and at best is often accomplished by lysis of cells and Western blots of total cellular material. Therefore, significant information on population variations that exist is missed, and advances in genomics and proteomic technologies that rely on lysate material do not access the heterogeneous subsets that exist in the immune system. Everyone who works in this area understands the limitations inherent in such studies—and the difficulties that arise when attempting to do such studies with rare cell subsets derived from primary patient material. The study of multiple activated signaling pathways in complex populations of cells, such as peripheral blood, at the single-cell level has not previously been possible. Multiparameter flow cytometric analysis allows small subpopulations to be discerned using cell-surface markers—representing different cellular subsets and their differentiation or activation states.

Autoimmune diseases such as RA or multiple sclerosis (MS) are extremely heterogeneous, both clinically and serologically. RA can present as a mild disease involving one or a few joints or as a spectrum of more severe diseases that may involve small joints of the hand, larger joints such as the knees and hips, and the axial skeleton. Some patients develop particular manifestations, including splenomegaly, neutropenia, vasculitis, nodulosis, and inflammatory eye disease. At the time of presentation, it is not possible to determine which RA patients will go on to develop severe disease or life-threatening manifestations. Similarly, it is not understood why MS strikes at various times in the life of the patient and remits or progresses aggressively. It is also not currently possible to determine which patients will respond to various therapeutic agents or to predict who will have adverse events related to specific therapeutic agents.

Clinicians have said that "every patient with autoimmune disease is unique." Underlying the immune system's inflammatory responses in autoimmunity are the signaling systems that drive the actions of individual components within the immune system. Current understandings of such autoimmune diseases point to an underlying fault with immune system processes. An imbalance between regulatory T cells, T_H1 and T_H2, coupled to B-cell disorders, are thought to be at the heart of the problem. Underlying the gross dysfunctionality of these immunocytes are the signaling systems that drive their actions. The last two decades of research have uncovered many

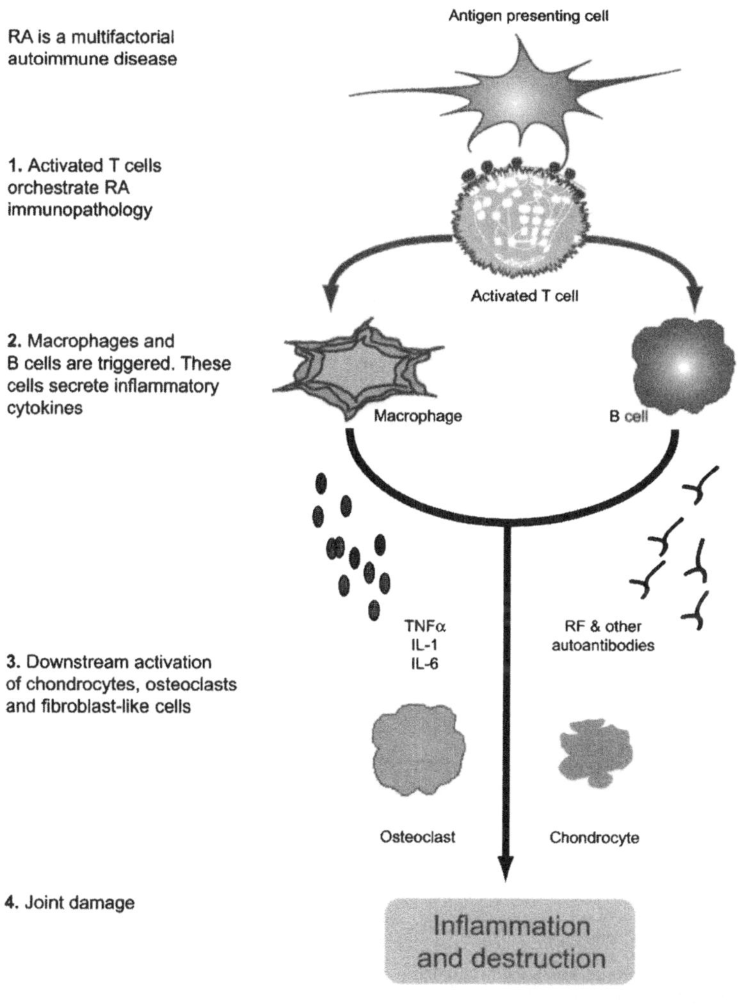

FIGURE 1. Complex cellular and chemical interactions involved in rheumatoid arthritis (RA). RA is a chronic systemic autoimmune disease that is multifactorial that can be viewed in four levels: (1) Activations of T cells by antigen-presenting cells harboring a self-antigen initiates T-cell activation. (2) Subsequent activation of macrophages and B cells is triggered, inducing secretion of proinflammatory cytokines such as TNF-α, IL-1, and IL-6, as well as production of autoantibodies. (3) Chondrocytes, osteoclasts, and fibroblast cells in the joint areas become activated and then cause localized inflammation and joint destruction. (4) Cartilage loss and bone erosion are physical manifestations of disease progression.

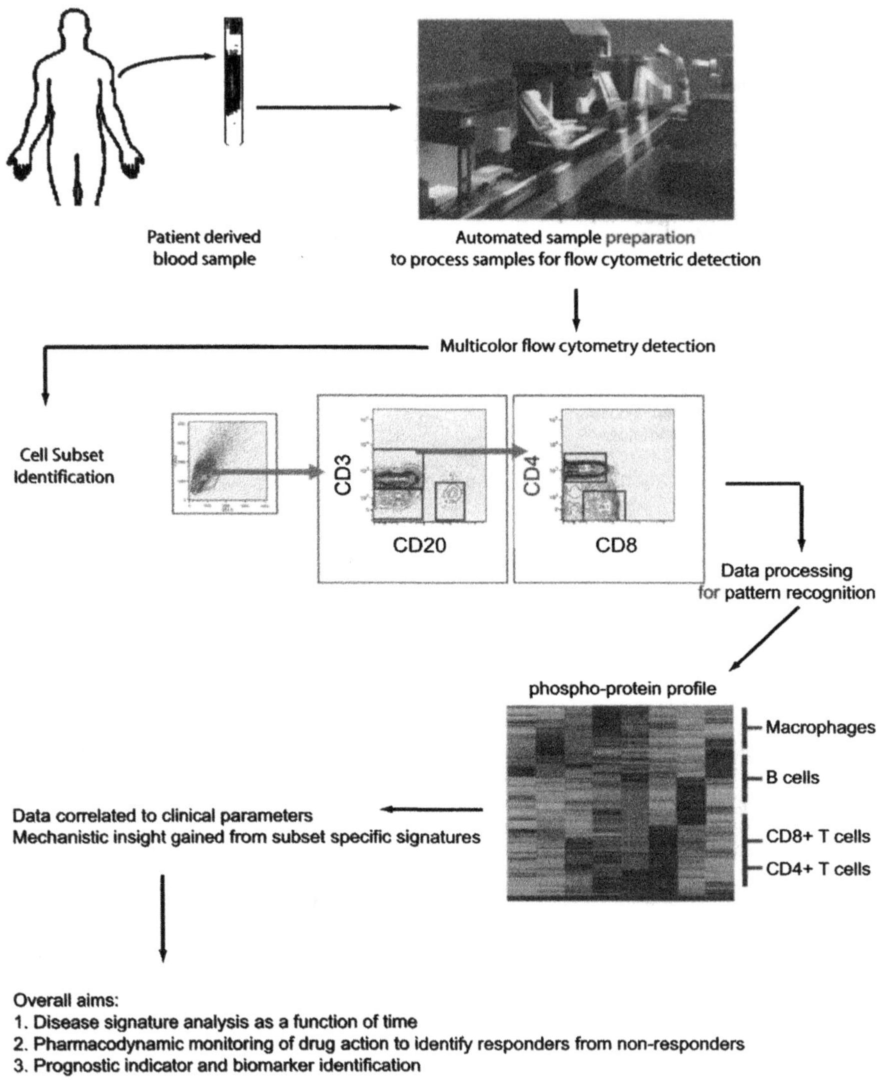

FIGURE 2. Processing of patient blood samples for phosphoepitope profiling by flow cytometry. Blood samples are acquired directly from the patient using standard operating protocols. Sample processing, staining, and flow cytometric staining are done using automated robotics platforms. Multicolor subset analysis is performed, and intracellular phosphosignals are processed by advanced algorithms for pattern recognition and hierarchical clustering. Subset-specific signaling responses are evaluated and correlated to clinical parameters. With sufficient sample profiling, disease biosignatures can be derived as a function of disease progression and may lead to the development of prognostic indicators or biomarker identification to monitor *in vivo* therapy efficacy.

pathways leading from surface receptors to gene regulation. Many if not all of these pathways pass signals through phosphorylation or dephosphorylation events on proteins or lipids. Integration of signaling events leads to relocalization of protein substituents within cells, such as with translocation to the nucleus. Until recently, measurement of such events has been limited to cell lines or bulk lysis assays. These are considered pale renditions of primary cell events, and therefore a true understanding of the nature of signaling dysfunctions during disease processes in patient samples or animal model systems has been beyond reach. To address this, we have developed a series of assay systems for flow cytometric–based biochemical analysis at the single-cell level for kinase and phosphoprotein profiling. These systems allow measurement on up to 12 simultaneous protein or kinase events per cell (and more with time) for studying signaling events in primary cells.[4,5] This development allows for unprecedented study of signaling in autoimmune diseases, as immunocytes are particularly amenable to the techniques we have developed.[6,7] Current work is focused on the identification of "autoimmune proteome biosignatures" to better understand the events that drive autoimmune disease in RA. Similarly, concurrent and parallel work is exploring other autoimmune diseases such as MS and lupus [as well as extreme examples of inflammation such as viral infection (human immunodeficiency virus and herpes simplex virus) and several forms of bacterial infection]. This, we believe, will allow us to determine procedures that can be applied in human samples to diagnose, prognosticate, and guide therapeutic approaches in the clinics. FIGURE 2 illustrates this in a flow diagram.

It is already clear that inflammatory events can be measured in the periphery. Ask yourself why individuals with diseases such as MS (focal diseases) or systemic lupus erythematosus (SLE) (disseminated) feel feverish or sick in ways distinct from the central autoimmune organ destruction. It is well accepted by autoimmune specialists that the general immune system knows there is something occurring and is reacting systemically, despite focal disease. We observe that the so-called cytokine storm of oncoming autoimmunity can be measured by the many cell subsets obtained from peripheral cells. In retrospect, this clearly should have been known: the immune system is a consummate carrier of information. The key to using this information is in understanding the distinction between the kinds of biosignatures one is measuring. The distinction is between functional and surrogate biomarkers as indicators of mechanism. We have observed that distinct subsets of cells carry the immune signature of inflammatory processes and that these can be revealed through potentiation. One must think of a cell as a miniature computational device, processing many inputs from the environment (e.g., cell-to-cell contact, chemical messengers). To observe the inner workings of the cell, you need it to process information. Analyzing the way signals are processed and comparing the capability of cells to respond to external stimuli provides a metric by which to contrast healthy and diseased extracted cells. This approach, when correlated with a clinical outcome, may provide a signal-based taxonomy of disease state.[8] The key is to determine which subsets of cells best reflect disease pathogenesis.

Rationale and Overall Approach

Autoimmune diseases such as RA are manifested at the level of the proteome and are associated with aberrancies in kinase pathways, cytokine expression, and autoantibody production. Kinase pathways play a critical role in immune regulation, and only a few kinases have been studied in RA, using primitive methods such as Western blotting or immunohistochemistry. Previous profiling techniques, such as individual autoantibody reactivity testing, provide clinically valuable information but have limited diagnostic applicability.[9] Combinations of autoantibody reactivities have greater diagnostic and prognostic utility for RA.[10,11] Similarly, it can be hypothesized that the underlying activation profiles of proteins such as kinases in immune system cells thought to be relevant to immune system function will show differences from "normal." Since it is hard to predict which kinases might be relevant in different cell subsets, this hypothesis has limited utility. However, if one could measure dozens of kinase activation profiles—or their target proteins—simultaneously, there is the opportunity to generate invaluable information about the role of signaling events in autoimmune disease, test hypotheses of signaling systems in response to various therapies, and develop diagnostic indicators.

Global kinase signaling pathways can be evaluated in human-derived blood cells based on the hypothesis that we can identify changes in relevant immune-cell subtypes that correlate with disease progression. We are determining, for instance, whether distinct profiles of kinase activation states are associated with the development, clinical progression, and response to therapy in autoimmune disease. Prior studies show that this is a reasonable hypothesis, as aberrant kinase expression and function are associated with autoimmune diseases such as SLE.[12] Therefore, this tests a most sensitive indicator of inflammation: that deregulation of kinase pathways plays a central role in the pathophysiology of RA and other inflammatory processes.

As noted previously, severe alterations in T_H1 and T_H2 balances, overproduction of autoantibodies, deregulation of cytokine production, and inappropriate responsiveness of T cells and B cells in general are hallmarks of RA and MS. It is well understood that intracellular signaling governs T- and B-cell function. Many of the signaling pathways involved use phosphoproteins as mediators of signaling. It is expected, then, that phosphoprotein balances will be disrupted in B cells and T cells during disease progression. Examples of kinase differences in B cells during autoimmune progression include abnormal signaling from the B-cell receptor (BcR) involving the Lyn kinase and the tyrosine phosphatase CD45.[13] In autoimmune SLE, T-cell expression of the T-cell receptor zeta chain is downregulated, but costimulation of such cells leads to unusually high global phosphorylation.[14] In 80% of patients with SLE, lymphocytes are profoundly deficient in the RIβ subunit of protein kinase A.[15] Thus, there are multiple examples of kinase modulation during autoimmune dysfunction. Specific cytokine profiles are also associated with pathogenic autoimmune responses.[16] Currently, we are testing the hypothesis that cytokine profiles have predictive value when correlated with activated kinase target profiling. Many have demonstrated that the efficacy of certain cytokine-blocking therapies is associated with reduction of autoreactive B-cell epitope spreading, deviation to production of non–tissue injuring autoantibody isotypes, and expression of protective cytokines.[17,18]

Thus, there is no better measure of immune inflammatory processes than the information at the single-cell level from the reacting cells themselves. Whether you are measuring direct mechanism of action or a surrogate at a distance, flow cytometric single-cell analysis of phosphoproteins in a multiparameter setting provides the most sensitive means to distinguish cell subsets as well as the real biochemistry of the cell's response.

BACKGROUND TECHNOLOGY DISCUSSIONS

Significance of Multiparameter Cell Analysis at the Single-Cell Level

The key to the power of flow cytometry and fluorescence-activated cell sorting is their ability to measure several independent properties on each cell and to use complex combinations of these quantitative measurements to classify and isolate cells of interest. Over the last 20 years, the number of measurements that can be made on each cell has increased dramatically, and this has produced waves of new discoveries.[19] These developments allow us to replace cell sorting and subsequent functional or biochemical assays with high-order multicolor analysis in the experiments we propose here. Paradoxically, the use of more fluorescence colors does not necessarily result in interpretations that are more complicated. Rather, the use of more colors, or parameters, per cell often simplifies the data by resolving previously unrecognized heterogeneities and subpopulations.

One can imagine, for instance, a one-dimensional protein gel versus a two-dimensional protein gel. Higher dimensionality separates overlapping protein components that would otherwise be missed. Patterns of protein posttranslational changes are readily observable as clusters of protein-staining bands in the two-dimensional architecture of the gel. Similarly, more dimensionality in simultaneous cell staining deconvolutes cellular subsets and makes functional characterization more precise. One becomes more able to focus on important, but perhaps numerically minor, subsets of cells without the "noise" introduced by the inclusion of other subsets that would not be resolved by four- or five-color immunophenotyping. Pairwise (or higher) gating of clustered cells in subpopulations means that an 11-color experiment on a single complex cell population (such as peripheral blood mononuclear cells) can identify many subpopulations "all at once" or in a gestaltic observation.

An important advantage of high-order multicolor fluorescence-activated cell-sorter technology is the ability to combine high-resolution immunophenotyping with single-cell functional analyses. To identify specific subsets of T cells, we often need five (or more) colors. For example, to uniquely identify naive T cells from memory T cells, cells must be simultaneously stained with CD3, CD4, and CD8 (to distinguish T-helper from T-cytotoxic cells), and then CD45RA, CD62L, CD28, CD27, and CD11a (to identify the differentiation stage). Standard flow cytometers, even specially upgraded commercially available instruments, are limited to eight fluorescence parameters; hence, no functional analysis can be performed on these subsets for other intracellular phenotypes such as phosphorylation events. With unique instrumentation and reagents, we can carry out comprehensive immunophenotyping and still devote several more colors to functional assays. Such assays include intracellular cytokines (e.g., simultaneous determination of IL-2, IL-4, and γ interferon expression),[6] apoptosis (intracellular caspase activation),[20] and cytotoxic T lymphocyte activity (by quantitating intracellular perforin or granzyme expression),[7] as well as specific phosphoprotein levels or nuclear translocation events.

Importantly, there is extraordinary statistical significance to the data collected (assuming the staining is done correctly and the machine appropriately calibrated). For instance, in a standard stain one is collecting information from as few as 5000–10,000 cells and up to 100,000 cells. Each cell is a distinct experimental subject, and thus can be used in statistical regimens to gain information of significant accuracy. Moreover, one can discern levels of expression within complex populations that are entirely lost during "bulk lysis" procedures such as Western blots or many other biochemical approaches. We show now that we can go beyond these types of analysis and access signaling systems more directly in primary cells. A significant problem in the study of complex biological phenomena, such as human disease, is the management and comparison of large and disparate data sets. Biological and clinical measurements of signaling processes or disease progression are tied to the experimental design. But single measurements of phenotype are often insufficient to give a rich picture of the underlying phenomena being studied. Often investigators resort to several independent measurements and then attempt to correlate outcomes to either prove a hypothesis or generate enough information to develop new hypotheses. The problem compounds with the advent of technologies capable of generating ultralarge datasets containing multiple parameters per measurement. Statistical regimens that allow verifiable claims to be made even on single datasets must be used and understood by the investigator(s). This has allowed us to use flow data at the single-cell level for an extraordinary application of machine learning using Bayesian networks to directly infer signaling diagrams from raw flow data.[21] We have shown that we can readily undertake sensitive studies on rare subsets of cells in response to physiological activation conditions.

Immune Deregulation in Genetic Diseases Can Be Revealed by Potentiated Signaling, a Model Using Human Leukemia

We hypothesized that variations in cell signaling found among leukemias could form the basis of a tumor classification system. We recently published this work, and it has now been commented upon and cited in reviews.[8] A primary goal in that work was developing a classification system by which one could determine whether responses of patients with acute myeloid leukemia to chemotherapy were significantly linked with a pattern of intracellular signaling in the leukemic blast cells. The potentiated model of cancer signaling states that changes during tumorigenesis impose alternative signaling outcomes based on epigenetic and genetic changes in these cells. A signal transduction–based classification would be especially useful if, in addition to stratifying patient risk, it indicated targets of opportunity for therapeutic intervention in patient subgroups or revealed mechanisms by which imposed genetic changes due to tumorigenesis affect cell signaling.

To meet a standard of measuring events simultaneously in a minimally perturbed context we applied intracellular phosphospecific flow cytometry,[4,22] to detect multiple phosphorylated, activated signaling molecules in primary leukemic cells drawn from such a cohort of acute myeloid leukemia patients. The hypothesis tested by this approach was that alterations to signaling common in leukemic cells would cause these cells to react in an inappropriate or sensitized manner to environmental inputs—and that this can be read out by single-cell flow cytometry.[8] Again, this is a key assumption, as it will be applied later to our studies on lymphoma cells and animal models.

CONCLUSION

Functional characterization of multifactorial autoimmune diseases will require interdisciplinary cell-based approaches that can access the primary patient material. The creation of flow cytometry was an interdisciplinary effort envisioned by Len Herzenberg at Stanford University, merging concepts from physics, engineering, and immunology, in the 1960s. Advances in hardware, software, and the development of specific reagents with cooperation from both the academic and private sectors have created instrumentation capable of measuring 12 simultaneous parameters currently, with pioneering individuals incorporating the latest advances in fluorescent technologies expanding that figure to 17.[23,24] However, flow cytometry still faces challenges in both the automation and software development arenas. An important aspect of flow cytometry is that it has already been widely accepted into the clinical arena, being one of the few technologies to have met clinical regulatory standards, with an approximate 30,000 machines installed throughout the world. This alone is apparent in that almost every hospital has a basic instrument that is used for surface phenotyping cancer patient samples or monitoring human immunodeficiency virus $CD4^+$ T-cell counts. A current obstacle for translational medicine is in the creation of facilities within hospitals to use advanced genomic and proteomic technologies in conjunction with investigators at nearby academic institutions to derive mechanistic information that can be used to either understand human disease pathogenesis or identify diagnostic biomarkers as indicators of disease progression. Data-management systems and standards and regulations for sharing machine-generated patient-specific information are still more obstacles to overcome in bridging research and development with clinical applications. Flow cytometric whole-blood assay systems that combine surface phenotyping in conjunction with functional assessment have a direct potential to be integrated into the current clinical environment.

ACKNOWLEDGMENTS

This work was supported by a Bristol-Meyer Squibb Irvington Fellowship, a Dana Foundation Human Immunology award, and National Heart, Lung, and Blood Institute proteomics contract N01-HV-28183I. Special thanks to Gina Jager and Khoua Vang for administrative assistance and Dennis Mitchell for technical support. O.D.P. acknowledges support from Robert Balderas and BD Biosciences-PharMingen.

[*Competing interests*: Consultant for BD-Bioscience, Bristol-Meyer Squibb, Clinical Advisors Group, and ODPCS; also, patents pending for the phospho-flow technologies.]

REFERENCES

1. Mor, A., S.B. Abramson & M.H. Pillinger. 2005. The fibroblast-like synovial cell in rheumatoid arthritis: a key player in inflammation and joint destruction. Clin. Immunol. **115:** 118–128.

2. SINGH, R., D.B. ROBINSON & H.S. EL-GABALAWY. 2005. Emerging biologic therapies in rheumatoid arthritis: cell targets and cytokines. Curr. Opin. Rheumatol. **17:** 274–279.
3. KOTZIN, B.L. 2005. The role of B cells in the pathogenesis of rheumatoid arthritis. J. Rheumatol. Suppl. **73:** 14–8; discussion 29–30.
4. PEREZ, O.D. & G.P. NOLAN. 2002. Simultaneous measurement of multiple active kinase states using polychromatic flow cytometry. Nat. Biotechnol. **20:** 155–162.
5. PEREZ, O.D., P.O. KRUTZIK & G.P. NOLAN. 2004. Flow cytometric analysis of kinase signaling cascades. Methods Mol. Biol. **263:** 67–94.
6. PEREZ, O.D., D. MITCHELL, G.C. JAGER, *et al.* 2003. Leukocyte functional antigen 1 lowers T cell activation thresholds and signaling through cytohesin-1 and Jun-activating binding protein 1. Nat. Immunol. **4:** 1083–1092.
7. PEREZ, O.D., D. MITCHELL, G.C. JAGER & G.P. NOLAN. 2004. LFA-1 signaling through p44/42 is coupled to perforin degranulation in CD56+CD8+ natural killer cells. Blood **104:** 1083–1093.
8. IRISH, J.M., R. HOVLAND, P.R. KRUTZIK, *et al.* 2004. Single cell profiling of potentiated phospho-protein networks in cancer cells. Cell **118:** 217–228.
9. HUEBER, W., P.J. UTZ, L. STEINMAN & W.H. ROBINSON. 2002. Autoantibody profiling for the study and treatment of autoimmune disease. Arthritis Res. **4:** 290–295.
10. ROBINSON, W.H., C. DIGENNARO, W. HUEBER, *et al.* 2002. Autoantigen microarrays for multiplex characterization of autoantibody responses. Nat. Med. **8:** 295–301.
11. ROBINSON, W.H., L. STEINMAN & P.J. UTZ. 2003. Protein arrays for autoantibody profiling and fine-specificity mapping. Proteomics **3:** 2077–2084.
12. KHAN, I.U. & G.M. KAMMER. 2004. Protein kinase A and signal transduction in T lymphocytes: biochemical and molecular methods. Methods Mol. Med. **102:** 73–85.
13. LIOSSIS, S.N., E.E. SOLOMOU, M.A. DIMOPOULOS, *et al.* 2001. B-cell kinase lyn deficiency in patients with systemic lupus erythematosus. J. Investig. Med. **49:** 157–165.
14. LIOSSIS, S.N., X.Z. DING, G.J. DENNIS & G.C. TSOKOS. 1998. Altered pattern of TCR/CD3-mediated protein-tyrosyl phosphorylation in T cells from patients with systemic lupus erythematosus. Deficient expression of the T cell receptor zeta chain. J. Clin. Invest. **101:** 1448–1457.
15. KHAN, I.U., D. LAXMINARAYANA & G.M. KAMMER. 2001. Protein kinase A RI beta subunit deficiency in lupus T lymphocytes: bypassing a block in RI beta translation reconstitutes protein kinase A activity and augments IL-2 production. J. Immunol. **166:** 7600–7605.
16. UTZ, P.J. 2005. Protein arrays for studying blood cells and their secreted products. Immunol. Rev. **204:** 264–282.
17. FELDMANN, M., F.M. BRENNAN, E. PALEOLOG, *et al.* 2004. Anti-TNFalpha therapy of rheumatoid arthritis: What can we learn about chronic disease? Novartis Found. Symp. **256:** 53–69; discussion 69–73, 106–111, 266–269.
18. VILCEK, J. & M. FELDMANN. 2004. Historical review: cytokines as therapeutics and targets of therapeutics. Trends Pharmacol. Sci. **25:** 201–209.
19. HERZENBERG, L.A., D. PARKS, B. SAHAF, *et al.* 2002. The history and future of the fluorescence activated cell sorter and flow cytometry: a view from Stanford. Clin. Chem. **48:** 1819–1827.
20. PEREZ, O.D., S. KINOSHITA, Y. HITOSHI, *et al.* 2002. Activation of the PKB/AKT pathway by ICAM-2. Immunity **16:** 51–65.
21. SACHS, K., O. PEREZ, D. PE'ER, *et al.* 2005. Causal protein-signaling networks derived from multiparameter single-cell data. Science **308:** 523–529.
22. KRUTZIK, P.O., J.M. IRISH, G.P. NOLAN & O.D. PEREZ. 2004. Analysis of protein phosphorylation and cellular signaling events by flow cytometry: techniques and clinical applications. Clin. Immunol. **110:** 206–221.
23. ROEDERER, M., J.M. BRENCHLEY, M.R. BETTS & S.C. DE ROSA. 2004. Flow cytometric analysis of vaccine responses: How many colors are enough? Clin. Immunol. **110:** 199–205.
24. PERFETTO, S.P., P.K. CHATTOPADHYAY & M. ROEDERER. 2004. Seventeen-colour flow cytometry: unravelling the immune system. Nat. Rev. Immunol. **4:** 648–655.

B-Cell Tolerance Checkpoints in Healthy Humans and Patients with Systemic Lupus Erythematosus

SERGEY YURASOV,[a,b] JOHANNA HAMMERSEN,[a] THOMAS TILLER,[a,c] MAKOTO TSUIJI,[a] AND HEDDA WARDEMANN[a]

[a]*Laboratory of Molecular Immunology, The Rockefeller University, New York, New York 10021, USA*

[b]*Department of Pediatrics, Memorial Sloan-Kettering Cancer Center, New York, New York 10021, USA*

[c]*Faculty of Medicine, Program in Molecular Medicine, University of Erlangen-Nuernberg, Erlangen, Germany*

ABSTRACT: Antibodies are protective effector molecules in the body's immune defense against pathogens. However, if directed against the body's own tissues or organs, antibodies can also play a role in the pathogenesis of autoimmune disease. Here, we discuss our data on how autoreactive antibodies are regulated in healthy humans and how a failure to establish self-tolerance during early B-cell development in patients with systemic lupus erythematosus may predispose to the development of this autoimmune disease.

KEYWORDS: B cell; tolerance; autoantibody; autoimmunity; SLE

The diversity of the antibody repertoire is generated by somatic recombination of immunoglobulin gene segments during early B-cell development in the bone marrow.[1] This random rearrangement process generates the basis for the diversity of the naïve antibody repertoire—including, however, antibodies that recognize self-antigens.[2,3] Many anti–self-immunoglobulin (Ig) transgenic mouse models have been generated to study the fate of B cells expressing autoreactive antibodies *in vivo*.[4–8] Although these models led to the discovery of the underlying mechanisms by which such autoreactive antibodies are regulated in bone marrow—deletion, anergy, and receptor editing—they did not allow determination of the frequency of self-reactive antibodies that are generated during normal B-cell development. Neither did they show where and when during B-cell development self-reactive antibodies are removed from a diverse naïve repertoire. To address these questions, we developed a method to clone and express antibodies from single human B cells that allowed us to test the recombinant antibodies for reactivity against self-antigens (FIG. 1).[2,9] Using fluorescence-activated cell sorting, we purified healthy human donor cells at dif-

Address for correspondence: Hedda Wardemann, Ph.D., The Rockefeller University, 1230 York Ave., New York, NY 10021. Voice: 212-327-8098; fax: 212-327-8370.
wardemh@rockefeller.edu

**Ann. N.Y. Acad. Sci. 1062: 165–174 (2005). © 2005 New York Academy of Sciences.
doi: 10.1196/annals.1358.019**

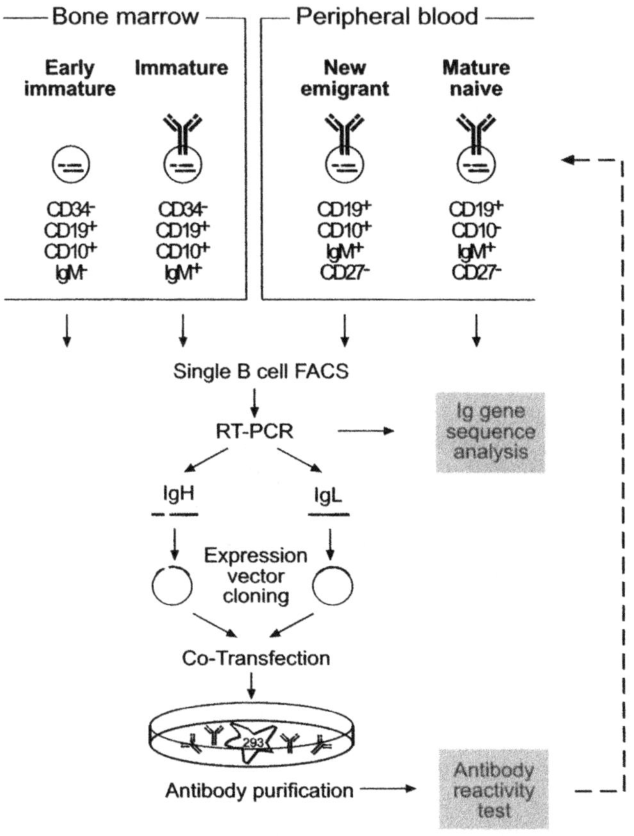

FIGURE 1. Strategy for cloning and *in vitro* expression of antibodies from single human B cells isolated at different stages of their development from bone marrow and peripheral blood. Early immature B cells displayed a pre–B-cell phenotype ($CD34^-$, $CD19^+$, $CD10^+$, IgM^-), but expressed functionally rearranged IgH and IgL chain gene transcripts. Immature B cells from bone marrow ($CD34^-$, $CD19^+$, $CD10^+$, IgM^+) resembled peripheral blood new emigrant B cells ($CD19^+$, $CD10^+$, IgM^+, $CD27^-$). Mature naïve cells from peripheral blood were $CD19^+$ and IgM^+, but lacked CD10 expression and were negative for the memory B-cell marker CD27. Ig genes from single fluorescence-activated cell sorter–purified B cells were amplified by reverse transcription–PCR, and products were sequenced to confirm the absence of somatic mutations. IgH chain and IgL chain PCR products amplified from the same cell were cloned into separate human Igγ1 and Igκ or Igλ expression vectors, respectively. For *in vitro* antibody expression, HEK293A cells were cotransfected with plasmids encoding the IgH and IgL chain regions amplified from the same cell. Antibodies were purified and tested for self-reactivity to determine the frequency of self-reactive and polyreactive antibodies in the different B-cell populations.

ferent stages of B-cell development based on cell-surface marker expression. These cells were from bone marrow (CD34$^-$, CD19$^+$, CD10$^+$, IgM$^-$ early immature B cells and CD34$^-$, CD19$^+$, CD10$^+$, IgM$^+$ immature B cells) and from peripheral blood (CD19$^+$, CD10$^+$, CD27$^-$, IgM$^+$ new emigrant B cells and CD19$^+$, CD10$^-$, CD27$^-$, IgM$^+$ mature naïve B cells).[2] For each B cell, Ig heavy (IgH) and Ig light (IgL) -chain gene transcripts were amplified by reverse transcription–polymerase chain reaction (PCR) and cloned into separate expression vectors. To produce the antibody *in vitro*, human embryonic kidney (HEK293) cells were cotransfected with the corresponding IgH- and IgL chain–encoding plasmids leading to antibody secretion. Significant amounts of antibody were purified from the tissue culture supernatant and tested for their reactivity against self-antigens. With this unbiased approach, many antibodies can be screened for their Ig gene repertoire and their reactivity profile at the same time. We cloned 248 antibodies from the four B-cell fractions and tested them for self-reactivity in two assays (FIG. 2).[2] In the first assay, which is used in clinical diagnostics as a standard assay to detect antinuclear antibodies (ANAs), we tested the antibodies for reactivity against self-antigens expressed by the human hepatocytoma cell line HEp-2 in enzyme-linked immunosorbent and indirect immunofluorescence assays. In the second assay, we determined the reactivity against specific antigens such as single-stranded DNA (ssDNA), double-stranded DNA (dsDNA), lipopolysaccharide (LPS), and insulin to assess whether some of the antibodies were polyreactive and bound several different antigens. Such antibodies could potentially be dangerous to the body, as they are not specific, and thus cannot discriminate between foreign and autoantigens. Our results showed that most (75%) newly generat-

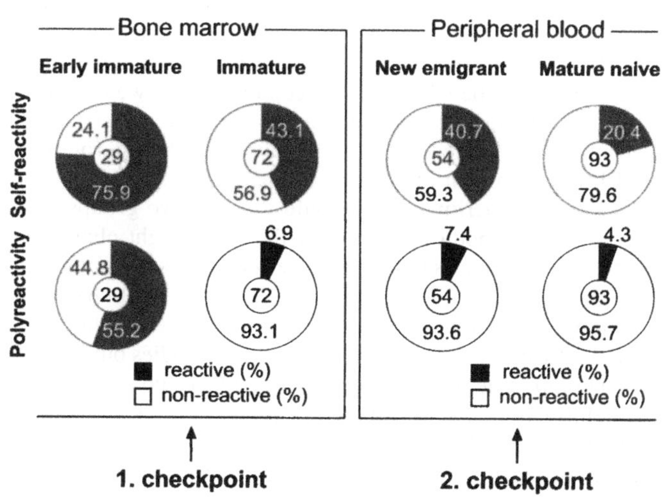

FIGURE 2. B-cell tolerance checkpoints during early B-cell development in bone marrow and periphery of healthy human donors. *Pie charts* show the frequency (%) of self-reactive and polyreactive antibodies in the four human B-cell populations. The absolute number of antibodies analyzed for each B-cell fraction is indicated in the pie chart center. Polyreactive antibodies are efficiently counterselected at the first B-cell tolerance checkpoint in the bone marrow. Self-reactive B cells are removed at two checkpoints: in the bone marrow and in the periphery.

ed early immature B cells express self-reactive antibodies, but such antibodies are lost from the repertoire at two checkpoints during B-cell development (FIG. 2).[2] The first checkpoint is in the bone marrow between the early immature (75% self-reactive) and immature B-cell stage (43% self-reactive; $P = .003$); the second checkpoint is in the periphery before maturation of new emigrant B cells (41% self-reactive) into naïve immunocompetent B lymphocytes (20% self-reactive; $P = .008$).

When the same antibodies were tested for reactivity against the specific antigens, 55% of early immature B-cell antibodies were polyreactive, but only 7% of antibodies from immature and new emigrant B cells and 4% from mature naïve B cells (FIG. 2).[2] From this finding we concluded that polyreactive antibodies are efficiently removed from the repertoire at the first checkpoint for self-reactivity in the bone marrow.[2]

When we analyzed the Ig gene sequences of the cloned antibodies, we found features previously shown to be associated with autoreactivity, such as long and positively charged IgH chain complementary determining region (CDR) 3 regions, to be enriched in self-reactive antibodies.[2,9–14] However, neither of these characteristics nor Ig gene usage itself was sufficient to predict whether an antibody was self-reactive. We think this finding reflects the enormous diversity of the Ig gene repertoire that has been selected over millions of years to protect us against invading pathogens while avoiding strong autoreactivity.

In mice, deletion, anergy, and receptor editing have been described as the mechanisms that silence autoreactive antibodies in the bone marrow, and it has been estimated that 25%–50% of naturally arising antibodies undergo receptor editing by light chain replacement.[15–17] However, besides the fact that most human Igλ-positive antibodies have functionally rearranged Igκ light chains, the relative contribution of receptor editing to silencing human autoreactive antibodies has not been determined.[18–20] To address the question of whether polyreactive antibodies from early immature B cells can be silenced by receptor editing, we exchanged the light chains from such antibodies with a collection of six Igκ and six Igλ light chains (FIG. 3).[21] All antibodies were expressed *in vitro* and tested for their reactivity against DNA, LPS, and insulin in comparison with the antibody with the original light chain. From these experiments, we could identify two groups of polyreactive early immature B-cell antibodies.[21] None of the tested light chains could silence highly polyreactive antibodies as measured by enzyme-linked immunosorbent assay (FIG. 3, upper right), whereas at least one of the exchange light chains could silence antibodies with low or moderate polyreactivity (FIG. 3, lower right). The first group represents around 10% of all early immature B-cell antibodies but is not found in the peripheral B-cell compartments. The second group makes up almost 45% of the early immature B-cell fraction, and few of these low polyreactive antibodies can escape the central tolerance mechanisms and are detectable at very low numbers in the new emigrant and mature naïve peripheral B-cell compartments (FIG. 3, lower right).[2] From this finding, we conclude that almost all autoreactive antibodies naturally generated during early human B-cell development can be silenced by light-chain receptor editing, and only a few highly polyreactive antibodies need to be deleted.[21]

Light chain replacement in these *in vitro* experiments efficiently silenced polyreactive antibodies, but many antibodies remained self-reactive as measured by HEp-2 cell reactivity.[21] This finding is consistent with our observation that significant numbers of immature and new emigrant B cells that passed the first checkpoint for

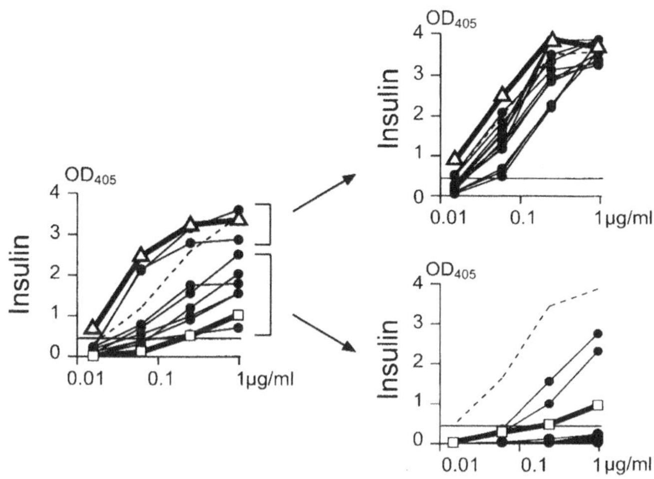

FIGURE 3. Silencing of naturally developing human polyreactive antibodies by light chain replacement *in vitro*. Polyreactive antibodies from early immature B cells fall into two groups (**left**). Highly polyreactive antibodies cannot be silenced by light chain replacement *in vitro* (**upper right**). Upper-right graph shows the reactivities of antibodies derived from a representative highly polyreactive early immature B-cell antibody (*triangles*) after light chain replacement (*circles*). Early immature B-cell antibodies with low or intermediate levels of polyreactivity can be silenced by light chain exchange (**lower right**). Lower-right graph shows the reactivities of antibodies derived from a representative low polyreactive early immature B-cell antibody (*squares*) after light chain replacement. Lines above the horizontal threshold line (*circles*) represent antibodies that were not silenced for polyreactivity by light chain replacement. Lines (*circles*) below the indicated horizontal threshold line represent antibodies with new light chains that silenced polyreactivity. Graphs show binding to insulin representative of polyreactivity with dsDNA, ssDNA, insulin, and LPS. *Dashed line* represents the highly polyreactive antibody ED38 as positive control.

B-cell tolerance in the bone marrow of healthy humans express HEp-2 self-reactive antibodies.[2] Half of these antibodies are lost at the second checkpoint for B-cell tolerance in the periphery before differentiation into mature naïve B cells, but the mechanisms involved in this selection process are not known. Thus, random Ig gene recombination leads to the generation of many autoreactive antibodies that must be removed from the initial repertoire to ensure self-tolerance, but most of the B cells producing such antibodies can be rescued by light-chain editing.[2,21]

How can a failure to establish B-cell tolerance at the two checkpoints be associated with the development of autoimmunity? A hallmark of systemic lupus erythematosus (SLE) is the production of high-affinity serum autoantibodies predominantly directed against nuclear self-antigens.[22,23] Although it has not been demonstrated that these serum antibodies are directly pathogenic, they form immune complexes and deposit in various target organs and the kidneys of the patients, often leading to fatal organ failure.[24,25] In mouse and human, several factors, such as FcγRIIb polymorphisms, cytokines, and apoptotic cell clearance, have been shown to play a role in the development of the disease, but the role of B-cell tolerance checkpoints has not been studied in this context.[26–28] Due to high titers of class-switched autoantibodies in serum from SLE patients, it appears obvious that B-cell tolerance is broken after activation of autoreactive B cells by antigen encounter and before their differentiation into memory and Ig-secreting plasma cells. After activation, somatic hypermutation and affinity maturation would then allow the differentiation and selection of B cells expressing strongly self-reactive antibodies. However, one can also imagine that SLE is associated with a failure to establish B-cell tolerance early during B-cell development at the first or second checkpoint in bone marrow or peripheral blood. In this scenario, increased numbers of self-reactive naïve B cells may predispose to the development of the disease and, if activated, lead to the development of clinical symptoms. To address the latter question, we cloned and expressed antibodies from new emigrant and mature naïve peripheral blood B cells of SLE patients and determined the frequency of self-reactive antibodies in these two B-cell compartments (FIG. 4).[29]

SLE is a multigene autoimmune disorder associated with many symptoms.[24] All three patients studied were diagnosed based on the revised classification criteria of the American College of Rheumatology, but their clinical diagnostic features reflected the broad spectrum of the disease.[29] However, most importantly, none of the patients had received any treatment prior to the analysis.[29]

Several studies have described Ig gene repertoire abnormalities in SLE.[30–33] Therefore, we performed detailed analyses of the Ig gene usage and IgH CDR3 chain characteristics of antibodies from new emigrant and mature naïve B cells of SLE patients and compared these with sequences obtained from antibodies of our healthy control subjects.[2,29] Although the analysis was limited to three patients, we observed some of the repertoire abnormalities described in the literature in individual patients.[29] These abnormalities included differences in VH gene usage, Vκ gene usage, and IgH CDR3 length, but we detected no signs of altered receptor editing as determined by changes in the representation of Jk gene families.[30,33] Overall, none of the Ig gene sequence abnormalities were consistent among patients and in some cases differed between antibodies cloned from new emigrant and mature naïve B cells of the same patient.[29]

Further, when we cloned the antibodies from SLE patients and expressed them *in vitro*, we found no correlation between the reactivity of an antibody and its IgH or IgL chain gene characteristic.[29] This finding is consistent with our previous observation in healthy humans that sequence analysis alone is not sufficient to predict whether an antibody is self-reactive.[2] This result is even more striking, as self-reactive antibodies were enriched in the naïve repertoire of the SLE patients.[29]

We expressed 222 antibodies from new emigrant and mature naïve SLE B cells and tested them for reactivity against HEp-2 cell self-antigens and polyreactivity with ssDNA, dsDNA, LPS, and insulin (FIG. 4).[29] Compared with our healthy controls, we detected no significant increase in the number of HEp-2 cell self-reactive antibodies cloned from new emigrant B cells (~40%–60% in SLE versus 43% in healthy humans; $P = .401$; FIG. 4A). However, 42%–50% of mature naïve SLE antibodies were HEp-2 self-reactive, but only 20% of the control subjects ($P = .0003$; FIG. 4B). When tested for binding against DNA, LPS, and insulin, about 24%–31% of the mature naïve antibodies were also considered polyreactive (FIG. 4B). This finding represents a consistent five- to sixfold increase in polyreactive antibodies in SLE patients compared with healthy control subjects (~5% polyreactivity in mature naïve B cells). Increased numbers of self- and polyreactive antibodies in mature

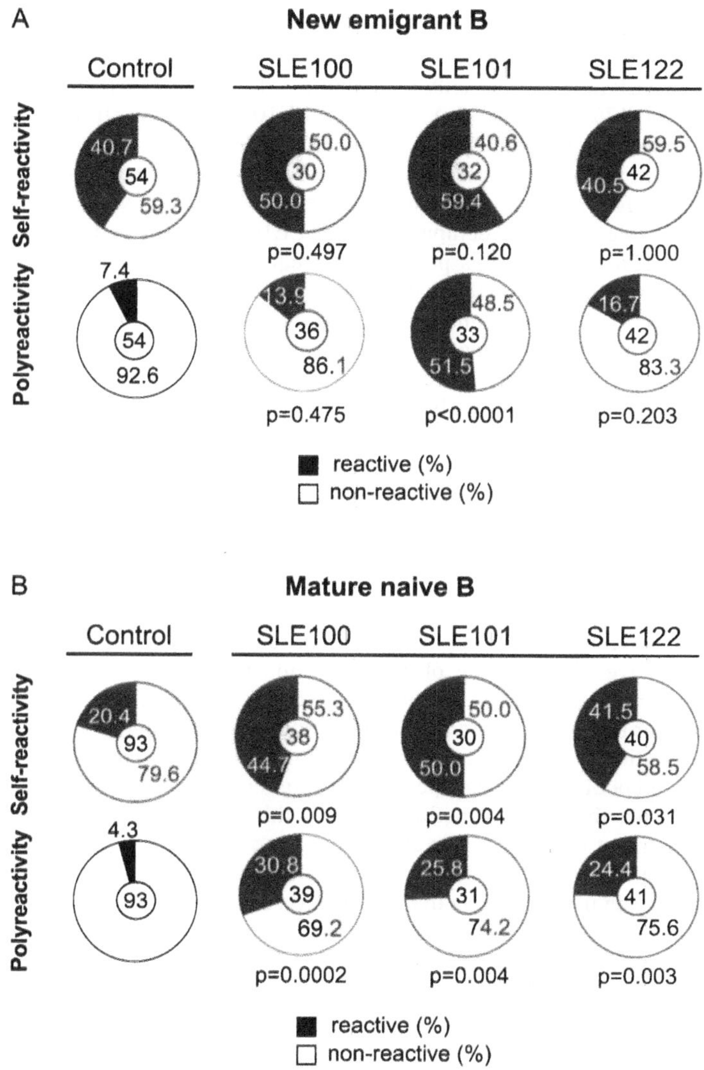

FIGURE 4. Defective early B-cell tolerance checkpoints in bone marrow and periphery of three untreated patients with SLE. *Pie charts* show the frequency (%) of self-reactive and polyreactive antibodies from new emigrant and mature naïve B cells of SLE patients and healthy control subjects. The absolute number of antibodies analyzed for each B-cell fraction is indicated in the pie chart center. New emigrant B cells from all three patients expressed normal numbers of self-reactive antibodies. Polyreactive antibodies were significantly increased in SLE101, but not in SLE100 and SLE122 compared with healthy control subjects. Self-reactive and polyreactive antibodies were significantly increased in the mature naïve B-cell compartment of all three patients with SLE.

naïve B cells from SLE patients can be due to a failure to establish B-cell tolerance at the first checkpoint in the bone marrow, the second checkpoint in the periphery, or both. Phenotypically and in their reactivity with self-antigens, new emigrant B cells in peripheral blood resemble immature B cells of the bone marrow and therefore directly reflect the central tolerance checkpoint. Two of the three patients (SLE100 and SLE122) showed only a moderate 2- to 2.5-fold increase in polyreactivity (14% and 17%, respectively), whereas SLE101 had many strongly polyreactive new emigrant B cells (51%) compared with healthy donors (FIG. 4A). Polyreactive antibodies are efficiently removed from the normal repertoire at the first checkpoint for self-reactivity in the bone marrow (FIG. 2).[2] Many such antibodies in the new emigrant B-cell compartment of SLE101 therefore reflect a central tolerance defect (FIG. 4).[29] In this patient, the frequency of polyreactive antibodies dropped with progression into the mature naïve B-cell compartment, suggesting that polyreactive antibodies are counterselected at the second checkpoint, but that this process is insufficient. The opposite effect was observed for SLE100 and SLE122, in whom the central tolerance mechanisms did not seem to be strongly affected (FIG. 4A). Instead, tolerance was broken at the second checkpoint in the periphery where self-reactive antibodies were favored at the transition between the new emigrant and mature naïve B-cell compartment (FIG. 4B). Thus, different checkpoints can be affected in different patients with SLE, but the common outcome of the failure to establish tolerance early during B-cell development is a significant increase in the number of self-reactive antibodies in the mature naïve B-cell repertoire.

Self-reactive naïve B cells do not secrete Igs and are therefore not directly involved in the pathogenesis of SLE. Also, we did not find self-reactive antibodies from mature naïve B cells of SLE patients enriched for anti–nuclear antigen specificities.[29] However, Ig-secreting plasma cells and memory B cells develop from naïve precursors after the cells become activated by antigen and participate in the germinal center response, where they acquire somatic hypermutations and undergo affinity maturation.[34] Thus, due to the high frequency of self-reactive antibodies in the naïve B-cell pool, antinuclear specificities might readily be generated, expanded, and selected once the cell becomes activated. In this context, many factors involved in the development of SLE—for example, impaired clearance of apoptotic material—altered signaling thresholds for B-cell activation, or soluble factors such as BAFF may play an important role in the activation or survival of self-reactive B cells and the development of clinical symptoms.[35–42]

Treatment of SLE patients includes steroid hormones and in very severe cases cytotoxic drugs, but so far there is no cure for the disease.[43] Restoration of early B-cell tolerance checkpoints might be a future goal in the treatment of SLE, but the effect of current therapies on the establishment of B-cell tolerance has not been determined.

So far, we have identified two checkpoints during B-cell development where self-reactive antibodies are removed from the naïve repertoire.[2] However, whether there are further checkpoints for self-tolerance after activation of naïve B cells still needs to be tested. After antigen-mediated activation, somatic hypermutation introduces random Ig gene mutations to increase the specificity of an antibody for its (foreign) antigen, but such mutations may also be potentially harmful and shift the antibody specificity toward anti-self.[34] One can therefore imagine that tolerance mechanisms play a role in the selection of activated B cells and that such a filter is defective in patients with SLE.

Autoantibodies are detected in many autoimmune diseases and can play an important role in their pathogenesis. To understand how autoantibodies are deregulated in autoimmunity and how B-cell tolerance checkpoints can be influenced will provide a foundation to establish new and more enduring therapies.

ACKNOWLEDGMENTS

This work was supported by grants from the Dana Foundation (H.W.), the Charles A. Dana Foundation (S.Y.), and the Studienstiftung des Deutschen Volkes (J.H.). One of the authors (S.Y.) is a Charles A. Revson Fellow in Biomedical Research.

[*Competing interests*: The authors declare that they have no competing financial interests.]

REFERENCES

1. TONEGAWA, S. 1983. Somatic generation of antibody diversity. Nature **302:** 575–581.
2. WARDEMANN, H., S. YURASOV, A. SCHAEFER, *et al.* 2003. Predominant autoantibody production by early human B cell precursors. Science **301:** 1374–1377.
3. JANKOVIC, M., R. CASELLAS, N. YANNOUTSOS, *et al.* 2004. RAGs and regulation of autoantibodies. Annu. Rev. Immunol. **22:** 485–501.
4. GAY, D., T. SAUNDERS, S. CAMPER, *et al.* 1993. Receptor editing: an approach by autoreactive B cells to escape tolerance. J. Exp. Med. **177:** 999–1008.
5. RADIC, M.Z., J. ERIKSON, S. LITWIN, *et al.* 1993. B lymphocytes may escape tolerance by revising their antigen receptors. J. Exp. Med. **177:** 1165–1173.
6. TIEGS, S.L., D.M. RUSSELL & D. NEMAZEE. 1993. Receptor editing in self-reactive bone marrow B cells. J. Exp. Med. **177:** 1009–1020.
7. NEMAZEE, D.A. & K. BURKI. 1989. Clonal deletion of B lymphocytes in a transgenic mouse bearing anti-MHC class I antibody genes. Nature **337:** 562–566.
8. GOODNOW, C.C., J. CROSBIE, S. ADELSTEIN, *et al.* 1988. Altered immunoglobulin expression and functional silencing of self-reactive B lymphocytes in transgenic mice. Nature **334:** 676–682.
9. MEFFRE, E., A. SCHAEFER, H. WARDEMANN, *et al.* 2004. Surrogate light chain expressing human peripheral B cells produce self-reactive antibodies. J. Exp. Med. **199:** 145–150.
10. KLONOWSKI, K.D., L.L. PRIMIANO & M. MONESTIER. 1999. Atypical VH-D-JH rearrangements in newborn autoimmune MRL mice. J. Immunol. **162:** 1566–1572.
11. ICHIYOSHI, Y. & P. CASALI. 1994. Analysis of the structural correlates for antibody polyreactivity by multiple reassortments of chimeric human immunoglobulin heavy and light chain V segments. J. Exp. Med. **180:** 885–895.
12. CROUZIER, R., T. MARTIN & J.L. PASQUALI. 1995. Heavy chain variable region, light chain variable region, and heavy chain CDR3 influences on the mono- and polyreactivity and on the affinity of human monoclonal rheumatoid factors. J. Immunol. **154:** 4526–4535.
13. AGUILERA, I., J. MELERO, A. NUNEZ-ROLDAN, *et al.* 2001. Molecular structure of eight human autoreactive monoclonal antibodies. Immunology **102:** 273–280.
14. NG, Y.S., H. WARDEMANN, J. CHELNIS, *et al.* 2004. Bruton's tyrosine kinase is essential for human B cell tolerance. J. Exp. Med. **200:** 927–934.
15. RETTER, M.W. & D. NEMAZEE. 1998. Receptor editing occurs frequently during normal B cell development. J. Exp. Med. **188:** 1231–1238.
16. CASELLAS, R., T.A. SHIH, M. KLEINEWIETFELD, *et al.* 2001. Contribution of receptor editing to the antibody repertoire. Science **291:** 1541–1544.
17. OBERDOERFFER, P., T.I. NOVOBRANTSEVA & K. RAJEWSKY. 2003. Expression of a targeted lambda1 light chain gene is developmentally regulated and independent of Igkappa rearrangements. J. Exp. Med. **197:** 1165–1172.

18. HIETER, P.A., S.J. KORSMEYER, T.A. WALDMANN, *et al.* 1981. Human immunoglobulin kappa light-chain genes are deleted or rearranged in lambda-producing B cells. Nature **290:** 368–372.
19. FARNER, N.L., T. DORNER & P.E. LIPSKY. 1999. Molecular mechanisms and selection influence the generation of the human V lambda J lambda repertoire. J. Immunol. **162:** 2137–2145.
20. BRAUNINGER, A., T. GOOSSENS, K. RAJEWSKY, *et al.* 2001. Regulation of immunoglobulin light chain gene rearrangements during early B cell development in the human. Eur. J. Immunol. **31:** 3631–3637.
21. WARDEMANN, H., J. HAMMERSEN & M.C. NUSSENZWEIG. 2004. Human autoantibody silencing by immunoglobulin light chains. J. Exp. Med. **200:** 191–199.
22. TAN, E.M. 1989. Antinuclear antibodies: diagnostic markers for autoimmune diseases and probes for cell biology. Adv. Immunol. **44:** 93–151.
23. HAHN, B.H. 1998. Antibodies to DNA. N. Engl. J. Med. **338:** 1359–1368.
24. KOTZIN, B.L. 1996. Systemic lupus erythematosus. Cell **85:** 303–306.
25. DAVIDSON, A. & B. DIAMOND. 2001. Autoimmune diseases. N. Engl. J. Med. **345:** 340–350.
26. THEOFILOPOULOS, A.N. & F.J. DIXON. 1985. Murine models of systemic lupus erythematosus. Adv. Immunol. **37:** 269–390.
27. KONO, D.H. & A.N. THEOFILOPOULOS. 2000. Genetics of systemic autoimmunity in mouse models of lupus. Int. Rev. Immunol. **19:** 367–387.
28. WAKELAND, E.K., K. LIU, R.R. GRAHAM, *et al.* 2001. Delineating the genetic basis of systemic lupus erythematosus. Immunity **15:** 397–408.
29. YURASOV, S., H. WARDEMANN, J. HAMMERSEN, *et al.* 2005. Defective B cell tolerance checkpoints in systemic lupus erythematosus. J. Exp. Med. **201:** 703–711.
30. DORNER, T., S.J. FOSTER, N.L. FARNER, *et al.* 1998. Immunoglobulin kappa chain receptor editing in systemic lupus erythematosus. J. Clin. Invest. **102:** 688–694.
31. DORNER, T., N.L. FARNER & P.E. LIPSKY. 1999. Ig lambda and heavy chain gene usage in early untreated systemic lupus erythematosus suggests intensive B cell stimulation. J. Immunol. **163:** 1027–1036.
32. HANSEN, A., T. DORNER & P.E. LIPSKY. 2000. Use of immunoglobulin variable-region genes by normal subjects and patients with systemic lupus erythematosus. Int. Arch. Allergy Immunol. **123:** 36–45.
33. DORNER, T. & P.E. LIPSKY. 2001. Immunoglobulin variable-region gene usage in systemic autoimmune diseases. Arthritis Rheum. **44:** 2715–2727.
34. WOLNIAK, K.L., S.M. SHINALL & T.J. WALDSCHMIDT. 2004. The germinal center response. Crit. Rev. Immunol. **24:** 39–65.
35. CASCIOLA-ROSEN, L.A., G. ANHALT & A. ROSEN. 1994. Autoantigens targeted in systemic lupus erythematosus are clustered in two populations of surface structures on apoptotic keratinocytes. J. Exp. Med. **179:** 1317–1330.
36. MEVORACH, D., J.L. ZHOU, X. SONG, *et al.* 1998. Systemic exposure to irradiated apoptotic cells induces autoantibody production. J. Exp. Med. **188:** 387–392.
37. LEADBETTER, E.A., I.R. RIFKIN & A. MARSHAK-ROTHSTEIN. 2003. Toll-like receptors and activation of autoreactive B cells. Curr. Dir. Autoimmun. **6:** 105–122.
38. MACKAY, F., S.A. WOODCOCK, P. LAWTON, *et al.* 1999. Mice transgenic for BAFF develop lymphocytic disorders along with autoimmune manifestations. J. Exp. Med. **190:** 1697–1710.
39. GROSS, J.A., J. JOHNSTON, S. MUDRI, *et al.* 2000. TACI and BCMA are receptors for a TNF homologue implicated in B-cell autoimmune disease. Nature **404:** 995–999.
40. KHARE, S.D., I. SAROSI, X.Z. XIA, *et al.* 2000. Severe B cell hyperplasia and autoimmune disease in TALL-1 transgenic mice. Proc. Natl. Acad. Sci. USA **97:** 3370–3375.
41. LESLEY, R., Y. XU, S.L. KALLED, *et al.* 2004. Reduced competitiveness of autoantigen-engaged B cells due to increased dependence on BAFF. Immunity **20:** 441–453.
42. THIEN, M., T.G. PHAN, S. GARDAM, *et al.* 2004. Excess BAFF rescues self-reactive B cells from peripheral deletion and allows them to enter forbidden follicular and marginal zone niches. Immunity **20:** 785–798.
43. MERRILL, J.T., D. ERKAN & J.P. BUYON. 2004. Challenges in bringing the bench to bedside in drug development for SLE. Nat. Rev. Drug. Discov. **3:** 1036–1046.

Potential Contribution of V_H Gene Replacement in Immunity and Disease

YANWEN LIU,[a,b] RUN FAN,[a,c] SONG ZHOU,[d] ZHIHONG YU,[a,b] AND ZHIXIN ZHANG[a–c]

[a]*Division of Developmental and Clinical Immunology, University of Alabama at Birmingham, Birmingham, Alabama 35294, USA*

[b]*Department of Medicine, University of Alabama at Birmingham, Birmingham, Alabama 35294, USA*

[c]*Department of Microbiology, University of Alabama at Birmingham, Birmingham, Alabama 35294, USA*

[d]*Department of Computer Sciences, University of Alabama at Birmingham, Birmingham, Alabama 35294, USA*

ABSTRACT: V_H replacement occurs through RAG-mediated recombination between a cryptic recombination signal sequence (cRSS) presented in a rearranged V_H gene and a 23-bp RSS from an upstream V_H gene. V_H replacement renews the entire V_H coding region and extends the immunoglobulin heavy-chain (IgH) CDR3 regions preferentially with charged amino acids. V_H replacement occurs in bone marrow–immature B cells and contributes significantly to the primary B-cell repertoire in humans. However, the biological significance of V_H replacement is not clear. Our recent studies revealed elevated frequencies of V_H replacement products in different autoimmune diseases, including rheumatoid arthritis, systemic lupus erythematosus, and Sjögren's syndrome. Moreover, elevated frequencies of V_H replacement products were also found in patients with human immunodeficiency virus or hepatitis C virus infections. These results provide the first clue that V_H replacement contributes to autoimmune disease and antiviral immunity, and they also suggest a potential link between viral infection and autoimmune disease.

KEYWORDS: V_H replacement; autoimmune disease; antiviral response

RAG-MEDIATED V(D)J RECOMBINATION

To protect our bodies against different infectious agents, such as bacteria or viruses, the immune system must generate virtually unlimited specificities of antibodies through somatic rearrangement of previously separated variable (V), diversity (D) (for heavy chain only), and joining (J) gene segments to form the variable domain exons of immunoglobulin genes, a process known as V(D)J recombination.[1–3]

Address for correspondence: Zhixin Zhang, Ph.D., University of Alabama at Birmingham, WTI378, 1824 6th Ave. S., Birmingham, AL 35294-3300. Voice: 205-974-6761; fax: 205-934-1875.

zhixin.zhang@ccc.uab.edu

**Ann. N.Y. Acad. Sci. 1062: 175–181 (2005). © 2005 New York Academy of Sciences.
doi: 10.1196/annals.1358.020**

The V(D)J recombination process is catalyzed by a pair of recombination activating gene products, namely, the RAG1 and RAG2 proteins.[4–6] Specific joining of the V, D, and J gene segments is directed by the recombination signal sequences (RSS) flanking these gene segments.[1] Each RSS is composed of a highly conserved heptamer (5′-CACTGTG-3′) and a nonamer (5′-ACAAAAACC-3′) separated by a nonconserved spacer region either 12 bp or 23 bp in length.[1,7] Both the heptamer and nonamer sequences are important for RAG1/2 binding and subsequent DNA cleavage, as modifications of the conserved heptamer or nonamer nucleotides profoundly compromise RAG-mediated recombination efficiency.[7–9] The length of the spacer region between the nonamer and the heptamer plays a crucial role in directing the joint formation. Known as the 12/23 rule, joint formation preferentially occurs through a gene segment tagged with a 12-bp spacer RSS and another gene segment tagged with a 23-bp spacer RSS.[1,7]

SECONDARY RECOMBINATION OF IMMUNOGLOBULIN GENES

During RAG-mediated V(D)J rearrangement, formation of the coding end joint is imprecise. This random feature provides the necessary diversity for the repertoire, but also leads to a significant amount of unwanted nonfunctional rearrangement products. On the other hand, the V(D)J recombination process will also generate other unwanted immunoglobulin products, such as μ heavy chains that fail to pair with surrogate or conventional light chains or antigen receptors that recognize self-antigens. In all these cases, B cells have to reinitiate the recombination process to rearrange the antigen receptor genes on heavy or light chain, a process known as receptor editing.[10–12]

Most previous studies of receptor editing have focused on the light-chain genes.[10–12] Secondary rearrangement of immunoglobulin light-chain (IgL) genes occurs by simply joining an upstream V_L with a downstream J_L gene segment to delete the primary V_L–J_L rearrangement. The organization of the V_L and J_L germline gene segments within the Ig κ or λ loci allows continuous IgL secondary rearrangement as long as the recombination machinery is operative, the locus remains accessible, and unrearranged gene segments are still available.[13] Also, cells with nonfunctional or dysfunctional κ rearrangements still have the opportunity to rearrange their λ light-chain genes.[12,13] Thus, immature B cells can generate a new variable region. This process, known as receptor editing, can be used to rescue an autoreactive B cell by changing its antigenic specificity.[10–12]

V_H GENE REPLACEMENT

Secondary rearrangement of an upstream V_H to a preformed $V_HD_HJ_H$ gene is apparently difficult, because all the intervening D_H gene segments were deleted during the primary V_H to D_HJ_H rearrangement, which leaves no 12-bp RSS to recombine with the 23-bp RSS flanked V_H genes.[10–12] However, functional IgH genes have been found to be generated in mouse pre–B-cell lines harboring nonfunctional IgH rearrangements, thus revealing a potential rearrangement process using a cryptic

RSS (cRSS) site embedded within the third framework region of the rearranged V_H gene, a process termed V_H gene replacement.[14–17]

The concept of V_H gene replacement has a long history. However, the molecular basis and natural occurrence of V_H replacement during B-cell development have only recently been demonstrated. EU12 cells, a B-lineage cell line established from a childhood acute lymphocytic leukemia, undergo continuous pro–B-cell to pre–B- and B-cell differentiation and generate intraclonal diversified repertoires using different V_H and V_L genes.[18] Detailed analysis of the IgH gene sequences identified sequence motifs within the V–D junctions that match with the 3′ end of other germline V_H genes.[19] These findings suggested a model of serial V_H gene replacement. This model was fully demonstrated by the detection of double-stranded DNA breaks at the cRSS border and by identification of the V_H replacement excision circles derived from each step of the V_H replacement reaction.[20]

The involvement of the heptameric cRSS site in RAG-mediated recombination was further confirmed by *in vitro* binding and cleavage assays using recombinant RAG1 and RAG2 core proteins. Recombinant RAG proteins bind efficiently to each of the cRSS sites derived from representative V_H germline genes.[20] Moreover, specific recombination between a cRSS and a 23-bp RSS was also tested in a coupled cleavage reaction, which occurs in the similar fashion as a pair of 12- and 23-bp RSS sites, despite the lower efficiency.[20]

Using ligation-mediated polymerase chain reaction (LM-PCR), we were also able to detect double-stranded DNA breaks at the cRSS border in immature B cells from the bone marrow, which provided the first evidence for the natural occurrence of V_H replacement during human B-cell development.[20] This finding is consistent with the inducible expression of the RAG genes in immature B cells and their ability to undergo secondary rearrangement of the IgL genes.[21–24] The occurrence of V_H replacement and light-chain gene secondary rearrangement in the bone marrow immature B cells further indicates that this is the preferential stage for receptor editing.

Immature B cells are generated throughout life in the bone marrow, and they migrate from the bone marrow into the circulation as they mature.[25] During inflammatory responses, however, cells at earlier stages of B-lineage development can be released from bone marrow in elevated numbers. Pro–B-, pre–B-, and immature B cells may thus migrate prematurely to secondary lymphoid organs, such as the spleen and lymph nodes, in response to inflammatory signals. Since these cells may still express the RAG genes, they have the potential to rearrange their light-chain genes in the periphery.[11,26] The capacity of these cells to undergo V_H replacement and generate new IgH genes outside of the bone marrow remains to be determined.

V_H REPLACEMENT CONTRIBUTES SIGNIFICANTLY TO THE PRIMARY B-CELL REPERTOIRE IN HUMANS

The remarkable diversity of the primary antibody repertoire generated during B-cell development is created through several different mechanisms. The random joining of the different V_H, D_H, and J_H genes provides the foundation of the diversification process.[1] The imprecise joint formation during the recombination mediated as a result of exonuclease activity or hairpin opening adds another layer of diversification.[7] The addition of nontemplate N nucleotides at the V–D and D–J joints and exonuclease activity by the different isoforms of TdT further contribute an almost unlimited diversification at the sites of V–D–J joining.[27,28] The subsequent use of similar diversification mechanisms to create light-chain genes provides another step of the primary repertoire diversification process. After generation of the functional IgH and IgL genes, editing these receptor genes by secondary rearrangements should also provide additional diversification to the repertoire.[13,23]

The elucidation of the V_H replacement process in the EU12 cells suggested a method to evaluate the contribution of V_H replacement to the diversification of primary B-cell repertoire by searching for the potential V_H replacement footprints within the V_H–D_H junction of IgH genes. Using this method, we could assign about 5% of the normal IgH sequences from 300 IgH sequences obtained from peripheral blood B cells as potential V_H replacement products,[20] suggesting a significant contribution of V_H replacement to the primary B-cell repertoire. Using a computer-based approach, we recently analyzed 15,000 IgH sequences from the IMGT database and revealed that the overall frequency of V_H replacement products is about 10%. These numbers already represented a significant contribution of V_H replacement to the B-cell repertoire; the actual frequency of V_H replacement is likely to be even higher. Our method for determining potential V_H replacement products relies on identification of the V_H replacement footprints, which could be nibbled away on both ends by exonuclease activity during coding joint formation, and they can later be mutated by somatic hypermutation. All these alterations would obscure the V_H replacement footprint sequences required for the analysis.

BIOLOGICAL SIGNIFICANCE OF V_H GENE REPLACEMENT

The biological significance of V_H gene replacement was first suggested by studies of a knock-in mouse carrying an IgH transgene encoding anti-DNA specificity in the J_H locus.[29] In such mice, the artificially inserted anti-DNA V_H gene was replaced by upstream V_H, D_H, or V_HD_H genes through recombination with the cRSS heptamer embedded at the 3′ end of the rearranged V_H genes. Sequence analysis identified three different types of recombination events, V_H→VDJ, D_H→VDJ, and V_H→D_H–VDJ.[29] The V_H replacement used to delete the anti-DNA specificity appeared to occur at the pre–B- to immature B–transitional stages in the bone marrow,[29] presumably after encountering self-antigens.

Our analysis of the amino acids contributed by the V_H replacement footprints indicates an unexpected consequence of V_H gene replacement, in which V_H replacement footprints preferentially contribute charged amino acids into the IgH CDR3 regions.[20] This feature contrasts sharply with the low frequency of charged amino acids encoded by germline D_H genes in both human and mouse or the N region sequences contributed by TdT activity.

The biological significance of the charged amino acids contributed by the V_H replacement "footprints" is unclear. Addition of charged amino acids into the CDR3 region could improve the antigen-binding affinity toward charged antigens, such as bacterial or viral antigens; however, it may also generate self-reactivity, as highly charged amino acids within the CDR3 regions are frequently seen in autoreactive antibodies. For example, Arg residues are frequently found within the IgH CDR3 regions of anti-DNA antibodies.[30] This line of reasoning indicates that V_H

replacement may contribute to the generation of autoreactive antibodies. Indeed, in mice carrying the knock-in anti-DNA IgH gene, other self-reactive antibodies may be generated through V_H replacement reaction.[31,32]

ELEVATED FREQUENCY OF V_H REPLACEMENT PRODUCTS IN AUTOIMMUNE DISEASES

The preferential contribution of charged amino acids into the IgH CDR3 regions suggested that V_H replacement contributes to the generation of autoreactive antibodies. Our analysis of many IgH sequences provided the first clue that the frequencies of V_H replacement products were higher in different autoimmune diseases, such as rheumatoid arthritis (RA) (30%) and Sjögren's syndrome (22%) or IgH genes encoding autoantibodies (22%) or anti-dsDNA antibodies (21%). In one early RA patient, we identified clonally related V_H replacement products in the lymphoid follicles of synovial tissue, which further suggested that V_H replacement contributes to the generation of autoreactive antibodies in RA. In systemic lupus erythematosus patients, it has been shown that a subgroup of plasma cells ($CD19^{low}CD27^{high}$) in the peripheral blood correlates with the disease activity and is responsible for the production of autoreactive antibodies.[33,34] Analysis of the IgH sequences obtained from this subgroup of plasma cells revealed a significantly higher frequency of V_H replacement products (48%), indicating that V_H replacement may contribute to the generation of autoreactive antibodies in SLE patients. Almost all the V_H replacement footprints contribute Arg residues into the IgH CDR3 regions, which may contribute to their anti-DNA specificities.

ELEVATED FREQUENCY OF V_H REPLACEMENT PRODUCTS IN ANTIVIRAL RESPONSE

It is difficult to believe that the often-occurring V_H replacement is used mainly to generate autoreactive antibodies. This powerful repertoire diversification process must have unexplored beneficial functions for our immune system. Our recent analysis of many IgH sequences from the IMGT database provided the first clue that V_H replacement may contribute to antiviral response, because the frequency of V_H replacement products is significantly higher (33%) in IgH genes encoding anti–human immunodeficiency virus (HIV) antibodies. This hypothesis was further supported by detailed analysis of 421 IgH sequences obtained from mucosal plasma cells of HIV-infected individuals. The frequency of V_H replacement products is 23%, which is significantly higher than that of normal peripheral B cells. Also, these V_H replacement products harbor somatic mutations, suggesting that these V_H replacement products participate in the anti-HIV immune response.

To determine whether V_H replacement also contributes in other antiviral responses, we also analyzed a limited number of IgH sequences obtained from patients with the hepatitis C virus. The overall frequency of V_H replacement in IgH genes from patients with hepatitis C virus is 38%, which is significantly higher than that of normal peripheral B cells.

These results provide the first evidence that V_H replacement contributes to antiviral response in general. Interestingly, the coincidence of elevated frequencies of V_H replacement products in patients with either viral infections or autoimmune diseases also suggested a potential link between viral infection and autoimmune diseases.

ACKNOWLEDGMENTS

Z.Z. is supported in part by a K01 grant (AR048592) from NIH/NIAMS and by the Human Immunology Program of the Dana Foundation.

[*Competing interests*: The authors declare that they have no competing financial interests.]

REFERENCES

1. Tonegawa, S. 1983. Somatic generation of antibody diversity. Nature **302:** 575–581.
2. Rajewsky, K. 1996. Clonal selection and learning in the antibody system. Nature **381:** 751–758.
3. Bassing, C.H., W. Swat, and F.W. Alt. 2002. The mechanism and regulation of chromosomal v(d)j recombination. Cell **109:** S45–S55.
4. Schatz, D.G. & D. Baltimore. 1988. Stable expression of immunoglobulin gene V(D)J recombinase activity by gene transfer into 3T3 fibroblasts. Cell **53:** 107–115.
5. Schatz, D.G., M.A. Oettinger & D. Baltimore. 1989. The V(D)J recombination activating gene, RAG-1. Cell **59:** 1035–1048.
6. Oettinger, M.A., D.G. Schatz, C. Gorka & D. Baltimore. 1990. RAG-1 and RAG-2, adjacent genes that synergistically activate V(D)J recombination. Science **248:** 1517–1523.
7. Lewis, S.M. 1994. The mechanism of V(D)J joining: lessons from molecular, immunological, and comparative analyses. Adv. Immunol **56:** 27–150.
8. Difilippantonio, M.J., C.J. McMahan, Q.M. Eastman, *et al.* 1996. RAG1 mediates signal sequence recognition and recruitment of RAG2 in V(D)J recombination. Cell **87:** 253–262.
9. Ramsden, D.A., J.F. McBlane, D. van Gent & M. Gellert. 1996. Distinct DNA sequence and structure requirements for the two steps of V(D)J recombination signal cleavage. EMBO J **15:** 3197–3206.
10. Radic, M. & M. Zouali. 1996. Receptor editing, immune diversification and self-tolerance. Immunity **5:** 505–511.
11. Nussenzweig, M.C. 1998. Immune receptor editing: revise and select. Cell **95:** 875–878.
12. King, L.B. & J.G. Monroe. 2001. Immunology. B cell receptor rehabilitation—pausing to reflect. Science **291:** 1503–1505.
13. Casellas, R., T.A. Shih, M. Kleinewietfeld, *et al.* 2001. Contribution of receptor editing to the antibody repertoire. Science **291:** 1541–1544.
14. Kleinfield, R., R.R. Hardy, D. Tarlinton, *et al.* 1986. Recombination between an expressed immunoglobulin heavy-chain gene and a germline variable gene segment in a Ly 1+ B-cell lymphoma. Nature **322:** 843–846.
15. Reth, M., P. Gehrmann, E. Petrac & P. Wiese. 1986. A novel VH to VHDJH joining mechanism in heavy-chain-negative (null) pre-B cells results in heavy-chain production. Nature **322:** 840–842.
16. Covey, L.R., P. Ferrier & F.W. Alt. 1990. VH to VHDJH rearrangement is mediated by the internal VH heptamer. Int. Immunol. **2:** 579–583.
17. Usuda, S., T. Takemori, M. Matsuoka, *et al.* 1992. Immunoglobulin V gene replacement is caused by the intramolecular DNA deletion mechanism. EMBO J. **11:** 611–618.

18. WANG, Y.H., Z. ZHANG, P.D. BURROWS, *et al.* 2003. V(D)J recombinatorial repertoire diversification during intraclonal pro-B to B-cell differentiation. Blood **101:** 1030–1037.
19. ZHANG, Z., Y.H. WANG, M. ZEMLIN, *et al.* 2003. Molecular mechanism of serial VH gene replacement. Ann. N.Y. Acad. Sci. **987:** 270–273.
20. ZHANG, Z., M. ZEMLIN, Y.-H. WANG, *et al.* 2003. Contribution of VH gene replacement to the primary B cell repertoire. Immunity **19:** 21–31.
21. HERTZ, M. & D. NEMAZEE. 1997. BCR ligation induces receptor editing in IgM+IgD- bone marrow B cells in vitro. Immunity **6:** 429–436.
22. MELAMED, D. & D. NEMAZEE. 1997. Self-antigen does not accelerate immature B cell apoptosis, but stimulates receptor editing as a consequence of developmental arrest. Proc. Natl. Acad. Sci. USA **94:** 9267–9272.
23. MELAMED, D., R.J. BENSCHOP, J.C. CAMBIER & D. NEMAZEE. 1998. Developmental regulation of B lymphocyte immune tolerance compartmentalizes clonal selection from receptor selection. Cell **92:** 173–182.
24. SANDEL, P.C. & J.G. MONROE. 1999. Negative selection of immature B cells by receptor editing or deletion is determined by site of antigen encounter. Immunity **10:** 289–299.
25. NUNEZ, C., N. NISHIMOTO, G.L. GARTLAND, *et al.* 1996. B cells are generated throughout life in humans. J. Immunol. **156:** 866–872.
26. NEMAZEE, D. & K.A. HOGQUIST. 2003. Antigen receptor selection by editing or downregulation of V(D)J recombination. Curr. Opin. Immunol. **15:** 182–189.
27. DESIDERIO, S.V., G.D. YANCOPOULOS, M. Paskind, *et al.* 1984. Insertion of N regions into heavy-chain genes is correlated with expression of terminal deoxytransferase in B cells. Nature **311:** 752–755.
28. THAI, T.H., M.M. PURUGGANAN, D.B. ROTH & J.F. KEARNEY. 2002. Distinct and opposite diversifying activities of terminal transferase splice variants. Nat. Immunol. **3:** 457–462.
29. CHEN, C., Z. NAGY, E.L. PRAK & M. WEIGERT. 1995. Immunoglobulin heavy chain gene replacement: a mechanism of receptor editing. Immunity **3:** 747–755.
30. RADIC, M.Z., J. MACKLE, J. ERIKSON, *et al.* 1993. Residues that mediate DNA binding of autoimmune antibodies. J. Immunol. **150:** 4966–4977.
31. SEKIGUCHI, D.R., S.M. JAINANDUNSING, M.L. FIELDS, *et al.* 2002. Chronic graft-versus-host in Ig knockin transgenic mice abrogates B cell tolerance in anti-double-stranded DNA B cells. J. Immunol. **168:** 4142–4153.
32. SEKIGUCHI, D.R., R.A. EISENBERG, & M. WEIGERT. 2003. Secondary heavy chain rearrangement: a mechanism for generating anti-double-stranded DNA B cells. J. Exp. Med. **197:** 27–39.
33. JACOBI, A.M., M. ODENDAHL, K. REITER, *et al.* 2003. Correlation between circulating CD27high plasma cells and disease activity in patients with systemic lupus erythematosus. Arthritis Rheum. **48:** 1332–1342.
34. DORNER, T. & P.E. LIPSKY. 2004. Correlation of circulating CD27high plasma cells and disease activity in systemic lupus erythematosus. Lupus **13:** 283–289.

Costimulatory Pathways in Rheumatoid Synovitis and T-Cell Senescence

JÖRG J. GORONZY,[a] GABRIELLA HENEL,[a,b] HIROKAZU SAWAI,[a] KARNAIL SINGH,[a] EUN BONG LEE,[a] SERGEY PRYSHCHEP,[a] AND CORNELIA M. WEYAND[a]

[a]*Kathleen B. and Mason I. Lowance Center for Human Immunology, Emory University, Atlanta, Georgia 30322, USA*

[b]*Department of Immunology, Mayo Graduate School, Rochester, Minnesota 55901, USA*

ABSTRACT: The pathogenesis of rheumatoid arthritis (RA) is determined by a complex interaction of genetic and environmental factors. Of all risk factors, age has the largest impact. RA occurs most often during the postmenopausal period of life, with incidence rates peaking in the eighth decade. While age is generally accepted as an etiologic factor for failure of immunocompetence, much less is understood about the role of T-cell senescence in autoimmunity. We have hypothesized that senescent T cells are particularly prone to be activated in specialized microenvironments, such as the synovial membrane. CD4 T cells in the senescence program were identified by the loss of CD28. Gene expression profiling documented that CD28⁻ T cells have acquired a spectrum of regulatory receptors that are usually seen only on NK cells. Such regulatory receptors include stimulatory and inhibitory members of the killer immunoglobulin–like receptor (KIR) family, the stimulatory c-type lectin receptor NKG2D, and CX_3CR1, the receptor for the chemokine fractalkine. Synovial fibroblasts express the relevant ligands, thus providing stimulatory signals to tissue-infiltrating T cells. The signaling pathways of these regulatory receptors are complex and dependent on the individual T cells, some of which express important adapter molecules such as DAP10 and DAP12. Inhibitory KIRs on T cells are often only partially functional. Our data suggest that, by virtue of altered receptor profiles, conventional tolerance mechanisms can be evaded in the aging host. By acquiring a new set of regulatory receptors, senescent CD4 T cells become responsive to novel environmental cues and find ideal stimulatory conditions in the synovial microenvironment.

KEYWORDS: rheumatoid arthritis; age; T-cell costimulation; autoimmunity; killer immunoglobulin–like receptor; NKG2D; synoviocyte

Rheumatoid arthritis (RA) is a systemic, chronic inflammatory disease that manifests itself predominantly as inflammation of diarthrodial joints. The last decade has seen a divergence between emergence of successful novel therapeutic approaches

Address for correspondence: Jörg J. Goronzy, M.D., Ph.D., Kathleen B. and Mason I. Lowance Center for Human Immunology, Emory University School of Medicine, Rm. 1003, Woodruff Memorial Research Bldg., 101 Woodruff Circle, Atlanta, GA 30322. Voice: 404-727-7310; fax: 404-727-7371.

jgoronz@emory.edu

Ann. N.Y. Acad. Sci. 1062: 182–194 (2005). © 2005 New York Academy of Sciences. doi: 10.1196/annals.1358.022

and lack in progress of pathogenetic understanding. Several biological reagents have been developed that have made inroads into clinical practice and have led to better control of the inflammatory response in many patients and the prevention of joint destruction. The introduction of tumor necrosis factor α (TNF-α) blockers into the therapeutic armamentarium in RA is one of the prime examples of how targeting a biological mediator can be successful.[1–3] Studies of human synovium from RA patients had led to the concept that TNF-α is positioned high in the hierarchy of inflammatory cytokines. This concept, which was not supported by arthritic animal models—with the later exception of the TNF-α transgenic mouse—was directly tested in clinical studies.[4] It is now known that TNF-α is an important effector molecule in many but not all steroid-responsive diseases and that RA is one of them.[5,6] However, TNF-α overproduction does not explain the pathogenesis of the disease, and anti–TNF-α treatment does not induce long-lasting remission, possibly excepting some patients with very early disease. Similarly, B-cell depletion was introduced into clinical studies when there was little pathogenetic evidence to support a unique role for B cells in RA.[7] Rheumatoid factor had been known for decades as an autoantibody with unique immunoregulatory properties;[8] however, it was not considered an important pathogenetic mechanism. Some clues came from studies in a human synovium–severe combined immunodeficient (SCID) mouse chimera model that had shown synovial inflammation to be partially B-cell dependent.[9] The exact mechanism of how B-cell depletion is efficacious remains unknown.[10]

Thus, although the landscape of treatment approaches in RA is changing, the dominant pathogenetic models of RA have undergone only minor modification. The synoviocyte-centric model that postulates a dedifferentiation of the fibroblast-like synoviocytes fails to explain the systemic complexity of the disease process. The T cell–centric model, originally based on the finding of the HLA-DRB1 association of the disease, is that of classical autoimmunity, namely, that RA is the consequence of an immune response toward arthritogenic self-antigens in restriction to disease-associated major histocompatibility complex genes. This model has been explored in many mouse models of increasing genetic sophistication but has failed to have a major clinical impact.

A reassessment of the pathogenetic models is therefore warranted. This appraisal has to start with the human disease itself and identify key determinants of epidemiology, clinical presentation, and treatment responses that could guide pathogenetic considerations. One of the key epidemiological features of the disease is that age is the strongest risk factor.

AGE AS A RISK FOR RHEUMATOID ARTHRITIS

RA is recognized as a disease that preferentially starts in women after menopause. More detailed epidemiologic population-based studies by Doran *et al.* have documented that the yearly incidence of RA continues to increase with age and peaks somewhere in the late 70s to early 80s.[11] The yearly incidence of RA around the age of 30 is about 10 per 100,000 individuals and about 10-fold higher at the age of 60 years. The finding that age is a risk factor for autoimmunity appears paradoxical. RA is considered an autoimmune disease that is initiated by the recognition of arthritogenic self-antigens in restriction to disease-associated HLA-DR molecules.

The ability of the immune system to respond to exogenous antigens, such as viral infections or vaccines, declines with age.[12] With increasing age, failing immune responses are a major reason for declining health. Signs of defective immunocompetence are already emerging in the sixth decade of life with increased morbidity and mortality from influenza infections and more frequent reactivation of varicella zoster infections. In healthy elderly people older than 65 years, only 15%–20% have an immune response to influenza vaccination that leads to an increase in serum antibody titers specific for influenza hemagglutinins.[13] How then can age favor priming and amplification of a self-antigen–specific immune response that leads to RA if T-cell responses to foreign antigens are compromised?

IMPACT OF AGE ON IMMUNE FUNCTION

The adaptive immune system undergoes complex changes with age. Understanding these changes will be pivotal for identifying the mechanisms underlying the age risk factor in RA and eventually provide insights into its pathogenesis. In particular, the T-cell system is highly dynamic with complex kinetics and therefore prone to systemic distortions and replicative senescence. Depending on the subpopulation of T cells and the presence or absence of stressors, T-cell survival times vary from half-times of a few hours to months or even close to 1 year. Naturally, the time span in which such T-cell dynamics occur, the size of the host, and the availability of space all have tremendous influences on the patterns that evolve as a consequence. Most rodents are therefore poor models that do not reflect characteristic findings in humans.

Surprisingly, the human naïve T-cell repertoire is relatively robust to the effects of aging, although generation of novel T cells through the thymus rapidly declines with age and is minimal to nonexistent after the ages of 40–50 years.[14] Despite this thymic demise, the size and diversity of the naïve repertoire is maintained up to the ages of 65–70 years,[15] after which it rapidly collapses.[16] Age-dependent changes are readily detected in the memory T-cell compartment.[17] CD4 and especially CD8 T cells undergo phenotypic changes, of which the loss of CD28 expression has been most widely studied.[18,19] At the age of 65 years, approximately 40% of all CD8 T cells and few percent of CD4 T cells lack the expression of CD28. Loss of CD28 is controlled at the level of transcriptional initiation and varies widely from person to person.[20]

AGE-DEPENDENT EXPRESSION OF REGULATORY RECEPTORS ON T CELLS

Comparison of $CD28^{+}$ and $CD28^{-}$ CD4 T memory cells yielded the surprising finding that transcriptional inactivation of CD28 was more prominently linked with a gain rather than a loss in gene expression (FIG. 1). Among the genes that are expressed on $CD28^{-}$ T cells are many regulatory cell surface receptors. A common theme of these receptors is that they serve to regulate the activation of NK cells.[21] Prime examples of cell surface molecules that can be expressed on $CD28^{-}$ CD4 T cells are the killer immunoglobulin–like receptors (KIRs),[22–24] ILT2 (CD85),

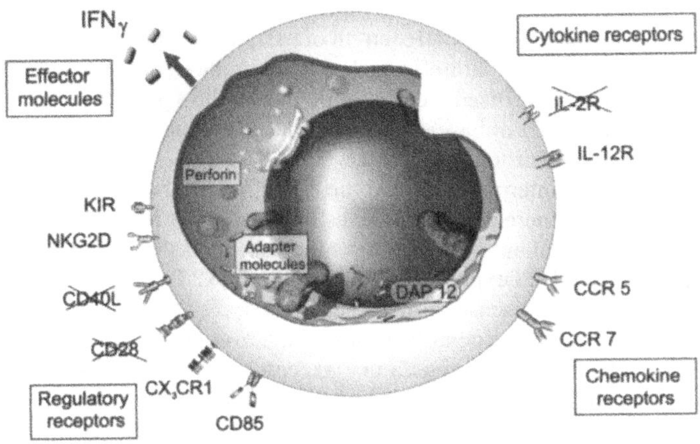

FIGURE 1. Gene expression in senescent CD4 memory T cells. Shown are differences between memory CD4 T cells in the young and end-differentiated senescent memory CD4 T cells that accumulate with aging. Of particular interest is the shift in regulatory cell surface receptors; CD40L and CD28 are lost, whereas several regulatory receptors that usually control the activation of NK cells can be newly expressed. (From Goronzy and Weyand.[15] Reproduced by permission.)

NKG2D,[25] and the fractalkine receptor CX_3CR1.[26] All of these receptors have in common that the expression of their ligands is not restricted to professional antigen-presenting cells (APCs), such as dendritic cells, but are found on various somatic cells. In fact, $CD28^-$ T cells have also lost the ability to express CD40 ligand on the surface,[27] the second costimulatory molecule that links T-cell activation to the activity of APCs. We have therefore concluded that ligands expressed on somatic cells can control the activation of these memory T cells and that this shift in the sensitivity of T cells to the microenvironment occurs to a variable degree with age and cellular senescence. This model could account for the finding of age as a risk factor for RA. Autoreactive T cells aberrantly express regulatory receptors that recognize ligands on various somatic cells such as synoviocytes. Costimulatory signals delivered by such nonprofessional APCs could break peripheral tolerance and sustain autoimmune responses.

PREMATURE AGING OF THE IMMUNE SYSTEM IN RA

To approach this hypothesis, we first examined how old the immune system is in RA patients and whether they have senescent cells. To phrase it more specifically: does the biological age of the immune system in RA patients correspond to its chronological age, or is the immune system better conserved than in age-matched control subjects, or is it even prematurely aged? One successful way to estimate the age of a cellular system is to determine telomeric length.[28] The structural unit of a telomere is a repetitive sequence that caps the end of linear chromosomes. During cell divisions, the 3' end of the telomere is not replicated. Telomere loss therefore reflects the number of cell cycles that have been completed as well as the efficiency of repair mechanisms. On the basis of telomere length of peripheral lymphocytes, the immune system of RA patients is prematurely aged.[29] Even in those few patients with seropositive RA that develop the disease early in life before the age of 30 years, telomeres are shortened by about 1 kilobase, indicating that RA patients by this age have already used up 50% of their telomeric reserve.[30]

Consistent with the interpretation that the T-cell repertoire in patients with RA is prematurely senesced, increased frequencies of T cells that have undergone phenotypic shifts are found. Patients with RA have increased frequencies of CD4 and CD8 T cells that have lost CD28 expression.[31,32] $CD4^+CD28^-$ T cells are associated with increased risk of erosive disease,[21] increased frequencies of extraarticular manifestations,[33] and cardiovascular complications of atherosclerotic disease.[34–36] A portion of these cells expressed regulatory receptors such as KIRs, NKG2D, or CX_3CR1. The biological function of the expression of these receptors for RA is determined by at least the following variables: Is the ligand for the receptor expressed in synovial tissue, in particular on fibroblast-like synoviocytes? What are the downstream signaling events in T cells of receptor triggering? What is the balance between negative and positive signals in T cells and how are the signals from different receptors integrated? These issues have been examined to different degrees for the different receptors.

BALANCE OF STIMULATORY AND INHIBITORY SIGNALS IN RA-PREFERENTIAL EXPRESSION OF STIMULATORY RECEPTORS

KIRs are a classical example for a family of structurally related receptors that can promote both activation and inhibition. This polymorphic gene family has only recently evolved and is not found in rodent genomes.[37] KIR isoforms have similar extracellular domains that recognize major histocompatibility complex class I molecules but differ in their cytoplasmic domains. Inhibitory KIRs have long cytoplasmic tails with two immunoreceptor tyrosine–based inhibitory motifs (ITIMs). Upon ligation of an inhibitory KIR to its ligand, the ITIMs are phosphorylated and recruit the phosphatase SHP-1, which is phosphorylated and activated.[38,39] Stimulatory KIRs bind to an adapter molecule DAP12[40,41] that contains two cytoplasmic immunotyrosine activation motifs (ITAMs) that are phosphorylated by Src family kinases. Similar to NK cells, KIR expression on T cells is clonally distributed; that is, each T cell can express one or more KIR genes stochastically.[23] The outcome of T-cell stimulation therefore depends on the balance between stimulatory and inhibitory receptors and their respective ligands. Selection of T-cell clones preferentially expressing stimulatory receptors could therefore be associated with autoimmunity. This appears to be indeed the case in patients with RA. Cloning of synovial T cells from RA patients showed a preponderance of clones expressing the stimulatory KIR2DS2,[22] often in the absence of inhibitory receptors of the KIR family and inhibitory c-type lectin receptors of the NKG family. Further support for a pathogenetic role of KIR2DS2 is given by the finding that the KIR2DS2 genotype is a genetic risk factor for vasculitic complications of RA.[24] This finding is consistent with the model that aberrant expression of stimulatory regulatory receptors on T cells promotes autoimmune disease. The ligand of KIR2DS2 is undetermined, and it is therefore unclear whether KIR2DS2 is selectively sensitive to cues in the synovial microenvironment or, given that KIR2DS2 is associated with vascular complications of RA, in the vascular microenvironment. KIR2DL2 and KIR2DL3, inhibitory homologs of KIR2DS2 with similar extracellular domains, recognize several HLA-C alleles; however, KIR2DS2 differs from these receptors by only three to four amino acids,[42,43] and this variation reduces the affinity to HLA-C. It cannot be excluded that KIR2DS2 has higher affinity to particular HLA-C–peptide complexes, and indeed, vascular complications of RA are associated with HLA-Cw3.[24]

BALANCE OF STIMULATORY AND INHIBITORY SIGNALS IN RA-LIMITED FUNCTION OF INHIBITORY RECEPTORS

Inhibitory KIRs are generally considered dominant over stimulatory signals. In NK cells, one of the major roles of inhibitory KIRs is to block the lipid raft movement to the NK cell–target cell contact area.[44,45] Lipid rafts contain most of the activating receptors and activating signaling molecules; KIRs in NK cells completely block cell activation. They do so by recruiting and activating SHP-1, which dephosphorylates Vav-1.[38] The inhibition of Vav-1 activation prevents actin cytoskeleton

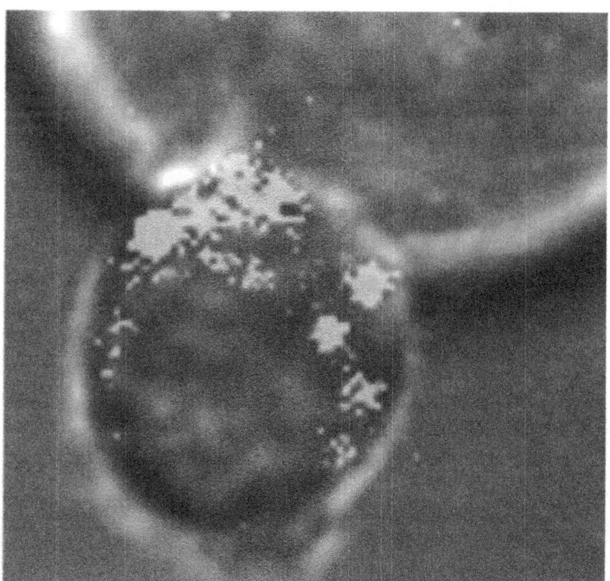

FIGURE 2. Incomplete activity of inhibitory regulatory receptors on senescent CD4 T cells. Regulatory receptors on senescent CD4 cells include inhibitory KIRs. Although these receptors suppress all NK cell function including cytotoxicity, their ability to interfere with T-cell receptor–mediated activation events is limited. Shown is a confocal photomicrograph from a CD4 T cell that undergoes granule expulsion after T-cell receptor stimulation despite cotriggering of an inhibitory KIR2DL2 molecule by its natural ligand. [Original magnification: ×100.]

reorganization and is therefore an efficacious mechanism to paralyze all effector functions in NK cells. By contrast, the inhibitory activity of KIRs is incomplete in T cells, as shown in the case of KIR2DL2. KIR2DL2 inhibits the transcriptional activation of some, but not all, genes after T-cell receptor activation.[46] More importantly, certain effector functions of T cells such as cytotoxicity and granule expulsion are completely unaffected (FIG. 2). One possible mechanism is that KIR2DL2 is initially excluded from the transient interaction platform between target cells and T cells.[46] In the presence of stimulatory KIRs, inhibitory KIRs do not inhibit the T-cell receptor–induced production of interferon γ. Thus, the function of inhibitory KIRs in T cells is more limited and focused than in NK cells, which at least for some effector functions again strike the balance in favor of stimulatory signals in senescent T cells from RA patients.

SIGNALING PATHWAYS OF KIRS IN T CELLS

Transmembrane signaling events after KIR stimulation have been well studied in NK cells. However, the cytoplasmic composition in T cells is sufficiently different from NK cells to create different functional outcomes. The adapter molecule DAP12 is ubiquitously expressed in NK cells but is absent in most T cells, even if they ex-

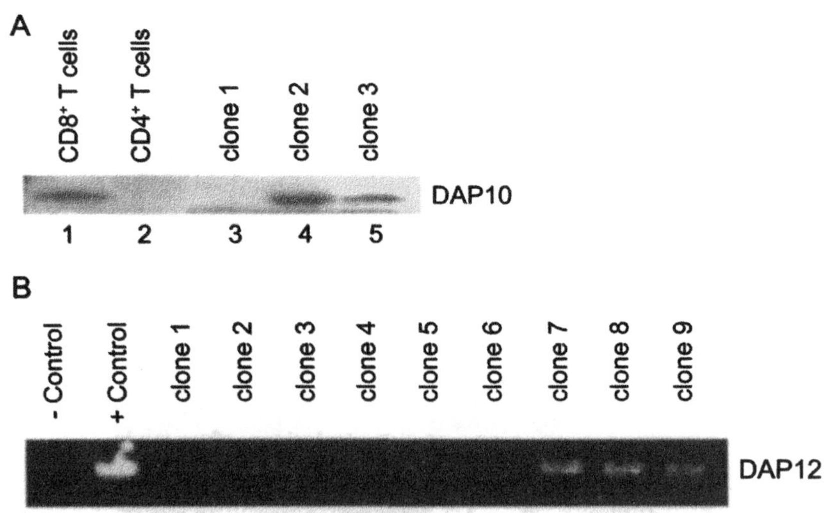

FIGURE 3. Expression of adapter molecules in senescent CD4 memory T cells. The function of stimulatory regulatory receptors on senescent CD4 T cells is influenced by variable expression of adapter molecules. Stimulatory KIRs signal through DAP12; NKG2D and possibly also stimulatory KIRs use DAP10 to signal. Both adapter molecules are not expressed in young memory T cells, but can be found in some senescent CD4 T cells. Shown is a Western blot for DAP10 (**A**) and a PCR for DAP12 (**B**) expression on a panel of CD4 T-cell clones from patients with rheumatoid arthritis. CD8$^+$ and CD4$^+$ T cells freshly isolated from peripheral blood served as positive and negative controls in (**A**).

press stimulatory KIRs. In NK cells, triggering of KIR2DS2 is sufficient to initiate a signaling cascade by recruiting signaling molecules with SH2 domains such as ZAP70 and Syk. By contrast, KIR2DS2 provides costimulatory and nonstimulatory signals in T cells.[47] The signaling pathway has been incompletely mapped but includes the activation of cJUN N-terminal kinases (JNK), possibly by means of the activation of the PI3K pathway.[47] KIR2DS2 in T cells might recruit the adapter molecule DAP10, which is known to activate the PI3K pathway. However, the affinity of DAP10 to KIR2DS2 is certainly much lower than to DAP12, and attempts to coprecipitate DAP10 and KIR2DS2 have failed.[47] DAP10 is not ubiquitously expressed in CD4 T cells but can be detected by Western blot if they senesce (FIG. 3). A small minority of T cells can even gain the expression of DAP12 (FIG. 3).[48] In these cells, KIR2DS2 is fully competent, and T-cell activation no longer requires the stimulation of small minority of T-cell receptor; stimulation of KIR2DS2 is sufficient to trigger cytotoxicity and transcriptional activation of cytokine genes.[48]

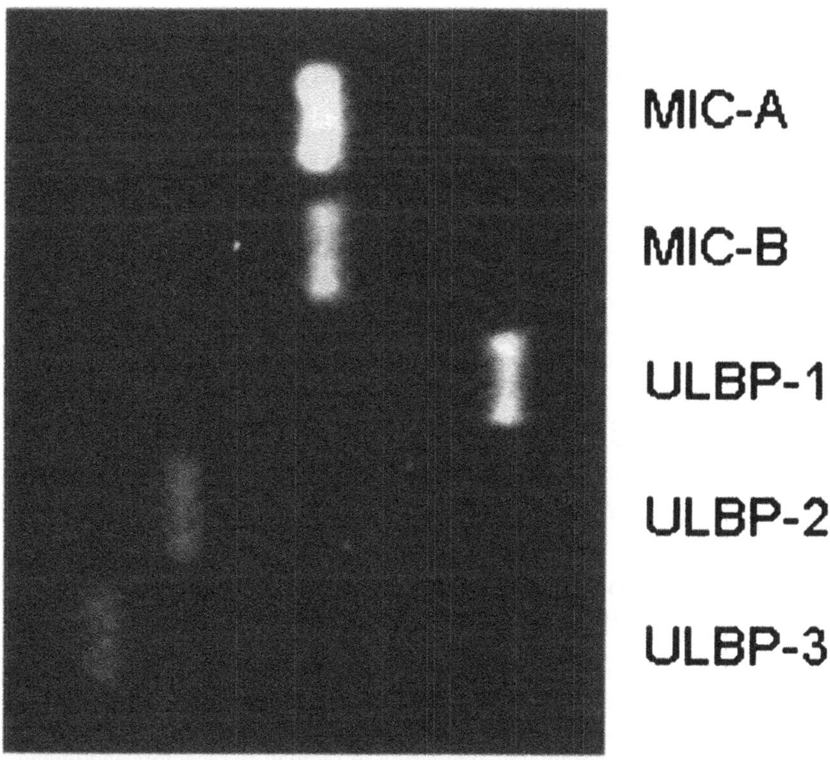

FIGURE 4. Expression of NKG2D ligands in rheumatoid synovitis. Fibroblast-like synoviocytes were obtained from patients with RA. Lines were established and examined for the expression of NKG2D ligands by PCR. Synoviocytes had transcripts for MIC-A, MIC-B, and the three different ULBP isoforms.

NKG2D-REGULATED RESPONSES IN RHEUMATOID SYNOVITIS

Like stimulatory KIRs, NKG2D is a stimulatory receptor that is usually expressed on NK cells and, in humans, also on CD8 T cells and is generally absent on CD4 T cells. However, subsets of senescent $CD4^{+}CD28^{-}$ T cells acquire the expression of NKG2D. NKG2D also signals through the DAP10–PI3K pathway and can provide costimulatory signals to upregulate cytokine transcription in response to T-cell receptor triggering. NKG2D recognizes several ligands, some of which are stress-induced in epithelial cells, and has therefore been implicated in gastrointestinal inflammatory diseases. Interestingly, expression and function of NKG2D appears to be partially controlled by interleukin 15,[25] a cytokine that has been found in the synovial inflammation of RA. Also, fibroblast-like synoviocytes express several ligands for NKG2D including MIC-A, MIC-B, and ULBP-1, -2, and -3 (FIG. 4).[25] Groh and colleagues have shown that the expression of NKG2D on CD4 T cells from RA patients is functional and that synovial fibroblasts provide costimulatory signals through triggering NKG2D, supporting the model that aberrant expression of regulatory molecules on T cells can sensitize these cells to cues in the synovial environment.

FRACTALKINE RECEPTOR AS A COSTIMULATORY MOLECULE IN RHEMATOID ARTHRITIS

Senescent $CD4^{+}$ T cells that accumulate in RA also express CX_3CR1, the receptor for the chemokine fractalkine.[26] Fractalkine exists as a cell-bound molecule with the chemokine domain sitting on an extended mucinlike stalk or as a soluble isoform and can mediate both adhesion and chemotaxis. It is found on cultured synovial fibroblasts and hyperplastic synoviocytes from RA patients. Membrane anchored on synoviocytes, fractalkine amplifies the retention and the proinflammatory functions of T cells. Like NKG2D and KIR2DS2, triggering of CX_3CR1 boosts interferon and TNF-α secretions, thus facilitating inflammation and tissue injury (FIG. 5).[26] Fractalkine-expressing synoviocytes also enhance the release of cytolytic granules from $CX_3CR1^{+}CD4^{+}$ T cells[26] and provide a survival signal for recruited T cells, thereby regulating T-cell longevity and turnover. Obviously, CX_3CR1, like all chemokine receptors, mediates signals through the activation of G proteins and has a different spectrum of costimulatory functions from that of NKG2D and stimulatory KIRs that activate the PI3K pathway.[49]

EXPRESSION OF COSTIMULATORY LIGANDS ON FIBROBLAST-LIKE SYNOVIOCYTES

The finding of regulatory ligands such as fractalkine and MIC-A expressed on synoviocytes reemphasizes their important roles in serving as accessory cells to invading lymphocytes and modulating several different aspects of chronic synovitis. Clearly there has to be a coordinated expression of regulatory receptors and ligands that involves the T cell as well as the synoviocyte. Through this expression, synoviocytes lower the threshold for T-cell stimulation and bias the local microenvironment against anergy and nonresponsiveness, thereby contributing critically to the break-

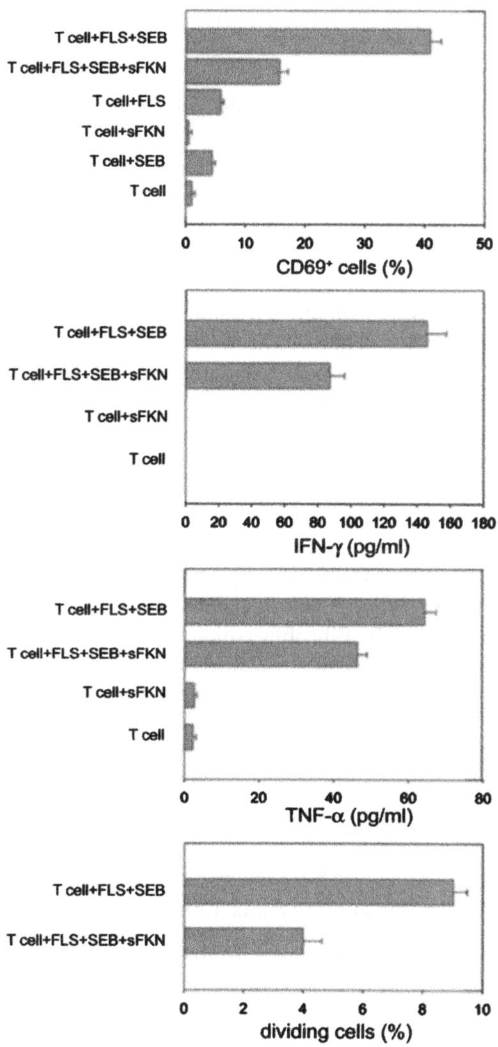

FIGURE 5. Costimulatory activity of fibroblast-like synoviocytes. $CD28^-CD4^+$ T cells from a patient with rheumatoid arthritis were stimulated with superantigen (SEB) and fibroblast-like synoviocytes (FLS) as APCs. Blocking the interaction between fractalkine (expressed on synoviocytes) and its receptor (expressed on senescent CD4 T cells) with soluble fractalkine (sFKN) partially inhibited T-cell activation, suggesting that this axis provided important costimulatory signals in the rheumatoid synovium. (From Sawai *et al.*[26] Modified and reproduced by permission.)

down of self-tolerance in the synovium. One other example for such a costimulatory function of synoviocytes is the production of thrombospondin 1. Thrombospondin binds to CD36 on synoviocytes and possibly endothelial cells. This cell-bound thrombospondin can cross-link CD47, thereby lowering the threshold for T-cell activation.[50] CD47 is expressed on all CD4 T cells; this costimulatory activity is therefore not restricted to subsets of T cells that emerge with senescence.

CONCLUSION

Progress in the understanding of disease comes from the interplay between clinical observations, epidemiological studies, and the understanding of basic biological principles. In RA, the age dependency of the disease has not been accounted for in any of the pathogenetic models, nor has it been incorporated in any of the animal models of the disease. Age is associated with complex changes in the adaptive immune system that provide important cues for understanding the pathogenesis of RA. Of particular interest is an age-related shift in the expression of regulatory receptors on memory T cells that redistributes the regulatory control of T-cell responses away from professional APCs and classical costimulatory ligands to certain types of somatic cells. The best example is the loss of CD28 on CD4 T cells that is associated with a gain of several cell surface molecules, which normally control the activation of NK cells. Control of T-cell activation depends on a fine balance between stimulatory and inhibitory receptors, and several mechanisms contribute to a dominance of stimulatory signals in RA. These include genetic predisposition with stimulatory receptors as susceptibility genes, stochastic expression of these receptors on individual cells, and the variable expression of adapter molecules that promote the transduction of positive and negative signals. Fibroblast-like synoviocytes express several molecules that can function as ligands for the stimulatory receptors, thereby providing fertile ground for the activation of such aged memory T cells in the synovium. These observations are not only important for the pathogenetic understanding of the disease but also identify new targets for therapeutic approaches.

ACKNOWLEDGMENTS

This work was funded by grants from the National Institutes of Health (AR41974, AR42527, and AG15043). The authors thank Tamela Yeargin for manuscript editing.

[*Competing interests*: The authors declare that they have no competing financial interests.]

REFERENCES

1. Feldmann, M. & R.N. Maini. 2001. Anti-TNF alpha therapy of rheumatoid arthritis: what have we learned? Annu. Rev. Immunol. **19:** 163–196.
2. Feldmann, M., R.N. Maini, J. Bondeson, *et al.* 2001. Cytokine blockade in rheumatoid arthritis. Adv. Exp. Med. Biol. **490:** 119–127.
3. Feldmann, M. & R.N. Maini. 2003. Lasker Clinical Medical Research Award. TNF defined as a therapeutic target for rheumatoid arthritis and other autoimmune diseases. Nat. Med. **9:** 1245–1250.

4. TAYLOR, P.C. 2001. Anti-tumor necrosis factor therapies. Curr. Opin. Rheumatol. **13:** 164–169.
5. TAYLOR, P.C., R.O. WILLIAMS & M. FELDMANN. 2004. Tumour necrosis factor alpha as a therapeutic target for immune-mediated inflammatory diseases. Curr. Opin. Biotechnol. **15:** 557–563.
6. WEGENER'S GRANULOMATOSIS ETANERCEPT TRIAL (WGET) RESEARCH GROUP. 2005. Etanercept plus standard therapy for Wegener's granulomatosis. N. Engl. J. Med. **352:** 351–361.
7. EDWARDS, J.C., L. SZCZEPANSKI, J. SZECHINSKI, *et al.* 2004. Efficacy of B-cell-targeted therapy with rituximab in patients with rheumatoid arthritis. N. Engl. J. Med. **350:** 2572–2581.
8. CARSON, D.A., P.P. CHEN & T.J. KIPPS. 1991. New roles for rheumatoid factor. J. Clin. Invest. **87:** 379–383.
9. TAKEMURA, S., P.A. KLIMIUK, A. BRAUN, *et al.* 2001. T cell activation in rheumatoid synovium is B cell dependent. J. Immunol. **167:** 4710–4718.
10. WEYAND, C.M., T.M. SEYLER & J.J. GORONZY. 2005. B cells in rheumatoid synovitis. Arthritis Res. Ther. **7**(Suppl. 3): S9–S12.
11. DORAN, M.F., G.R. POND, C.S. CROWSON, *et al.* 2002. Trends in incidence and mortality in rheumatoid arthritis in Rochester, Minnesota, over a forty-year period. Arthritis Rheum. **46:** 625–631.
12. GRUBECK-LOEBENSTEIN, B., P. BERGER, M. SAURWEIN-TEISSL, *et al.* 1998. No immunity for the elderly. Nat. Med. **4:** 870.
13. GORONZY, J.J., J.W. FULBRIGHT, C.S. CROWSON, *et al.* 2001. Value of immunological markers in predicting responsiveness to influenza vaccination in elderly individuals. J. Virol. **75:** 12182–12187.
14. GORONZY, J.J. & C.M. WEYAND. 2005. T cell development and receptor diversity during aging. Curr. Opin. Immunol. **17:** 468–475.
15. GORONZY, J.J. & C.M. WEYAND. 2005. Rheumatoid arthritis. Immunol. Rev. **204:** 55–73.
16. NAYLOR, K., G. LI, A.N. VALLEJO, *et al.* 2005. The influence of age on T cell generation and TCR diversity. J. Immunol. **174:** 7446–7452.
17. VALLEJO, A.N., C.M. WEYAND & J.J. GORONZY. 2004. T-cell senescence: a culprit of immune abnormalities in chronic inflammation and persistent infection. Trends Mol. Med. **10:** 119–124.
18. VALLEJO, A.N. 2005. CD28 extinction in human T cells: altered functions and the program of T-cell senescence. Immunol. Rev. **205:** 158–169.
19. VALLEJO, A.N., E. BRYL, K. KLARSKOV, *et al.* 2002. Molecular basis for the loss of CD28 expression in senescent T cells. J. Biol. Chem. **277:** 46940–46949.
20. VALLEJO, A.N., C.M. WEYAND & J.J. GORONZY. 2001. Functional disruption of the CD28 gene transcriptional initiator in senescent T cells. J. Biol. Chem. **276:** 2565–2570.
21. WARRINGTON, K.J., S. TAKEMURA, J.J. GORONZY & C.M. WEYLAND. 2001. CD4+,CD28– T cells in rheumatoid arthritis patients combine features of the innate and adaptive immune systems. Arthritis Rheum. **44:** 13–20.
22. NAMEKAWA, T., M.R. SNYDER, J.H. YEN, *et al.* 2000. Killer cell activating receptors function as costimulatory molecules on CD4+CD28null T cells clonally expanded in rheumatoid arthritis. J. Immunol. **165:** 1138–1145.
23. SNYDER, M.R., L.O. MUEGGE, C. OFFORD, *et al.* 2002. Formation of the killer Ig-like receptor repertoire on CD4+CD28null T cells. J. Immunol. **168:** 3839–3846.
24. YEN, J.H., B.E. MOORE, T. NAKAJIMA, *et al.* 2001. Major histocompatibility complex class I-recognizing receptors are disease risk genes in rheumatoid arthritis. J. Exp. Med. **193:** 1159–1167.
25. GROH, V., A. BRUHL, H. EL-GABALAWY, *et al.* 2003. Stimulation of T cell autoreactivity by anomalous expression of NKG2D and its MIC ligands in rheumatoid arthritis. Proc. Natl. Acad. Sci. USA **100:** 9452–9457.
26. SAWAI, H., Y.W. PARK, J. ROBERSON, *et al.* 2005. T cell costimulation by fractalkine-expressing synoviocytes in rheumatoid arthritis. Arthritis Rheum. **52:** 1392–1401.
27. WEYAND, C.M., J.C. BRANDES, D. SCHMIDT, *et al.* 1998. Functional properties of CD4+ CD28– T cells in the aging immune system. Mech. Ageing Dev. **102:** 131–147.

28. LANSDORP, P.M. 2005. Major cutbacks at chromosome ends. Trends Biochem. Sci. **30:** 388–395.
29. KOETZ, K., E. BRYL, K. SPICKSCHEN, *et al.* 2000. T cell homeostasis in patients with rheumatoid arthritis. Proc. Natl. Acad. Sci. USA **97:** 9203–9208.
30. SCHONLAND, S.O., C. LOPEZ, T. WIDMANN, *et al.* 2003. Premature telomeric loss in rheumatoid arthritis is genetically determined and involves both myeloid and lymphoid cell lineages. Proc. Natl. Acad. Sci. USA **100:** 13471–13476.
31. WAASE, I., C. KAYSER, P.J. CARLSON, *et al.* 1996. Oligoclonal T cell proliferation in patients with rheumatoid arthritis and their unaffected siblings. Arthritis Rheum. **39:** 904–913.
32. BRYL, E., A.N. VALLEJO, E.L. MATTESON, *et al.* In press. Modulation of CD28 expression with anti-tumor necrosis factor-alpha therapy in rheumatoid arthritis. Arthritis Rheum. **52:** 2996–3003.
33. MARTENS, P.B., J.J. GORONZY, D. SCHAID & C.M. WEYAND. 1997. Expansion of unusual CD4+ T cells in severe rheumatoid arthritis. Arthritis Rheum. **40:** 1106–1114.
34. LIUZZO, G., J.J. GORONZY, H. YANG, *et al.* 2000. Monoclonal T-cell proliferation and plaque instability in acute coronary syndromes. Circulation **101:** 2883–2888.
35. WARRINGTON, K.J., P.D. KENT, R.L. FRYE, *et al.* 2005. Rheumatoid arthritis is an independent risk factor for multi-vessel coronary artery disease: a case control study. Arthritis Res.Ther. **7:** R984–R991.
36. NAKAJIMA, T., S. SCHULTE, K.J. WARRINGTON, *et al.* 2002. T-cell-mediated lysis of endothelial cells in acute coronary syndromes. Circulation **105:** 570–575.
37. PARHAM, P. 2005. MHC class I molecules and KIRs in human history, health and survival. Nat. Rev. Immunol. **5:** 201–214.
38. STEBBINS, C.C., C. WATZL, D.D. BILLADEAU, *et al.* 2003. Vav1 dephosphorylation by the tyrosine phosphatase SHP-1 as a mechanism for inhibition of cellular cytotoxicity. Mol. Cell. Biol. **23:** 6291–6299.
39. VYAS, Y.M., H. MANIAR, C.E. LYDDANE, *et al.* 2004. Ligand binding to inhibitory killer cell Ig-like receptors induce colocalization with Src homology domain 2-containing protein tyrosine phosphatase 1 and interruption of ongoing activation signals. J. Immunol. **173:** 1571–1578.
40. LANIER, L.L., B.C. CORLISS, J. WU, *et al.* 1998. Immunoreceptor DAP12 bearing a tyrosine-based activation motif is involved in activating NK cells. Nature **391:** 703–707.
41. TOMASELLO, E., L. OLCESE, F. VELY, *et al.* 1998. Gene structure, expression pattern, and biological activity of mouse killer cell activating receptor-associated protein (KARAP)/DAP-12. J. Biol. Chem. **273:** 34115–34119.
42. SAULQUIN, X., L.N. GASTINEL & E. VIVIER. 2003. Crystal structure of the human natural killer cell activating receptor KIR2DS2 (CD158j). J. Exp. Med. **197:** 933–938.
43. WINTER, C.C., J.E. GUMPERZ, P. PARHAM, *et al.* 1998. Direct binding and functional transfer of NK cell inhibitory receptors reveal novel patterns of HLA-C allotype recognition. J. Immunol. **161:** 571–577.
44. DAVIS, D.M., I. CHIU, M. FASSETT, *et al.* 1999. The human natural killer cell immune synapse. Proc. Natl. Acad. Sci. USA **96:** 15062–15067.
45. FASSETT, M.S., D.M. DAVIS, M.M. VALTER, *et al.* 2001. Signaling at the inhibitory natural killer cell immune synapse regulates lipid raft polarization but not class I MHC clustering. Proc. Natl. Acad. Sci. USA **98:** 14547–14552.
46. HENEL, G., K. SINGH, D. CUI, *et al.* Uncoupling of T-cell effector functions by inhibitory killer immunoglobulin-like receptors. Submitted for publication.
47. SNYDER, M.R., M. LUCAS, E. VIVIER, *et al.* 2003. Selective activation of the c-Jun NH2-terminal protein kinase signaling pathway by stimulatory KIR in the absence of KARAP/DAP12 in CD4+ T cells. J. Exp. Med. **197:** 437–449.
48. SNYDER, M.R., T. NAKAJIMA, P.J. LEIBSON, *et al.* 2004. Stimulatory killer Ig-like receptors modulate T cell activation through DAP12-dependent and DAP12-independent mechanisms. J. Immunol. **173:** 3725–3731.
49. SNYDER, M.R., C.M. WEYAND & J.J. GORONZY. 2004. The double life of NK receptors: stimulation or co-stimulation? Trends Immunol. **25:** 25–32.
50. VALLEJO, A.N., H. YANG, P.A. KLIMIUK, *et al.* 2003. Synoviocyte-mediated expansion of inflammatory T cells in rheumatoid synovitis is dependent on CD47-thrombospondin 1 interaction. J. Immunol. **171:** 1732–1740.

Vascular Dendritic Cells in Giant Cell Arteritis

CORNELIA M. WEYAND,[a] WEI MA-KRUPA,[a] OLGA PRYSHCHEP,[a] STEFAN GRÖSCHEL,[a] ROBERTO BERNARDINO,[b] AND JÖRG J. GORONZY[a]

[a]*Kathleen B. and Mason I. Lowance Center for Human Immunology, Department of Medicine, Emory University School of Medicine, Atlanta, Georgia 30322, USA*

[b]*Department of Ophthalmology, Emory University School of Medicine, Atlanta, Georgia 30322, USA*

ABSTRACT: Giant cell arteritis (GCA) is a granulomatous vasculitis that selectively targets medium-sized and large arteries, especially the cranial branches of the aorta. The inflammatory activity of vascular lesions is driven by adaptive immune responses, with CD4 T cells undergoing clonal expansion in the vessel wall and releasing interferon γ. Recent studies have described a distinctive population of dendritic cells (DCs) localized at the adventitia–media border of normal medium-sized arteries that appear to play a critical role in the initiation of vasculitis. Immune effector functions of this DC population are being examined in human artery–severe combined immunodeficient (SCID) mouse chimeras. In their constitutive form, $CD11c^+$ $fascin^+$ adventitial DCs are not recognized by alloreactive T cells. Triggering with Toll-like receptor (TLR) ligands is sufficient to break this state of tolerance and initiate DC activation, T-cell recruitment, T-cell activation, and T-cell retention in the arterial wall. Systemic administration of ligands for TLR2 or -4 in human artery–SCID chimeras drives differentiation of adventitial DCs into chemokine-producing effector cells with high-level expression of both CD83 and CD86 and mediates T-cell regulatory function through release of interleukin 18. In established vasculitis, fully matured DCs retain antigen-presenting function; antibody-mediated DC depletion disrupts T-cell and macrophage activation and has marked anti-inflammatory effects. We conclude that adventitial DCs, an indigenous cell population of the arterial wall, are responsive to pathogen-derived macromolecules and have gatekeeper function in regulating T-cell recruitment and retention to the arterial adventitia. A switch of adventitial DCs from being nonstimulatory to T-cell activating emerges as a critical event in the initiation of vasculitis.

KEYWORDS: vasculitis; arteritis; dendritic cell; Toll-like receptors; T-cell activation; chemokines

Address for correspondence: Cornelia M. Weyand, M.D., Ph.D., Kathleen B. and Mason I. Lowance Center for Human Immunology, Emory University School of Medicine, Rm. 1003, Woodruff Memorial Research Bldg., 101 Woodruff Cir., Atlanta, GA 30322. Voice: 404-727-7310; fax: 404-727-7371.
cweyand@emory.edu

**Ann. N.Y. Acad. Sci. 1062: 195–208 (2005). © 2005 New York Academy of Sciences.
doi: 10.1196/annals.1358.023**

INTRODUCTION

The relationship between blood vessels and the immune system is intimate. Immune cells rely upon traveling with the bloodstream to reach their destination and must transmigrate through the vessel wall to enter the tissue.[1] Even under steady-state conditions, dendritic cells (DCs), monocytes/macrophages, and lymphocytes must all be able to enter tissues, patrol for damaged cells and structures, and respond appropriately. Endothelial cells and resident cells of the blood vessel wall are thus constantly exposed to bypassing immune cells. The potential for immune recognition events should therefore be particularly high in vascular walls.

However, the host cannot afford to jeopardize the integrity of vascular structures since a breakdown of blood vessels causes hemorrhage, a potentially life-threatening event. Inflammatory blood vessel diseases are, in fact, feared for the high risk of serious and possibly fatal complications.[2] In the interest of the host's well-being and survival, it is particularly important to prevent vessel wall inflammation, even if this comes at the price of suppressing immune recognition. It is likely no coincidence that inflammatory vasculopathies occur infrequently.

In atherosclerosis, which is now emerging as an inflammatory syndrome,[3–5] somewhat different rules may apply. In most patients with this disease, the intensity of the inflammatory process remains low and appears to smolder over decades. If inflammatory cells accumulate in the atherosclerotic plaque, however, they cause vessel wall damage and elicit atherothrombotic occlusion of the lumen. This scenario is instantly dangerous and is thought to give rise to the acute coronary syndromes, including sudden cardiac death, unstable angina, and myocardial infarction.[6]

When vasculitis affects small vessels, such as capillaries and small arterioles, the vessel wall itself is too thin to become the target of inflammatory attack. Instead, inflammatory infiltrates cluster around the vessel, with the inflammatory response unfolding in the perivascular tissue. Vascular destruction leads to small areas of hemorrhage. Capillaries, arterioles, and venules can also respond with occlusion, thereby causing ischemic damage in dependent tissue. Fortunately, tissue areas supplied by such small vessels are also limited in size. Classic examples include the small-vessel vasculitides that preferentially target the skin, the capillary beds of the kidney, and the lung.[7]

In contrast, medium-sized and large arteries supply critical organ structures and entire organ systems.[8] Inflammation in the wall of medium-sized and large arteries thus has profound clinical consequences.[9] A typical example is giant cell arteritis (GCA), a granulomatous vasculitis of medium-sized and large arteries. GCA targets the aorta and its major branches, with granulomatous infiltrates occupying the artery wall layers. Hemorrhage almost never occurs in GCA. Rather, inflammatory injury of the arterial wall induces a "response to injury" in which excessive proliferation of myofibroblasts leads to thickening of the intima. Eventually, the vessel lumen becomes occluded, blood flow is disrupted, and dependent organ structures suffer from ischemia. Occlusion of large arteries has immediate consequences for the patient, often with massive ischemic damage of vital organs, such as the brain, the eye, and the heart. In GCA, immune responses driving the disease process unfold within the wall layers of the arteries, not in the perivascular tissue. This places arterial resident cells at the center of pathogenic events.

THE PROBLEM

GCA is the most common vasculitis in the Western world.[10] Incidence rates are estimated at 5–25 cases per 100,000 persons and are highest in individuals of Northern European origin. The disease can start insidiously or abruptly, leaving the patient with the clinical manifestations of a systemic inflammatory syndrome as well as the consequences of vascular insufficiency. Most patients seek clinical evaluation because of malaise, weight loss, depression, and painful stiffness of shoulder and pelvic girdle muscles. This combination of symptoms is diagnosed as polymyalgia rheumatica (PMR). Clinical evaluation demonstrates that the patient has high levels of acute-phase proteins, such as a highly elevated sedimentation rate or elevated levels of interleukin 6 (IL-6) and C-reactive protein. Anemia is often encountered. This systemic inflammatory syndrome substantially limits the patient's ability to function in daily activities. Localized symptoms of vasculitis include headaches, visual loss, temporal tenderness, claudication in the masseter muscles, and, less often, diminished pulse or unequal blood pressure measurements in different extremities. Clinically most disastrous is ischemia of the eye or central nervous system.

GCA is an ophthalmologic emergency because it can cause sudden blindness in one or both eyes if not diagnosed and treated promptly.[11,12] The diagnosis is established by a biopsy of the affected blood vessels, usually taken from the temporal artery.[13] The histology shows panarteritis with mononuclear cells arranged in granulomatous infiltrates. About 50% of patients have multinucleated giant cells, hence, the name "giant cell arteritis." Treatment includes large doses of corticosteroids, which promptly relieve the symptoms associated with the inflammatory syndrome and prevent further ischemic damage. Most patients can be withdrawn from corticosteroids after about 2 years. Low-grade inflammatory activity persists in such patients, and it is not known whether this inflammatory activity requires continuous immunosuppressive therapy.[14]

CLUES FROM THE PATIENT

Host risk factors conferring susceptibility to GCA have been well characterized.[15] Most patients are females. Incidence rates are the highest in Scandinavian populations; African-Americans have low risk. The risk of developing GCA is reduced in patients diagnosed with rheumatoid arthritis, for reasons not yet understood.[18] Most significantly, GCA has an almost absolute age requirement. The disease occurs in individuals who are aged 50 years and older, and the median age of onset is about 75 years. Incidence rates increase with age, and no convincing cases have been reported in those younger than 50 years.[16] Selected HLA-DR haplotypes are associated with this disease and seem to function as risk but not as progression factors.[17,18]

CLUES FROM THE LESION

GCA displays a stringent tissue tropism. Certain vascular beds are targeted, whereas other blood vessels of similar size and diameter are apparently ignored. The

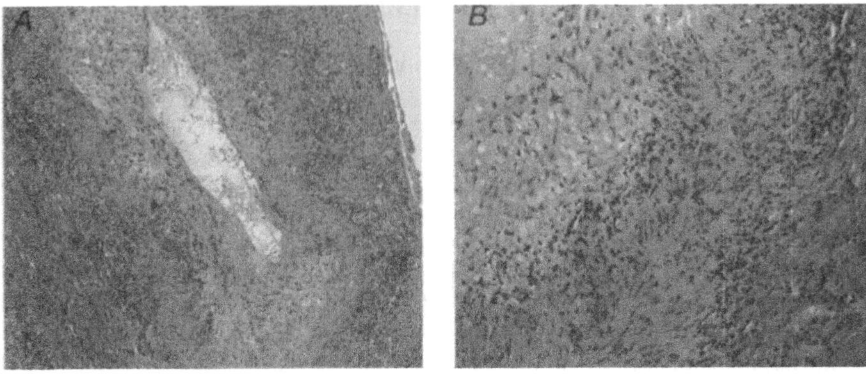

FIGURE 1. Giant cell arteritis. (**A**) Cross section of the temporal artery showing transmural inflammatory infiltrates with granulomatous arrangements. The medial smooth muscle cell layer is damaged; the vessel lumen is compromised by hyperplastic intima (hematoxylin and eosin stain, ×100). (**B**) Enlarged view of a media segment with several multinucleated giant cells near fragments of the lamina elastica interna (hematoxylin and eosin stain, ×200). (From Weyand and Goronzy.[8] Reproduced by permission.)

most likely sites of GCA are the second to fifth branches of the aorta, particularly the extracranial branching vessels of the carotid arteries. Also included are vertebral arteries and the extracranial part of the basilar artery. Granulomatous inflammation can manifest in the subclavian arteries and the axillary arteries. Femoral arteries and coronary arteries are rarely affected. Despite similarities in the gross anatomy of mesenteric and intracerebral arteries, these vascular territories appear to be spared from the disease. A common target for GCA is the aortic wall, with the highest likelihood of aortitis in the thoracic aorta.[2]

Vascular lesions are composed of CD4 T cells, macrophages, and DCs (FIG. 1).[19] B cells are explicitly uncommon. Granulocytes are not often represented in the vessel wall infiltrates.[20] Multinucleated giant cells are preferentially positioned at the junction between the media and the intima. The lamina elastica externa, which separates the intimal and medial layers, is typically fragmented, and giant cells have been described to lie adjacent to such fragments.[21] Granulomatous formations characteristically spread throughout the media.

Careful analysis of tissue-infiltrating CD4 T cells has demonstrated that they undergo clonal expansion in the vessel wall.[22,23] Dominant clonotypes with identical T-cell receptor sequences have been isolated from the right and the left temporal arteries of affected patients. The repertoire of tissue-infiltrating CD4 T cells was found to be restricted, which suggests that selection mechanisms, such as vasculogenic antigens, are at work.[24,25] Tissue extracts drove the proliferation of tissue-derived T-cell lines, supporting the concept that antigen recognition drives T-cell activation *in situ*. Interferon γ (IFN-γ) appears to play a key role in the vasculitic response, as IFN-γ tissue levels closely correlate with clinical manifestations.[26,27] IFN-γ transcript levels in arteries from patients with ischemic complications are 10-fold higher than in biopsy specimens from patients lacking restricted blood flow.[28] In tissue samples from patients with PMR, IL-2 production has been reported to be particularly high.[29] Taken together, these data support the model that T-cell differentiation in the vascular lesions is directly connected to the clinical course of disease.

IMMUNOLOGIC NICHES IN MEDIUM-SIZED AND LARGE ARTERIES

The first hint of biologically relevant compartmentalization in the wall of human temporal arteries came from studies showing that IFN-γ–producing CD4 T cells were located exclusively in the adventitia.[30] Also, T cells expressing CCR5 and CXCR3 predominantly cluster in the adventitia.[31] Data accumulated over the last decade strongly support the model that immune functions in both healthy and inflamed arteries are strictly regulated and that distinctive microenvironments support characteristic immune reactions.[32,33] Information is emerging on how such microenvironments are defined and which determinants shape cell–cell and cell–matrix interactions. Particular interest has focused on the adventitia, which contains several unique structures that are critically involved in regulating the immunogenicity of the arterial wall. In healthy arteries, the adventitia is the only region of the vessel wall that is vascularized. Vasa vasorum are exclusively encountered in the adventitia, surrounded by fibroblast-rich stroma. A population of DCs is positioned at the adventitia–media border, often arranged around the outer side of the lamina elastica externa.[34] Immunoregulatory functions of these adventitial DCs should be critical in disease states leading to panarteritis.

FUNCTIONAL ACTIVITY OF ADVENTITIAL DCs IN HEALTHY MEDIUM-SIZED ARTERIES

Temporal arteries, subclavian arteries, vertebral arteries, and the aorta all hold a population of DCs in the adventitia.[35] Immunohistochemical analysis shows the following marker profile: CD11c, the actin-bundling molecule fascin, S-100, and CD68. DCs are negative for the activation marker CD83, and they lack expression of CD1a, distinguishing them from classical Langerhans cells. By immunohistochemical staining, CD11c$^+$ DCs in the adventitia are negative for HLA-DR.

To address the function of these adventitial DCs, we have established an experimental system in which we can test the biologic activity of DCs in attracting and stimulating T cells. In this experimental system, human medium-sized arteries are collected from donors that are free of vasculitis and implanted into NOD-Rag1$^{-/-}$ mice.[35] After engraftment, alloreactive human T cells are adoptively transferred into the chimeras. The arterial grafts are explanted and analyzed for DC and T-cell function. As summarized in FIGURE 2, implanted temporal arteries can elicit allorecognition. Alloreactive CD4 T cells are recruited to the adventitia as indicated by the accumulation of T-cell receptor transcripts. Low concentrations of CCL19-specific sequences are detected in the vascular grafts, and CCL19 may be involved in attracting human T cells to the adventitial layer. However, recruited alloreactive T cells do not undergo activation. Both early (CD40 ligand) and late (IFN-γ) markers of T-cell activation remain undetectable.

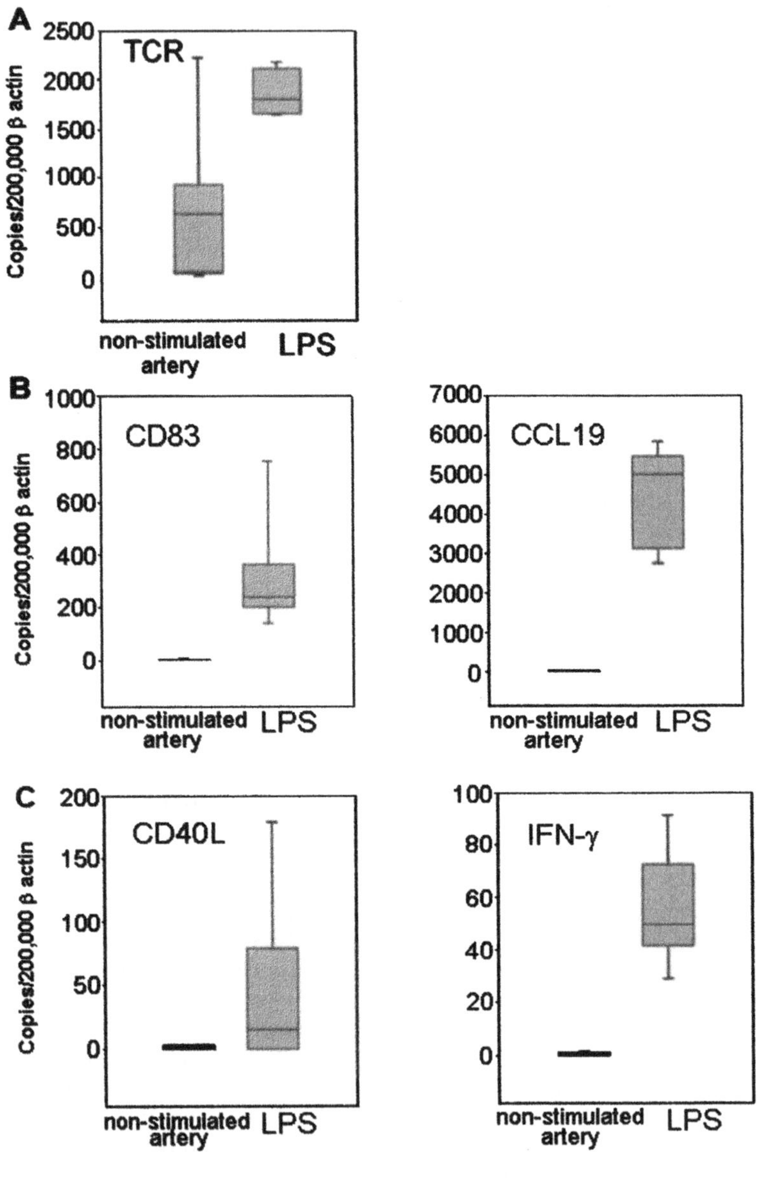

FIGURE 2. Vascular dendritic cells and immunogenicity of human medium-sized arteries. Human temporal arteries were implanted into SCID mice. On day 6 after implantation, the artery–SCID chimeras were injected with either LPS (3 ng/mouse) or sham-treated (nonstimulated artery). One day later they received an adoptive transfer of allogeneic human CD4 T cells. Human arteries were explanted and tissue extracts were analyzed for markers of T-cell recruitment (TCRα), dendritic cell activation (CD83, CCL19), and T-cell activation (IFN-γ, CD40L). T cells were recruited to the nonstimulated arteries (**A**), but did not under-

In an effort to discover how adventitial DCs can function as immunogenic partners for CD4 T cells, we have explored whether activation of DCs is sufficient to overcome their nonstimulatory state.[35,36] Injection of proinflammatory cytokines, such as tumor necrosis factor α, into human artery–severe combined immunodeficient (SCID) mouse chimeras induced partial activation of the adventitial DCs but could not facilitate activation of alloreactive T cells. Notably, upon triggering with tumor necrosis factor α, adventitial DCs responded with production of CCL21 but failed to upregulate CCL19, CCL18, and IL-18—products typically seen with full differentiation of this DC population. Conversely, injection of the bacterial macromolecule lipopolysaccharide (LPS) mediated a complete activation program of the adventitial DCs. When exposed to LPS, the DCs in the human arteries produce CCL21, CCL19, CCL18, and IL-18, and they become strongly positive for the activation marker CD83 (FIG. 3). After infusion of alloreactive CD4 T cells, these T cells accumulated at the adventitia–media border. Moreover, such tissue-infiltrating T cells undergo activation, thereby initiating production of CD40 ligand and IFN-γ.

ACTIVATION OF ARTERIAL WALL DCs AS AN EARLY EVENT IN VASCULITIS

To test the hypothesis that the adoptive transfer model in the human artery–SCID chimeras could truly mimic some of the steps occurring in the early phases of GCA, we made use of the fact that PMR represents a forme fruste of GCA.[35,37] Patients with PMR and GCA share many clinical features of disease, but temporal artery biopsy samples in PMR patients are free of vasculitis.[38] We examined temporal artery tissues from patients with PMR and found that the adventitial DCs had left their physiologic state of immaturity. Instead, they expressed CD83 and actively produced chemokines, including CCL19 and CCL21 (FIG. 3). To demonstrate that PMR arteries could principally support T-cell recruitment and activation, we devised an experimental setup that would allow for testing the functional capabilities of tissue-resident DCs. Temporal arteries from three different clinical sources were coimplanted into SCID mice. These temporal arteries were derived from a patient with PMR, a patient with GCA, and a donor without vasculitis; the samples were matched for sharing the HLA-DR4 haplotype. Chimeras carrying only one artery type each served as controls. Activated T cells were presented in the GCA arteries, but absent in the PMR and normal control arteries. Once coimplanted, activated T cells migrated from the GCA arteries to the PMR arteries, but avoided the normal arteries. These data clearly demonstrated that the functional status of arterial DCs was altered in PMR patients and that such DCs could support local T-cell triggering once T cells

go activation (**C**). Vascular DCs remained immature (**B**) and did not express CD83 or produce CCL19. Following LPS triggering, T-cell recruitment was amplified (**A**) and DCs upregulated CD83 and began to produce CCL19 (**B**). LPS injection was also followed by *in situ* activation of the recruited T cells, which began to transcribe IFN-γ and CD40L (**C**). Results are shown as box plots with medians, 25th and 75th percentiles as *boxes*, and 10th and 90th percentiles as *whiskers*. Data shown were derived from nine independent experiments.

with vasculogenic potential were available. DCs in normal temporal arteries remained nonstimulatory. These experiments also lend strong support to the concept that a change in the functional status of the adventitial DC is an early event in the disease process, preceding the invasion of T cells into the vessel wall.

DENDRITIC CELL FUNCTION IN CHRONIC GCA

Since attracting T cells and their *in situ* activation are necessary elements of initiating the disease process in vasculitis, a role for wall-residing DCs is intuitive. It is much less clear whether DCs continue to play a part in vasculitis once the initial steps of establishing disease have been taken. Immunohistochemical studies have revealed that many DCs are present in the vessel wall infiltrates. DCs are present in the adventitia, but can also be found in the media. Some multinucleated giant cells stain positive with S-100 antibodies, suggesting that DCs participate in the fusion process of phagocytes, which leads to giant cell formation.[35] Phenotyping of DCs in temporal arteries with panarteritis has established the following molecular profile: S-100, fascin, CD83, thereby classifying them as activated DCs (FIG. 3).[36] Gene profiling has failed to detect CD1a, and DC-SIGN–specific sequences have been seen only in a small group of vasculitic arteries. Thus, DCs participating in vasculitic lesions express a unique pattern of molecules, distinct from those described for other DC populations. Also in contrast to DCs in normal, noninflamed arteries, DCs in vasculitis stain strongly positive for CD86 and HLA-DR, providing indirect evidence for their capability to present antigens and activate T cells. Also, DCs express CCR7 and are the single cellular source for CCL19 and CCL21 in established disease.[34] It has been proposed that the expression of CCR7 and the secretion of CCR7-binding chemokines create a scenario in which the highly activated DCs are trapped in the lesions and cannot migrate to lymphoid tissues. The disease-sustaining function of arterial DCs was confirmed in depletion studies using anti-CD83 antibodies in human artery–SCID chimeras. Injection of anti-CD83 antibodies had profound inhibitory effects on T-cell activation in vasculitic arteries. Also, IL-1β declined markedly, demonstrating downstream inhibition of macrophage function. Taken together; these data confirm that CD83-expressing DCs assume a crucial role as antigen-presenting and T-cell stimulatory cells in vasculitis. Although the vessel wall lesions include several cell populations that could theoretically serve as antigen-presenting cells, such as fibroblasts, vascular smooth muscle cells, endothelial cells, and macrophages, experimental data indicate that that function is limited to DCs. Thus, DCs appear to regulate disease initiation as well as disease maintenance.[35]

DCs IN VASCULAR HEALTH AND DISEASE

Studies exploring the functional activity of vascular DCs have gone beyond DCs that participate in maintaining chronic inflammation and have started to examine the concept that DCs have an important place in protecting vascular health. Positioned at the junction between the fibroblast-rich, vascularized adventitia and the avascular media, DCs appear to be the guardians of the vessel wall. Under physiologic conditions, they remain in an immature state (FIG. 3). Indeed, in an allorecognition model,

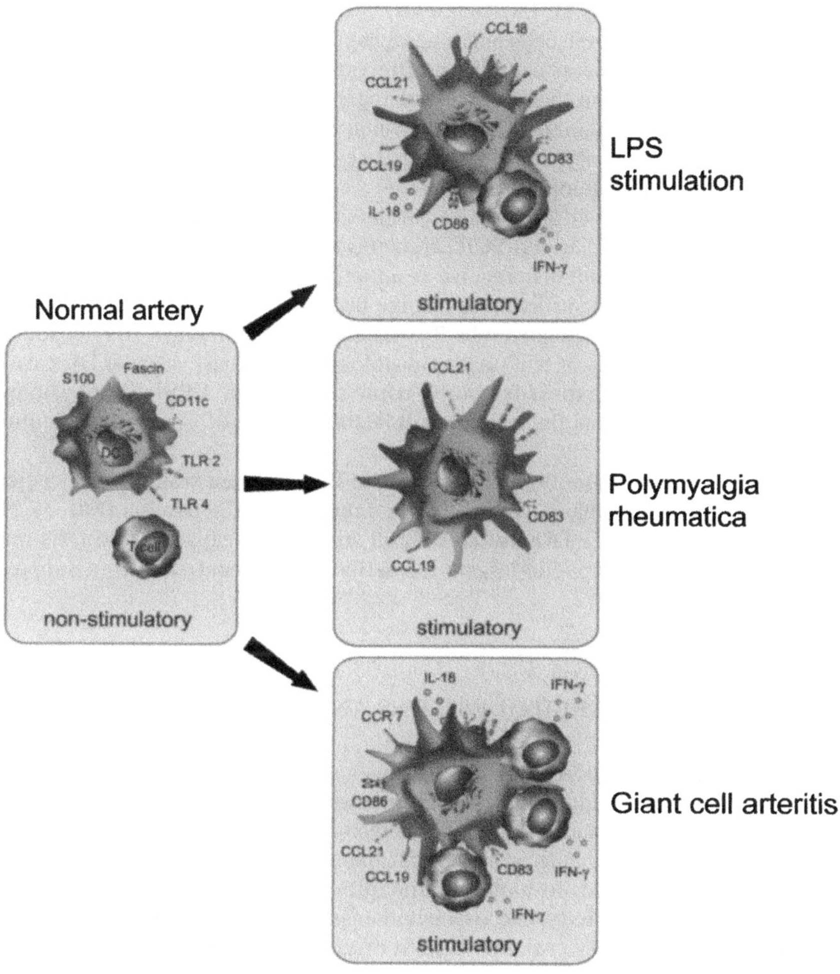

FIGURE 3. Functional profile of arterial dendritic cells in healthy arteries and in vasculitis. In medium-sized arteries, a population of dendritic cells (DCs) is positioned at the adventitia–media border. Under physiologic conditions, these DCs recruit small numbers of T cells and do not support T-cell activation (**A**). When triggered with TLR ligands, such as LPS, adventitial DCs effectively attract and stimulate T cells (**B**). Two disease states have been identified in which adventitial DCs are fully matured and acquire T-cell stimulatory capacity. In patients with polymyalgia rheumatica (**C**), adventitial DCs produce T-cell–attracting chemokines and express CD83; yet the patients appear to lack T cells responsive to these activated adventitial DCs, and T-cell migration to the artery is prevented. In patients with giant cell arteritis (**D**), highly activated DCs sustain T-cell recruitment and *in situ* activation.

T cells are recruited to the adventitia, but not activated. In patients with PMR, DCs enter the activation program, increase production of chemokines, and can attract and stimulate T cells. In nearly all PMR patients, DC activation alone is insufficient to promote the recruitment of T cells and macrophages to the vessel wall. Results from human artery–SCID chimeras examining different stages of the disease process are compatible with the notion that an essential ingredient of vasculitis is also T cells capable of promoting vascular inflammation and that this component is lacking in PMR. Thus, vascular DC activation plus a disease-prone repertoire of T cells appear to be prerequisites for developing GCA.

Early steps in the interaction between wall-positioned DCs and circulating T cells can be mimicked in human artery–SCID chimeras that are implanted with normal arteries, treated with LPS, and then receive an adoptive transfer of human T cells. LPS injection is necessary and sufficient to change the functional state of vascular DCs so that the vessel wall is recognized by T cells and supports their *in situ* activation. These experiments document that under physiologic conditions, vascular DCs avoid T-cell stimulation. When exposed to blood-borne stimuli (e.g., LPS), this physiologic function is abolished and the arterial wall becomes a site of immune recognition events.

In fully established vasculitis, DCs persist in the inflamed wall and are critical antigen-presenting cells that sustain T-cell and macrophage activation (FIG. 3). No other cell type can replace DCs in their T-cell stimulatory capacity, and DCs may well represent ideal therapeutic targets for antibody treatment studies to suppress vasculitis.

UNANSWERED QUESTIONS AND CHALLENGES

The ultimate goal of dissecting the pathogenesis of vasculitis is to understand how certain at-risk individuals develop an intense granulomatous inflammation in at-risk arteries, eventually causing vessel occlusion and organ ischemia.[39] Research conducted over the last decade promises that the impact of these studies are farther reaching, opening our eyes to biologic principles governing the function of blood vessels, their immunogenicity, and tissue homeostasis in these organ structures that are critical for host survival. Another benefit of examining the relationship between the immune system and medium-sized arteries relates to atherosclerosis, the major cause of mortality in developed countries. Inflammation of the atherosclerotic lesion has emerged as a principal disease component of atherosclerosis and its clinical complications.

Surprising findings have come from studying temporal arteries of patients diagnosed with GCA.[40,41] Careful histologic evaluation of vasculitic lesions predicted that the granulomatous reactions reflected the cross-communication between highly activated T cells and macrophages. Intimal hyperplasia leading to vessel stenosis could have been predicted as a maladaptive "healing" response of the artery. However, detailed evaluation of the vasculitic arteries collected from patients revealed several unanticipated and promising clues[36] that have the potential to cross-fertilize the fields of vascular biology and immunology. The most important discoveries and questions arising from these insights are the following:

(1) The principal antigen-presenting cells in vasculitis are DCs. In a lesion filled with activated macrophages, endothelial cells, fibroblasts, and vascular smooth muscle cells, choices for antigen-presenting cells should be quite broad. However, blocking DCs with anti-CD83 essentially abolishes T-cell function. Why do DCs hold this unique position, and why are they required to sustain T-cell activation?

(2) DCs are an indigenous population in the adventitia of medium-sized blood vessels. This observation identified the arterial adventitia as an immunologic surveillance zone, comparable to mucosal surfaces and the skin. How are such vascular DCs related to other DC populations in peripheral lymphoid tissues?[42] What are the physiologic functions of DCs sitting in this tissue region and to which signals do they respond? Answers to these questions will be essential in understanding blood vessel wall function in general.

(3) Functional studies *in vitro* and *in vivo* strongly support the notion that adventitial DCs function primarily by preventing vessel wall inflammation. Do adventitial DCs represent tolerogenic DCs?[43–45] Do they use mechanisms previously described in tolerogenic DCs,[46,47] or do they rely on novel pathways in avoiding T-cell recruitment and activation in the vessel wall?

(4) Triggering of adventitial DCs that is sufficient to initiate wall inflammation can be achieved through blood-borne stimuli. This finding has widened the search for vasculogenic antigens from the vessel wall itself to systemically distributed triggers. Specifically, infectious events far from the blood vessel could potentially initiate vascular inflammation. Indeed, any episode of bacterial infection leading to the release of LPS should stimulate adventitial DCs and might lay the groundwork for vasculitis. How does the host protect itself from widespread vascular DC activation in the face of infectious episodes?

(5) Spatial context is critical in regulating vessel wall inflammation. Positioning of DCs and their relationship to the capillary network is critical. Also, the functional commitment of macrophages in the vasculitic infiltrates is closely correlated with their placement in the wall layers.[32,40,48–51] The effect of the three-dimensional arrangement of cells in their local microenvironment also stresses the need to faithfully recapitulate the special conditions of the medium-sized artery when studying GCA, DC function in the adventitia, and the response of resident vessel wall cells to systemic stimuli.

(6) The challenge of studying human arteries and arteritis. The structure of the vessel wall is intimately related to the size dimensions of the blood vessel and only arteries with a certain wall thickness require a capillary network to supply oxygen to the wall itself.[52–54] Spatial conditions of the vessel wall structure thus change dramatically with the size of the host. This imposes an enormous challenge, as rodents do not possess arteries that resemble human medium-sized vessels in size and layering. Considering the importance of scale in studying the dialogue between the immune system and the vessel wall, certain questions can be asked and answered only by studying humans.

ACKNOWLEDGMENTS

This work was funded by grants from the Dana Foundation and the National Institutes of Health (R01 EY 11916). The authors thank Dr. Sergey Pryshchep for help with preparing the figures, and Tamela Yeargin for manuscript editing.

[*Competing interests*: The authors declare that they have no competing financial interests.]

REFERENCES

1. Springer, T.A. 1995. Traffic signals on endothelium for lymphocyte recirculation and leukocyte emigration. Annu. Rev. Physiol. **57:** 827–872.
2. Hoffman, G.S. 2004. Determinants of vessel targeting in vasculitis. Clin. Dev. Immunol. **11:** 275–279.
3. Liuzzo, G. 2001. Atherosclerosis: an inflammatory disease. Rays **26:** 221–230.
4. Hansson, G.K. 2005. Inflammation, atherosclerosis, and coronary artery disease. N. Engl. J. Med. **352:** 1685–1695.
5. Mullenix, P.S., C.A. Andersen & B.W. Starnes. 2005. Atherosclerosis as inflammation. Ann. Vasc. Surg. **19:** 130–138.
6. Mulvihill, N.T. & J.B. Foley. 2002. Inflammation in acute coronary syndromes. Heart **87:** 201–204.
7. Falk, R.J. & J.C. Jennette. 2004. Thoughts about the classification of small vessel vasculitis. J. Nephrol. **17**(Suppl. 8): S3–S9.
8. Weyand, C.M. & J.J. Goronzy. 2003. Medium- and large-vessel vasculitis. N. Engl. J. Med. **349:** 160–169.
9. Salvarani, C. 2003. Large vessel vasculitis. Clin. Exp. Rheumatol. **21:** S133–S134.
10. Weyand, C.M. & J.J. Goronzy. 2003. Giant-cell arteritis and polymyalgia rheumatica. Ann. Intern. Med. **139:** 505–515.
11. Chin, R.L. & N. Latov. 2005. Central nervous system manifestations of rheumatologic diseases. Curr. Opin. Rheumatol. **17:** 91–99.
12. Schmidt, W.A. & D. Blockmans. 2005. Use of ultrasonography and positron emission tomography in the diagnosis and assessment of large-vessel vasculitis. Curr. Opin. Rheumatol. **17:** 9–15.
13. Nordborg, E. & C. Nordborg. 2004. Giant cell arteritis: strategies in diagnosis and treatment. Curr. Opin. Rheumatol. **16:** 25–30.
14. Weyand, C.M., J.W. Fulbright, G.G. Hunder, *et al.* 2000. Treatment of giant cell arteritis: interleukin-6 as a biologic marker of disease activity. Arthritis Rheum. **43:** 1041–1048.
15. Weyand, C.M. 2000. The Dunlop-Dottridge Lecture: the pathogenesis of giant cell arteritis. J. Rheumatol. **27:** 517–522.
16. Langford, C.A. 2005. Vasculitis in the geriatric population. Clin. Geriatr. Med. **21:** 631–647.
17. Weyand, C.M., N.N. Hunder, K.C. Hicok, *et al.* 1994. HLA-DRB1 alleles in polymyalgia rheumatica, giant cell arteritis, and rheumatoid arthritis. Arthritis Rheum. **37:** 514–520.
18. Weyand, C.M., K.C. Hicok, G.G. Hunder & J.J. Goronzy. 1992. The HLA-DRB1 locus as a genetic component in giant cell arteritis. Mapping of a disease-linked sequence motif to the antigen binding site of the HLA-DR molecule. J. Clin. Invest. **90:** 2355–2361.
19. Weyand, C.M. & J.J. Goronzy. 1995. Giant cell arteritis as an antigen-driven disease. Rheum. Dis. Clin. North Am. **21:** 1027–1039.
20. Cid, M.C., E. Campo, G. Ercilla, *et al.* 1989. Immunohistochemical analysis of lymphoid and macrophage cell subsets and their immunologic activation markers in temporal arteritis. Influence of corticosteroid treatment. Arthritis Rheum. **32:** 884–893.

21. SPIERA, R. & H. SPIERA. 2004. Inflammatory disease in older adults. Cranial arteritis. Geriatrics **59:** 25–29; quiz 30.
22. WEYAND, C.M., J. SCHONBERGER, U. OPPITZ, *et al.* 1994. Distinct vascular lesions in giant cell arteritis share identical T cell clonotypes. J. Exp. Med. **179:** 951–960.
23. WEYAND, C.M. & J.J. GORONZY. 2002. Pathogenic mechanisms in giant cell arteritis. Clevel. Clin. J. Med. **69**(Suppl. 2): SII28–SII32.
24. WEYAND, C.M. & J.J. GORONZY. 1996. The pathogenic role of T lymphocytes in vasculitis. Sarcoidosis Vasc. Diffuse Lung Dis. **13:** 217–220.
25. MARTINEZ-TABOADA, V., N.N. HUNDER, G.G. HUNDER, *et al.* 1996. Recognition of tissue residing antigen by T cells in vasculitic lesions of giant cell arteritis. J. Mol. Med. **74:** 695–703.
26. GORONZY, J.J. & C.M. WEYAND. 2002. Cytokines in giant-cell arteritis. Clevel. Clin. J. Med. **69**(Suppl. 2): SII91–SII94.
27. BLAIN, H., I. ABDELMOUTTALEB, J. BELMIN, *et al.* 2002. Arterial wall production of cytokines in giant cell arteritis: results of a pilot study using human temporal artery cultures. J. Gerontol. A. Biol. Sci. Med. Sci. **57:** M241–M245.
28. WEYAND, C.M., N. TETZLAFF, J. BJORNSSON, *et al.* 1997. Disease patterns and tissue cytokine profiles in giant cell arteritis. Arthritis Rheum. **40:** 19–26.
29. BRACK, A., V. MARTINEZ-TABOADA, A. STANSON, *et al.* 1999. Disease pattern in cranial and large-vessel giant cell arteritis. Arthritis Rheum. **42:** 311–317.
30. WAGNER, A.D., J. BJORNSSON, G.B. BARTLEY, *et al.* 1996. Interferon-gamma-producing T cells in giant cell vasculitis represent a minority of tissue-infiltrating cells and are located distant from the site of pathology. Am. J. Pathol. **148:** 1925–1933.
31. BRUHL, H., V. VIELHAUER, M. WEISS, *et al.* 2005. Expression of DARC, CXCR3 and CCR5 in giant cell arteritis. Rheumatology (Oxford) **44:** 309–313.
32. WEYAND, C.M., A.D. WAGNER, J. BJORNSSON & J.J. GORONZY. 1996. Correlation of the topographical arrangement and the functional pattern of tissue-infiltrating macrophages in giant cell arteritis. J. Clin. Invest. **98:** 1642–1649.
33. RITTNER, H.L., M. KAISER, A. BRACK, *et al.* 1999. Tissue-destructive macrophages in giant cell arteritis. Circ. Res. **84:** 1050–1058.
34. KRUPA, W.M., M. DEWAN, M.S. JEON, *et al.* 2002. Trapping of misdirected dendritic cells in the granulomatous lesions of giant cell arteritis. Am. J. Pathol. **161:** 1815–1823.
35. MA-KRUPA, W., M. KWAN, J.J. GORONZY & C.M. WEYAND. 2004. Activation of arterial wall dendritic cells and breakdown of self-tolerance in giant cell arteritis. J. Exp. Med. **199:** 173–183.
36. MA-KRUPA, W., M. KWAN, J.J. GORONZY & C.M. WEYAND. 2005. Toll-like receptors in giant cell arteritis. Clin. Immunol. **115:** 38–46.
37. WEYAND, C.M., W. MA-KRUPA & J.J. GORONZY. 2004. Immunopathways in giant cell arteritis and polymyalgia rheumatica. Autoimmun. Rev. **3:** 46–53.
38. SALVARANI, C., F. CANTINI, L. BOIARDI & G.G. HUNDER 2004. Polymyalgia rheumatica. Best Pract. Res. Clin. Rheumatol. **18:** 705–722.
39. HOFFMAN, G.S. 2003. Large-vessel vasculitis: unresolved issues. Arthritis Rheum. **48:** 2406–2414.
40. RITTNER, H.L., V. HAFNER, P.A. KLIMIUK, *et al.* 1999. Aldose reductase functions as a detoxification system for lipid peroxidation products in vasculitis. J. Clin. Invest. **103:** 1007–1013.
41. WEYAND, C.M., K.C. HICOK, G.G. HUNDER & J.J. GORONZY. 1994. Tissue cytokine patterns in patients with polymyalgia rheumatica and giant cell arteritis. Ann. Intern. Med. **121:** 484–491.
42. STEINMAN, R.M., L. BONIFAZ, S. FUJII, *et al.* 2005. The innate functions of dendritic cells in peripheral lymphoid tissues. Adv. Exp. Med. Biol. **560:** 83–97.
43. STEINMAN, R.M., D. HAWIGER, K. LIU, *et al.* 2003. Dendritic cell function *in vivo* during the steady state: a role in peripheral tolerance. Ann. N.Y. Acad. Sci. **987:** 15–25.
44. STEINMAN, R.M., D. HAWIGER & M.C. NUSSENZWEIG. 2003. Tolerogenic dendritic cells. Annu. Rev. Immunol. **21:** 685–711.
45. STEINMAN, R.M. & M.C. NUSSENZWEIG. 2002. Avoiding horror autotoxicus: the importance of dendritic cells in peripheral T cell tolerance. Proc. Natl. Acad. Sci. USA **99:** 351–358.

46. TARBELL, K.V., S. YAMAZAKI, K. OLSON, *et al.* 2004. CD25+ CD4+ T cells, expanded with dendritic cells presenting a single autoantigenic peptide, suppress autoimmune diabetes. J. Exp. Med. **199:** 1467–1477.
47. DHODAPKAR, M.V. & R.M. STEINMAN. 2002. Antigen-bearing immature dendritic cells induce peptide-specific CD8(+) regulatory T cells in vivo in humans. Blood **100:** 174–177.
48. KAISER, M., B. YOUNGE, J. BJORNSSON, *et al.* 1999. Formation of new vasa vasorum in vasculitis. Production of angiogenic cytokines by multinucleated giant cells. Am. J. Pathol. **155:** 765–774.
49. WAGNER, A.D., J.J. GORONZY & C.M. WEYAND. 1994. Functional profile of tissue-infiltrating and circulating CD68+ cells in giant cell arteritis. Evidence for two components of the disease. J. Clin. Invest. **94:** 1134–1140.
50. KAISER, M., C.M. WEYAND, J. BJORNSSON & J.J. GORONZY. 1998. Platelet-derived growth factor, intimal hyperplasia, and ischemic complications in giant cell arteritis. Arthritis Rheum. **41:** 623–633.
51. BORKOWSKI, A., B.R. YOUNGE, L. SZWEDA, *et al.* 2002. Reactive nitrogen intermediates in giant cell arteritis: selective nitration of neocapillaries. Am. J. Pathol. **161:** 115–123.
52. AGLIANO, M., G. SACCHI, E. WEBER, *et al.* 1997. Vasa vasorum of superficial collecting lymphatics of human thigh. Lymphology **30:** 116–121.
53. WILLIAMS, J.K. & D.D. HEISTAD. 1996. [The vasa vasorum of the arteries]. J. Mal. Vasc. **21**(Suppl. C): 266–269.
54. OKUYAMA, K., G. YAGINUMA, T. TAKAHASHI, *et al.* 1988. The development of vasa vasorum of the human aorta in various conditions. A morphometric study. Arch. Pathol. Lab. Med. **112:** 721–725.

Immunologic Role of the Cholinergic Anti-Inflammatory Pathway and the Nicotinic Acetylcholine α7 Receptor

MARGOT GALLOWITSCH-PUERTA AND KEVIN J. TRACEY

Feinstein Institute for Medical Research, Manhasset, New York 11030-3816, USA

ABSTRACT: Cytokines are small protein molecules that facilitate communication between cells of the immune system and other tissues. Their messenger function elicits responses in other cells, ranging from DNA binding and tissue remodeling to coordinating the local cellular response to inflammation. The magnitude of the cytokine response is regulated closely, because an over- or underabundance of cytokine activity can impair organ function and cause shock and tissue injury. Counterregulatory molecular and humoral mechanisms protect the host from cytokine excess, including the pituitary–adrenal–glucocorticoid system, and the anti-inflammatory cytokine system. These humoral systems are protective, but they are relatively slow-acting, concentration-gradient dependent, and not integrated. We recently discovered that the "cholinergic anti-inflammatory pathway," a nervous system–based, rapid, and locally acting mechanism, can inhibit the cytokine response. Signals transmitted via the vagus nerve converge on cytokine-producing cells that express the nicotinic acetylcholine receptor alpha 7 (nAChR α7). The α7 receptor is an essential component of the cholinergic anti-inflammatory pathway, because activation of this receptor prevents cytokine release. Advances in understanding the molecular structure and function of α7 have begun to provide a better understanding of potential mechanisms regarding its assembly, expression, and cytokine-inhibiting functions. It may be possible to exploit this pathway to therapeutic advantage for diseases caused by excessive cytokine activity.

KEYWORDS: cholinergic anti-inflammatory pathway; nAChR7; macrophage; vagus nerve

INTRODUCTION

Injury, infection, or ischemia activate immune cells to produce cytokines, small proteins that function as intracellular messengers to coordinate the immunological and metabolic response. Low levels of proinflammatory cytokine activity are beneficial to the host, but high levels can cause shock, tissue injury, organ failure, and death (FIG. 1). Individual cytokines can cause specific pathological effects. This "cytokine theory of disease" is that the development of some disease syndromes requires the activity of a specific cytokine. The systemic release of tumor necrosis fac-

Address for correspondence: Kevin J. Tracey, Feinstein Institute for Medical Research, 350 Community Drive, Manhasset, NY 11030-3816. Voice: 516-562-2416; fax: 516-562-2356.. kjtracey@nshs.edu

Ann. N.Y. Acad. Sci. 1062: 209–219 (2005).
doi: 10.1196/annals.1358.024

tor (TNF) causes septic shock with disseminated vasculitis, adrenal necrosis and hemorrhage, and acute inflammatory damage in the intestines, lungs, brain, and other organs.[1,2] Another potentially lethal cytokine, high-mobility group box one (HMGB1), causes a different severe sepsis syndrome with minimal tissue injury or cell death, and no shock.[3–5] Thus, the systemic activity of specific cytokines can mediate distinct pathophysiological responses. Both of these cytokines have been implicated in the pathogenesis of arthritis, highlighting the importance of understanding that the response to cytokine activity in tissues may be different from the response to systemic overproduction. As other cytokines continue to be discovered, it is likely that the list of associated disease syndromes will continue to expand.

To limit the damaging effects of proinflammatory cytokines, the immune response is controlled closely by molecular and humoral mechanisms that keep cytokine activity in check. Humoral anti-inflammatory factors that suppress cytokine synthesis include glucocorticoids, interleukin-10 (IL-10), transforming growth factor beta (TGF-β), and soluble receptors that neutralize the activity of cytokines. These factors are critical in modulating the cytokine response, but they are also inherently slow-acting, concentration-gradient dependent, and cannot be integrated. Here, we review the actions of the "cholinergic anti-inflammatory pathway," a

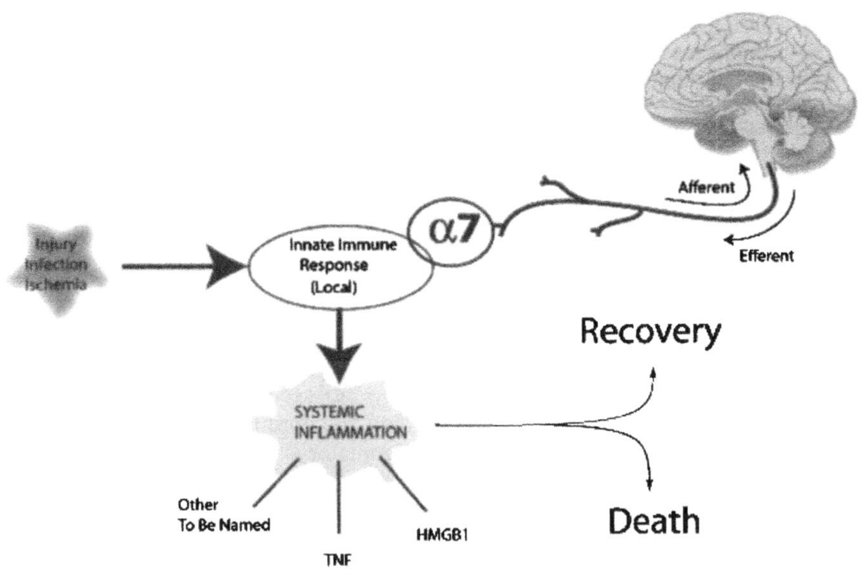

FIGURE 1. In the cytokine theory of disease, cytokines mediate the signs and symptoms of specific diseases. Inciting events such as injury, infection, or ischemia cause a local innate immune response; cytokine levels are transiently and appropriately elevated to combat infection and promote healing. Levels subsequently return to normal and the patient recovers. However, if cytokine levels become too high they can cause disease, including shock, tissue injury, arthritis, severe organ failure, and death. The cholinergic anti-inflammatory pathway, via the vagus nerve, can counterregulate the proinflammatory cytokine response through the α7 receptor.

neural-based cytokine counterregulatory mechanism that is fast, local, and can be integrated.[6] Signals transmitted via the vagus nerve converge on cytokine-secreting cells that express the nicotinic cholinergic receptor alpha 7 (nAChR α7) to inhibit cytokine release. Vagus nerve stimulation with small pacemaker devices or pharmacological activation of the α7 pathway confer significant protection against cytokine-mediated diseases.[6]

CHOLINERGIC ANTI-INFLAMMATORY PATHWAY

The vagus nerve, the tenth cranial nerve, originates in the brain stem. Its name is derived from the Latin word *vagus*, meaning "to meander"; the nerve follows an indirect path to the major body organs from the brain to the colon. Its function is traditionally associated with maintaining balance in the autonomic nervous system by controlling heart rate, blood pressure, digestion, and other systems. Acetylcholine, the principle neurotransmitter of the vagus nerve, interacts with peripheral muscarinic receptors to modulate organ functions.

We recently identified a previously unrecognized role of the vagus nerve in the control of cytokine release by the immune system. Electrical stimulation of the vagus nerve of animals exposed to endotoxin, a potent activator of cytokine release, significantly inhibited the release of TNF and other proinflammatory cytokines, and prevented the development of lethal shock and tissue injury.[7] Vagus nerve stimulation also inhibited cytokine release in an animal model of ischemia reperfusion; vagus nerve stimulation prevented shock and inhibited TNF production in serum, heart, and liver.[8,9] In a model of local inflammation, vagus nerve stimulation significantly decreased the recruitment of inflammatory cells into a carrageenan air pouch, and reduced the activation of the endothelial cells lining the pouch.[10] Together, these studies reveal that signaling via the vagus nerve can protect significantly against the development of harmful inflammation.

The molecular basis of cytokine inhibition in the cholinergic anti-inflammatory pathway requires the nicotinic acetylcholine receptor α7 subunit.[11] Animal experiments using α7 knockout mice showed that vagus nerve stimulation failed to inhibit TNF production, indicating that α7 is required for the interaction of the vagus nerve with the cytokine-producing arm of the immune system. Alpha 7 knockout animals develop a higher TNF response to endotoxin as compared with wild-type animals, suggesting that vagus nerve activity contributes to the tonic, protective anti-inflammatory regulation of systemic cytokine release.[11] Addition of α7 agonists to stimulated cytokine-producing macrophages significantly decreases the activation of nuclear factor kappa B (NFκB), a transcription factor that regulates cytokine release.[12] Nicotine binding to the α7 receptor also activates recruitment and phosphorylation of the JAK2 receptor; subsequent Stat3 phosphorylation and translocation to the nucleus is associated with a decreased downstream response to TNF, macrophage inflammatory protein 2 (MIP-2), and interleukin 6 (IL-6).[13] These anticytokine effects of α7 signaling are specific, because ligation of α7 does not alter the endotoxin-induced activation of p38, c-JUN NH2-terminal protein kinase (JNK), or extracellular signal-regulated kinase (ERK). Thus, in the absence of α7 stimulation, production of endotoxin, TNF, or other factors that activate macrophages culminate in the translocation of activated NFκB to the nucleus, which increases the

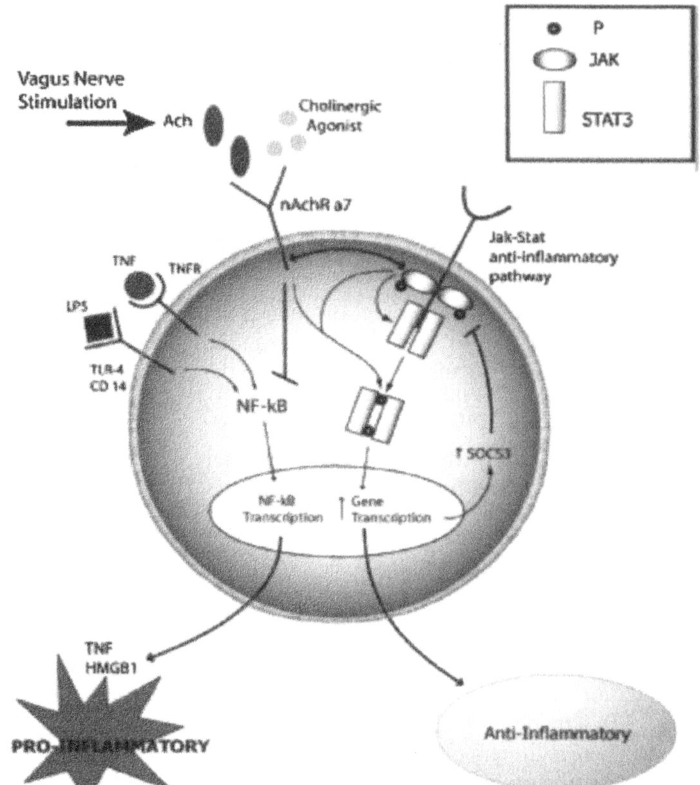

FIGURE 2. The molecular basis of inhibiting cytokine release via α7. Endotoxin or TNF binds to toll-like receptor 4 (TLR-4), or CD-14 or TNF receptors, respectively. This induces NFκB to translocate to the nucleus, thereby increasing the release of TNF and HMGB1. Acetylcholine and nicotine bind to the α7 subunit receptor on macrophages and prevent the translocation of NFκB to the nucleus as well as initiate the JAK/STAT pathway, which subsequently reduces proinflammatory cytokine release.[6,7,9,11–14]

production of proinflammatory cytokines. Acetylcholine, nicotine, or cholinergic agonists that bind to α7 on macrophages both prevent the translocation of NFκB to the nucleus and activate the JAK/STAT pathway, thereby reducing proinflammatory cytokine release (FIG. 2).[6–9,11–14]

NEUROTRANSMISSION AND α7

Otto Loewi originally formulated the neurotransmitter hypothesis after he dreamed about an isolated frog heart submerged in a saline chamber with the vagus nerve intact. He then performed the now-famous experiments in which he stimulated the vagus nerve of the isolated frog heart from his dream, and observed that the heart rate slowed. Then, when he irrigated a second isolated frog heart with the solution bathing the first heart, the second heart also slowed. Loewi named this mysterious factor "Vagusstoff," now known as acetylcholine, the principal neurotransmitter of the vagus nerve that regulates heart rate by instantaneously slowing the time between successive heart beats.[15,16] The mechanism of neurotransmission was not understood until Ehrlich and Langley developed the concept of the receptor in the late nineteenth century; they coined the term "receptor" in 1913. They studied the effects of atropine (an antagonist of cholinergic receptors) and pilocarpine (a plant alkaloid that is a cholinergic agonist) on salivary flow in cats. Langley inhibited salivary flow by administering atropine, and reversed the inhibition by giving pilocarpine. Readministration of atropine again blocked the effects of pilocarpine. In 1905, Langley described the effects as working through a "receptive substance"; a century later we know this substance as an acetylcholine receptor.[17] Acetylcholine receptors are divided functionally into two groups, muscarinic and nicotinic. Muscarinic receptors are metabotropic and consist of five receptor subtypes; nicotinic receptors are ionotropic hetero- or homopentamers composed from combinations of various subunits. Each of these receptor types has been identified in the central nervous system and in peripheral tissues. Recent studies of the molecular basis of the cholinergic anti-inflammatory pathway indicate that α7 nicotinic receptors occupy a critical role in mediating the anti-inflammatory cytokine-suppressing effects.[18]

The human nicotinic cholinergic receptor α7 subunit was first isolated from a human fetal brain cDNA library using a rat α7 probe.[19] The Subcommittee on Nicotinic Acetylcholine Receptors of the International Union of Pharmacology (IUPHAR) Committee on Receptor Nomenclature and Drug Classification (NC-IUPHAR) has recommended the use of the Greek letter–based nomenclature for nicotinic acetylcholine receptor subunits. Subscripts are used to define the number of particular subunits within a pentamer; for example, $\alpha7_5$ represents the homopentamer α7.[20]

Little is known about the expression, function, or activity of the nAChR α7 in macrophages, but a great deal is known about this receptor in other cell types. Nicotinic acetylcholine receptors are ligand-gated ion channels of the cys-loop superfamily, which includes glycine, GABA, and serotonin receptors.[21] The structure of the α7 receptor includes an extracellular N-terminal region, four transmembrane domains, and an extracellular C terminus. Cys-loops, which are highly conserved and are located in the N-terminal domain of the receptors,[22] are believed to contribute to protein structure.[23,24] The loops are composed of 13 amino acids positioned between two cysteine residues, which form a disulfide bridge.[20] The region between the cysteine residues is unique to each subunit.[20]

The classic α7 nAChR is a homomeric pentamer composed of five individual α7 subunits. Each individual subunit includes 10 exons, with the four transmembrane domains located in exons 7 to 10,[25] three putative glycosylation sites located extracellularly in exons 2, 4, and 5,[25,26] and three competitive agonist-binding sites in exons 4, 6, and 7.[27] Phosphorylation sites located in the cytosolic portion of exon 10 (between transmembrane domains 3 and 4) may be involved in signaling cascades subsequent to ligand binding.[28] Human, rat, and mouse nAChR α7 are more than 90% homologous.[29] The assembled subunits form a central pore, with ligand binding at subunit junctions responsible for changes in the state of the receptor. The molecular weight of the complete α7 is 56.4 kDa, and the full length of the individual α7 gene is estimated to be greater than 75 kb in size. Brejc *et al.* crystallized and constructed a model of recombinant acetylcholine-binding protein (AChBP), a novel protein derived from the snail *Lymnaea stagnalis*.[30] AChBP aligns with the N-terminal extracellular portion of nicotinic receptors and when expressed in yeast, forms stable homopentamers. AChBP includes the amino acid residues necessary for ligand binding and shares similar pharmacology with the neuronal nicotinic receptor α7, suggesting a homology between AChBP and nicotinic receptors. Their model also revealed that AChBP consists of five subunits, with dimensions that match electron microscopy findings from nAChRs. Ligand binding sites have been found to exist at the junctions of the subunits as binding pockets formed by loops in the structure.

In 2003, Miyazawa *et al.* expanded on the data of Brejc *et al.* and created crystal structures from *Torpedo marmorata* membranes that revealed the pore of the nicotinic receptor.[31] Confirming observations by Brejc *et al.*, Miyazawa found that the N-terminal region of the receptor was composed predominantly of β-sheet folds, but switched to α-helical domains in the four transmembrane segments, M1, M2, M3, and M4. This sterologic transformation occurs about 10 Å distal to the cell membrane, enabling elongation of the hydrophobic core lumen. The inner pore of the channel is lined by the M2 helices from each individual α7 subunit, which tilt radially inward toward the central axis of the structure. The M2 helices from each subunit are referred to collectively as the inner helices. In contrast, the outer helices (M1, M3, and M4) tilt radially toward and around the central axis of the channel. Miyazawa *et al.* suggested that the outer helices protect the inner ring of helices from the surrounding lipids, and staining supports this theory. Moreover, the inner M2 helices do not form thorough van der Waals forces with M1 or M3, suggesting that the space between them is filled with water. Additionally, only the inner helices change their conformation upon activation by the ligand, allowing ions to pass through the channel, while the outer helices remain fairly unchanged.[32] There is currently no detailed data describing the intracellular cytoplasmic loop region to such levels as can be found with the extracellular and transmembrane domains. However, studies using site-directed mutagenesis have found that the intracellular cytoplasmic loop is necessary for the assembly and expression of functional receptors.[33,34]

α7 GENE AND DUPLICATION

The human nAChR α7 gene has been mapped to chromosome 15q14.[28,29,35] An additional variant of the α7 gene is a hybrid of the wild-type α7 gene and the novel gene FAM7A. The hybrid gene, CHRFAM7A, also known as the α7 duplicate gene, (Gene ID 89832, Entrez Gene) has been mapped to 15q13.1. A potentially significant aspect of the α7 receptor is the existence of at least two α7 homologues. The wild-type gene plays a critical role in the cholinergic anti-inflammatory pathway in mice; therefore, it is plausible that a duplicate gene, which has the potential to produce a structurally similar receptor, may also play a role in controlling inflammation. It is unknown whether the duplicate gene protein is expressed in humans, and its function and importance are unknown.

In 1998, Gault *et al.* reported the structure of the original full-length human α7 receptor subunit gene and promoter region.[28] The original wild-type α7 gene consists of 10 exons. In addition to the wild type, Gault detected six mRNA splice variants. Of the six splice variants, one, which lacks exon 3, maintains the reading frame and does not include a premature stop codon. Theoretically, this could produce a functional receptor, but there is no evidence that this is expressed. Variants with a premature stop codon presumably would produce a truncated product lacking the ability to bind the ligand and disabling receptor functionality. To date, it remains uncertain whether any of the splice variants are expressed in cytokine-producing cells.

Gault cited evidence for a partial duplication of the α7 gene, also identified by Riley *et al.*,[36] and found that exons 5 to 10 of the wild-type α7 gene were duplicated within 1 Mb from the original nAChR α7 gene. The duplicated gene has been found in human postmortem brain tissue and includes four novel exons derived from the FAM7A gene, also located near the nAChR α7 gene.[36] The gene described as "duplicated α7" is likely to be the product of two partially duplicated genes that combined to form a hybrid gene. Riley *et al.* termed this hybrid gene the "cholinergic receptor family with sequence similarity 7A" (CHRFAM7A, Gene ID 89832, Entrez Gene).[36] Alternative splicing has been observed in the duplicated gene (CHRFAM7A); there is also a variant that lacks an entire exon.[28] The large open reading frames on CHRFAM7A and its splice variant predict that the products could have a truncated N-terminal region lacking the majority of the ligand-binding domain, but retaining the transmembrane region that forms the ion channel. This may lead to a receptor missing the signal peptide that in other nicotinic receptors is necessary for assembly and surface expression.[23] There is evidence that CHRFAM7A is transcribed, but evidence of translation is lacking (Entrez Gene). There are variants and single nucleotide polymorphisms (snp) of CHRFAM7A; as many as 21 variants have been observed (Gault, 2003).[37] A 2-bp deletion has been detected in the duplicate gene; it varies between ethnic groups (60% white, 80% Malays, 10% African Bantus), but even within the groups, the frequencies vary.[36] The presence of the duplicated gene may be more common than its absence, leading to the hypothesis that this region of the chromosome is unstable and may be relevant to the neuropsychiatric disorders that map here, such as schizophrenia and epilepsy.[36]

In 2004, Severance *et al.* reported evidence that two isoforms of the α7 receptor in rat contribute to the ion channel function *in vivo*.[38] The first isoform was the wild-type α7, whereas the second isoform incorporated an additional 87 bases near the N terminus in exon 4 that preserved the reading frame, an isoform termed α7-2. Basic Local Alignment Search Tool (BLAST) searches showed that the 87-bp insert mapped to intron 4 of the nAChR α7 gene in both mouse and rat. Both isoforms were detected in rat autonomic neurons, had slow rates of desensitization, and were reversibly blocked by α bungarotoxin. Expression of the α7-2 receptor coincided with mRNA expression. The α7-2 receptor was shown to form functional homomeric ion channels that were activated by acetylcholine and blocked by α bungarotoxin when expressed in *Xenopus laevis* oocytes. It is therefore possible that functional variants of the α7 receptor can be expressed.

REGULATION

Regulatory sites for CHRNA7 have been identified, although their usage and downstream effects remain somewhat enigmatic. The promoter region of the α7 gene was identified and sequenced from P1 artificial chromosomes (PAC).[28] The GC rich region (77%) lacks a TATA box and includes four transcription-factor binding sites, Sp-1, Ap-2, Erg-1, and CREB. The four transcription sites identified in humans are positioned at approximately the same region relative to the protein coding sequence in the bovine α7. The promoter region of the CHRFAM7A duplicate gene has not been identified or sequenced to date, and the regulatory mechanisms underlying α7 expression are largely unknown. Recent studies have implicated a role for glucocorticoids in transcriptional activation of α7.[39] Glucorticoids mediated increased expression of α7 transcripts and activation of the α7 promoter in chromaffin cells that coexpressed human glucocorticoid receptor and α7 promoter-luciferase.[39] Although there are no glucocorticoid binding sites in the α7 promoter, there is an Egr-1 site, which has been shown to interact with other stimuli.[40] Carrasco-Serrano and Criado postulated that dexamethasone was acting indirectly through the Egr-1 binding site.[39] Mutations on two of the three Egr-1 binding sites reduced dexamethasone induction of the α7 promoter, whereas mutations on either one or three of the binding sites did not alter dexamethasone induction significantly. When the two effective mutations were combined with a mutation at a site required for transcription (USF), then activation was eliminated completely. These results indicate that Egr-1 sites are necessary for maximal activation of the α7 promoter in response to glucocorticoids. It is plausible to consider that if dexamethasone increases α7 promoter activity in cells involved in the cholinergic anti-inflammatory pathway, signaling through this neural pathway may be enhanced by glucocorticoids.

POSTTRANSLATIONAL MODIFICATION

To our knowledge, there are no data on posttranslational modifications of the α7 receptor in macrophages or other cytokine-secreting cells that are part of the cholinergic anti-inflammatory pathway. Data from other sources however, can be reviewed to consider whether modifications exist. Drisdel *et al.* showed that in neuronal α bungarotoxin–sensitive receptors of PC12 cells, palmitoylation during assembly plays a role in the expression of functional receptors.[41] Inhibiting palmitoylation blocked receptor expression, whereas cells deficient in α7 receptor expression, such as HEK cells, were not significantly palmitoylated. Additional evidence of modification of the α7 receptor comes from Rakhilin *et al.*[42] They showed that the α7 subunit can fold and assemble by two independent pathways. Subunits assembled in a single conformation are inserted into the membrane but are not functional, as they do not bind α bungarotoxin. Subunits in specialized cells undergo additional processes, presumably in the endoplasmic reticulum, to produce functional α bungarotoxin–binding receptors with two α7 conformations, both of which are expressed in the functional receptors. Rakhilin suggests that a posttranslational mechanism regulates α7 subunit variety, which is necessary for functional homomeric receptors. Differential processing of α7 subunits also was studied further by Drisdel and Green,[43] who used anti-α7 antibodies to detect labeled and purified receptors run on protein gels. Samples subjected to isoelectric focusing, which produced multiple spots from a single band, were all recognized by anti-α7 antibodies, indicating differentially processed α7 subunits. This was found in rat brain as well as PC12 cells and indicates the existence of α7 pentamers containing differentially processed α7 subunits.

Blumenthal *et al.*[44] showed that PC12 cells with high levels of α7 mRNA could be negative for α bungarotoxin binding, even though they may have other nicotinic receptors. Analysis revealed no defects in the α7 RNA in the non–α bungarotoxin–binding cells. Moreover, they showed that the nonbinding cells contained full-length protein, but at lower levels when compared with α bungarotoxin–binding cells. After transfecting PC12 cells lacking native toxin-binding receptors with α7 gene constructs, they noticed the cells could not produce α7 receptors, whereas other transfected gene constructs were produced. Blumenthal *et al.* suggest that these receptors necessitate supplementary gene products to aid assembly and stabilization of the receptors. Williams *et al.*[45] found that exposure of HEK293 cells expressing α7 to nicotine did not cause a current detectable by whole-cell patch-clamp recording; however, cells coexpressing α7 and hric3 exhibited detectable currents with the kinetics of endogenous α7 receptor-expressing cells. Immunoprecipitation experiments showed coassociation of α7 and hric3, but α bungarotoxin staining was visible only on cells coexpressing α7 and hric3. The levels of α7 expressed on the cell surface do not change significantly when hric3 is present, leading to the hypothesis that hric3 participates in folding and/or assembly of the functional receptor.

SUMMARY

The cholinergic anti-inflammatory pathway is a neural pathway that utilizes α7 receptors to control cytokine synthesis. It confers significant protection against cytokine production and toxicity in animal models of inflammation, and therapeutic approaches targeting the nicotinic α7 receptor in this pathway are being prepared for clinical trials. The activity of α7 receptors on macrophages and other cytokine-secreting cells is a new and rapidly expanding field of study, and research is beginning to reveal potential mechanisms regarding α7 receptor assembly, expression, and function in the cholinergic anti-inflammatory pathway. Ongoing research is likely to provide additional insights into the role of variants and duplicates of α7 and whether this molecular knowledge can be used to develop future therapeutics for cytokine diseases under the control of the cholinergic anti-inflammatory pathway.

[*Competing interests*: Kevin Tracey declares that he has competing interests as consultant to Critical Therapeutics, which has licensed rights to technology that he invented.]

REFERENCES

1. Tracey, K.J., B. Beutler, S.F. Lowry, *et al.* 1986. Shock and tissue injury induced by recombinant human cachectin. Science **234:** 470–474.
2. Tracey, K.J., S.F. Lowry & A. Cerami. 1987. Physiological responses to cachectin. Ciba Found. Symp. **131:** 88–108.
3. Wang, H., O. Bloom, M Zhang, *et al.* 1999. HMG-1 as a late mediator of endotosin lethality in mice. Science **285:** 248–251.
4. Yang, H., M. Ochani, J. Li, *et al.* 2004. Reversing established sepsis with antagonists of endogenous high-mobility group box 1. Proc. Natl. Acad. Sci. USA **101:** 296–301.
5. Lotze, M.T. & K.J. Tracey. 2005. High-mobility group box 1 protein (HMGB1): nuclear weapon in the immune arsenal. Nat. Rev. Immunol. **5:** 331–342.

6. TRACEY, K.J. 2002. The inflammatory reflex. Nature **420:** 853–859.
7. BOROVIKOVA, L.V., S. IVANOVA, M. ZHANG, *et al.* 2000. Vagus nerve stimulation attenuates the systemic inflammatory response to endotoxin. Nature **405:** 458–462.
8. BERNIK, T.R., S.G. FRIEDMAN, M. OCHANI, *et al.* 2002. Cholinergic antiinflammatory pathway inhibition of tumor necrosis factor during ischemia reperfusion. J. Vasc. Surg. **36:** 1231–1236.
9. BERNIK, T.R., S.G. FRIEDMAN, M. OCHANI, *et al.* 2002. Pharmacological stimulation of the cholinergic antiinflammatory pathway. J. Exp. Med. **195:** 781–788.
10. SAEED, R.W., S. VARMA, T. PENG-NEMEROFF, *et al.* 2005. Cholinergic stimulation blocks endothelial cell activation and leukocyte recruitment during inflammation. J. Exp. Med. **201:** 1113–1123.
11. WANG, H., M. YU, M. OCHANI, *et al.* 2003. Nicotinic acetylcholine receptor alpha7 subunit is an essential regulator of inflammation. Nature **421:** 384–388.
12. WANG, H., H. LIAO, M. OCHANI, *et al.* 2004. Cholinergic agonists inhibit HMGB1 release and improve survival in experimental sepsis. Nat. Med. **10:** 1216–1221.
13. DE JONGE, W.J., E.P. VAN DER ZANDEN, F.O. THE, *et al.* 2005. Stimulation of the vagus nerve attenuates macrophage activation by activating the Jak2-STAT3 signaling pathway. Nat. Immunol. **6:** 844–851. Erratum in: Nat. Immunol. **6:** 954.
14. METZ, C.N. & K.J. TRACEY. 2005. It takes nerve to dampen inflammation. Nat. Immunol. **6:** 756–757.
15. NOBEL LECTURES, PHYSIOLOGY OR MEDICINE 1922-1941. 1965. Elsevier. Amsterdam. http://www.nobelprize.org/medicine/laureates/1936/loewi-bio.html (Accessed Nov. 15, 2005.)
16. WIKIPEDIA. 2005. Otto Loewi. Wikipedia, The Free Encyclopedia. http://en.wikipedia.org/wiki/Otto_Loewi (Accessed Nov. 15, 2005.)
17. COLQUHOUN, D. & B. SAKMANN. 1998. From muscle endplate to brain synapses: a short history of synapses and agonist-activated ion channels. Neuron **20:** 381–387.
18. PAVLOV, V.A. & K.J. TRACEY. 2005. The cholinergic anti-inflammatory pathway. Brain Behav. Immun. **19:** 493–499.
19. DOUCETTE-STAMM, L., L.M. MONTEGGIA, D. DONNELLY-ROBERTS, *et al.* 1993. Cloning and sequence of the human alpha-7 nicotinic acetylcholine receptor. Drug Dev. Res. **30:** 252–256.
20. LUKAS, R.J., J.P. CHANGEUX, N. LE NOVERE, *et al.* 1999. International Union of Pharmacology XX. Current status of the nomenclature for nicotinic acetylcholine receptors and their subunits. Pharmacol. Rev. **51:** 397–401.
21. KARLIN, A. 2002. Emerging structure of the nicotinic acetylcholine receptors. Nat. Rev. Neurosci. **3:** 102–114.
22. LEITE, J.F., M.P. BLANTON, M. SHAHGHOLI, *et al.* 2003. Conformation-dependent hydrophobic photolabeling of the nicotinic receptor: electrophysiology-coordinated photochemistry and mass spectrometry. Proc. Natl. Acad. Sci. USA **100:** 13054–13059. Epub, Oct. 20, 2003.
23. BLOUNT, P. & J.P. MERLIE. 1990. Mutational analysis of muscle nicotinic acetylcholine receptor subunit assembly. J. Cell Biol. **111**(Pt. 1): 2613–2622.
24. GREEN, W.N. & C.P. WANAMAKER. 1997. The role of the cystine loop in acetylcholine receptor assembly. J. Biol. Chem. **272:** 20945–20953.
25. SEGUELA, P., J. WADICHE, K. DINELEY-MILLER, *et al.* 1993. Molecular cloning, functional properties, and distribution of rat brain alpha 7: a nicotinic cation channel highly permeable to calcium. J. Neurosci. **13:** 596–604.
26. SCHOEPFER, R., W.G. CONROY, P. WHITING, *et al.* 1990. Brain alpha-bungarotoxin binding protein cDNAs and MAbs reveal subtypes of this branch of the ligand-gated ion channel gene superfamily. Neuron **5:** 35–48.
27. GALZI, J.L., F. REVAH, F. BOUET, *et al.* 1991. Allosteric transitions of the acetylcholine receptor probed at the amino acid level with a photolabile cholinergic ligand. Proc. Natl. Acad. Sci. USA **88:** 5051–5055.
28. GAULT, J., M. ROBINSON, R. BERGER, C. DREBING, *et al.* 1998. Genomic organization and partial duplication of the human alpha7 neuronal nicotinic acetylcholine receptor gene (CHRNA7). Genomics **52:** 173–185.

29. Chini, B., E. Raimond, A.B. Elgoyhen, *et al.* 1994. Molecular cloning and chromosomal localization of the human alpha 7-nicotinic receptor subunit gene (CHRNA7). Genomics **19:** 379–381.
30. Brejc, K., W.J. van Dijk, R.V. Klaassen, *et al.* 2001. Crystal structure of an ACh-binding protein reveals the ligand-binding domain of nicotinic receptors. Nature **411:** 269–276.
31. Miyazawa, A., Y. Fujiyoshi & N. Unwin. 2003. Structure and gating mechanism of the acetylcholine receptor pore. Nature **423:** 949–955.
32. Unwin, N. 1995. Acetylcholine receptor channel imaged in the open state. Nature **373:** 37–43.
33. Yu, X.M. & Z.E. Hall. 1994. A sequence in the main cytoplasmic loop of the alpha subunit is required for assembly of mouse muscle nicotinic acetylcholine receptor. Neuron **13:** 247–255.
34. Valor, L.M., J. Mulet, F. Sala, *et al.* 2002. Role of the large cytoplasmic loop of the alpha 7 neuronal nicotinic acetylcholine receptor subunit in receptor expression and function. Biochemistry **41:** 7931–7938.
35. Orr-Urtreger, A., M.F. Seldin, A. Baldini & A.L. Beaudet. 1995. Cloning and mapping of the mouse alpha 7-neuronal nicotinic acetylcholine receptor. Genomics **26:** 399–402.
36. Riley, B., M. Williamson, D. Collier, *et al.* 2002. A 3-Mb map of a large segmental duplication overlapping the alpha7-nicotinic acetylcholine receptor gene (CHRNA7) at human 15q13-q14. Genomics **79:** 197–209.
37. Gault, J., J. Hopkins, R. Berger, *et al.* 2003. Comparisons of polymorphisms in the alpha7 nicotinic receptor gene and its partial duplication in schizophrenic and control subjects. Am. J. Genet. B. Neuropsychiatr. Genet. **123:** 39–49.
38. Severance, E.G., H. Zhang, Y. Cruz, *et al.* 2004. The alpha7 nicotinic acetylcholine receptor subunit exists in two isoforms that contribute to functional ligand-gated ion channels. Mol. Pharmacol. **66:** 420–429.
39. Carrasco-Serrano, C. & M. Criado. 2004. Glucocorticoid activation of the neuronal nicotinic acetylcholine receptor alpha7 subunit gene: involvement of transcription factor Egr-1. FEBS Lett. **566:** 247–250.
40. Beckmann, A.M. & P.A. Wilce. 1997. Egr transcription factors in the nervous system. Neurochem. Int. **31:** 477–510.
41. Drisdel, R.C., E. Manzana & W.N. Green. 2004. The role of palmitoylation in functional expression of nicotinic alpha7 receptors. J. Neurosci. **24:** 10502–10510.
42. Rakhilin, S., R.C. Drisdel, D. Sagher, *et al.* 1999. alpha-bungarotoxin receptors contain alpha7 subunits in two different disulfide-bonded conformations. J. Cell Biol. **146:** 203–218.
43. Drisdel, R.C. & W.N. Green. 2000. Neuronal alpha-bungarotoxin receptors are alpha7 subunit homomers. J. Neurosci. **20:** 133–139.
44. Blumenthal, E.M., W.G. Conroy, S.J. Romano, *et al.* 1997. Detection of functional nicotinic receptors blocked by alpha-bungarotoxin on PC12 cells and dependence of their expression on post-translational events. J. Neurosci. **17:** 6094–6104.
45. Williams, M.E., B. Burton, A. Urrutia, *et al.* 2005. Ric-3 promotes functional expression of the nicotinic acetylcholine receptor alpha7 subunit in mammalian cells. J. Biol. Chem. **280:** 1257–1263.

Pathogenic T-Cell Recruitment into the Airway in Human Disease

BENJAMIN D. MEDOFF,[a,b] SEDDON Y. THOMAS,[a] ALEENA BANERJI,[a] JOHN C.WAIN,[c] HUI ZHANG,[d] CRAIG M. LILLY,[e] LEO C. GINNS,[b] AND ANDREW D. LUSTER[a]

[a]*Center for Immunology and Inflammatory Diseases, Division of Rheumatology, Allergy and Immunology, Massachusetts General Hospital and Harvard Medical School, Charlestown, Massachusetts, 02129 USA*

[b]*Pulmonary and Critical Care Unit, Massachusetts General Hospital and Harvard Medical School, Boston, Massachusetts, 02114 USA*

[c]*Division of Thoracic Surgery, Massachusetts General Hospital and Harvard Medical School, Boston, Massachusetts, 02114 USA*

[d]*Biostatistics Center, Massachusetts General Hospital and Harvard Medical School, Boston, Massachusetts, 02114 USA*

[e]*Pulmonary Division, Brigham and Women's Hospital, Boston, Massachusetts 02115, USA*

ABSTRACT: Effector T cells significantly contribute to inflammatory diseases. These cells are recruited into tissue, where they orchestrate an inflammatory response that can either protect against infection or sometimes stimulate human disease. The recruitment of T cells into tissue from the blood and lymphoid compartments is an active process controlled by chemokines and the chemokine receptors expressed on distinct effector T-cell subsets. Thus, the chemokines secreted in the tissue will determine the specific types of T lymphocyte recruited into that tissue based on the chemokine receptors expressed on these cells. It follows that the chemokine receptor profile on T cells isolated from the lungs of patients with inflammatory pulmonary disease will define the subtype of pathogenic T lymphocytes mediating the disease process and will identify the mechanisms that recruit these cells into the lung. This article reviews data from both human and animal studies that define the chemokine receptors involved in the recruitment of T lymphocytes into the lung in various inflammatory pulmonary diseases, including asthma, obliterative bronchiolitis, sarcoidosis, and chronic eosinophilic pneumonia. We then speculate on the potential role of these chemokine receptors in the pathogenesis of these disorders and potential novel therapeutic approaches suggested by these data.

KEYWORDS: T cells; lung inflammation; sarcoidosis; asthma; lung transplantation; chemokines; chemokine receptors

Address for correspondence: Andrew D. Luster, M.D., Ph.D., Center for Immunology and Inflammatory Diseases, Division of Rheumatology, Allergy and Immunology, Massachusetts General Hospital, Bldg. 149-8301, 13th St., Charlestown, MA 02129. Voice: 617-726-5710; fax: 617-726-5651.

luster.andrew@mgh.harvard.edu

Ann. N.Y. Acad. Sci. 1062: 220–241 (2005). © 2005 New York Academy of Sciences. doi: 10.1196/annals.1358.026

INTRODUCTION

T lymphocytes are important mediators of the adaptive immune response and are vital for the integrity of host defense against infection. The lung is one of the most frequent sources of microbial infection and antigen exposure; thus, the mechanisms that control T-lymphocyte trafficking into the lung are crucial for immune surveillance. Studies in animal models of pulmonary infections and experience with patients with defects in adaptive immunity have demonstrated the importance of T-lymphocyte recruitment into the lungs for control of infectious diseases.[1,2] Although important for host defense, aberrant accumulation of T cells in the lung is seen in many noninfectious pulmonary inflammatory diseases. In many of these diseases, such as asthma and sarcoidosis, it is thought that the T lymphocytes in the lung orchestrate the abnormal inflammatory process.[3,4] It follows that a better understanding of the mechanisms that control the accumulation of T cells in the lung would provide insight into the pathogenesis of these disorders and potentially identify novel therapeutic targets.

The lung has a large network of lymphatics that aid in antigen presentation to T cells in associated lymph nodes located within the lung parenchyma and mediastinum. Also, the adult lung contains many memory T cells residing in the alveoli, airway (bronchial) lumen, intraepithelial layer, submucosa, and interstitium.[5] These T cells accumulate with age in the lung, suggesting that antigen exposure leads to memory T-cell migration into the lung to aid in surveillance and immune function. It is thought that lymphocytes home to tissues in response to specific molecular signals generated by the target organs. This is a tightly regulated and complex process that involves expression of many different adhesion molecules and chemokines.[6] These signals allow T cells to arrest on endothelial cells and migrate into the tissue. Further signals generated from chemokine gradients can then guide T cells into specific microcompartments, such as the alveoli or bronchial lumen.[7] Thus, the signals that determine the migration and homing of T cells into the lung are crucial for effective immune function. However, inappropriate homing of T cells into the lung may also be a cause or component of noninfectious inflammatory diseases. In this article we will explore the chemotactic mechanisms that control T-cell accumulation in the lung during inflammatory pulmonary disease.

BASIC PRINCIPLES

Chemokines, Lipid Chemoattractants, and Their Receptors

The active movement of leukocytes toward a site of antigen challenge, infection, or tissue damage represents a central aspect of the establishment of both the inflammatory and immune responses.[8,9] The movement of cells toward a chemical gradient of a particular stimulus or chemotactic factor is called chemotaxis. The chemotactic factors, which induce the directional movement of leukocytes, include the chemokines, a superfamily of proteins 8–10 kDa in size, and various lipid-derived chemoattractants. Approximately 50 chemokines have now been identified that share 20%–70% homology in amino acid sequence identity. Chemokine families are defined and named on the basis of the spacing of the first two cysteine amino acids in the mature protein. Based on this system, four families of chemokines exist: CC, CXC, C, and CXXXC.[8–10]

In addition to the chemokines, there are several lipid-derived mediators that have potent chemotactic activity. These include membrane-derived mediators such as prostaglandin D_2 (PGD_2) and leukotriene B_4 (LTB_4), both of which can have chemotactic effects on T cells recruited into the lung.[11,12]

The chemokines and various lipid-derived chemoattractants stimulate chemotaxis by signaling through seven-transmembrane G protein–coupled cell surface receptors (GPCRs),[13,14] which are named based on the type of chemokines to which they bind. The binding of chemokine to receptor causes a complex signaling cascade, which then leads to directed cell movement, cell activation, and sometimes differentiation and/or proliferation.[8–10]

Chemokine Receptor Expression on T Cells, Relationship to Inflammatory Response, Localization, and Chemokine Secretion

Chemokine receptor expression profiles can define functional subsets of leukocytes and can provide insights into the tissue localization and functional interactions in cellular immunity. There are two overlapping models of chemokine-induced T-cell trafficking: tissue-specific homing of T cells as part of basic immune surveillance and an inflammation-specific model of T-cell trafficking. Well-characterized examples of tissue-specific homing include the trafficking of T cells into lymphoid tissue and the movement of T cells into the skin or gut. In lymphoid-specific homing, naïve and central memory T cells that express CCR7 and CD62L are directed to lymph nodes by means of high endothelial venules. Effector memory T cells lose CD62L expression, downregulate CCR7 expression, and gain tissue-specific homing receptors. However, $CCR7^+$ T cells have also been observed at high levels in "effector" tissue sites, suggesting that some of these cells can also gain access to the lymphoid compartment by trafficking through the afferent lymph vessels in tissue.[15] Recent data from our group suggest that CCR7 expression on T cells in peripheral sites denotes T cells capable of recirculation to the lymphoid organs.[111] CCR7 expression is probably dynamically regulated *in vivo* and may be responsible for the return of peripheral tissue effector T cells to the lymph node during the process of antigen surveillance. In T-cell trafficking to the gut or skin, specific chemokine receptors are believed to orchestrate tissue-specific homing. For example, the chemokine receptors CCR4 and CCR10 seem to direct T cells into the skin.[16,17] Consistent with this finding, the ligands for CCR4 and CCR10, CCL17, and CCL27, respectively, are found on the luminal surface of postcapillary venules during cutaneous inflammation.[16,18] Also, CCL27 is expressed by keratinocytes in the skin. Similar to the tissue-specific homing receptors for the skin, the chemokine receptor CCR9 is associated with small intestine–homing memory T cells.[19,20] As expected, expression of the ligand for CCR9, CCL25, is found in epithelial cells in the crypts of the small intestine. These tissue-specific homing receptors support a role for chemokine receptors in homeostatic trafficking of T cells and determine the distribution of T cells at baseline. However, a lung-specific chemokine receptor has not been identified, suggesting that in some organs combinations of chemokine receptors determine the trafficking patterns of T cells into the lung.

Inflammatory Chemokine and Lipid Chemoattractant Receptor Expression and T-Cell Trafficking

In addition to tissue-specific trafficking, an inflammation-specific model of T-cell trafficking has been proposed, which focuses on effector T-cell populations. This model does not exclude a homeostatic role for tissue-specific lymphocyte trafficking but suggests that during inflammation, inflammatory chemokines and their receptors play an important role in effector T-cell trafficking. Thus, in Th1-type inflammation, NF-κB–inducible and STAT1-inducible chemokines and their receptors (CXCR3, CCR5, and CXCR6), which are found on Th1 cells and effector CD8 T cells, play a dominant role in effector T-cell recruitment.[21–24] Other chemokine receptors, which are expressed at lower levels on T cells, such as CCR2, CX_3CR1, CXCR1, and CXCR2, may also play a role in Th1-type inflammation.[25–28] In contrast, in Th2-type inflammation, STAT6-inducible chemokines and their cognate receptors, which are found on Th2-cells, such as CCR3, CCR4, and CCR8, play a dominant role in effector T-cell recruitment.[29]

Although CCR6 is not associated specifically with either Th1- or Th2-associated cells, this receptor is highly enriched on memory T cells and may be important for trafficking to sites of inflammation.[30] The ligand for CCR6, CCL20 (MIP-3α), is highly expressed on inflamed epithelium.[31,32] Since CCR6 is expressed on immature, but not mature, dendritic cells, this receptor may play an important role in the interaction of memory T and immature dendritic cells in the tissue.[32]

In addition to chemokines, lipid chemoattractants, such as LTB_4 and PGD_2, are produced in response to inflammatory stimuli and recruit T cells through the use of their cognate receptors, BLT1 and DP2. These lipid chemoattractants can be produced more rapidly than the peptide-based chemokines and play a critical role in early effector T-cell recruitment to sites of inflammation.[33,34]

These data indicate that the chemokine and lipid chemoattractant receptor profile of T cells that accumulate in the lung during inflammation may provide insight into the mechanisms that recruit these cells into the tissue as well as the nature of the inflammatory response. Furthermore, the identification of specific chemokine receptors expressed on T cells in the lung during pulmonary inflammation may identify potential therapeutic targets for intervention in these disorders.

T CELLS AND CHEMOKINE RECEPTORS IN PATHOGENESIS

Asthma

Human allergic asthma is a chronic inflammatory disease characterized by airway eosinophilia, production of allergen-specific immunoglobulin E (IgE), Th2 cytokine, and mucus production, airway hyperresponsiveness, and airway remodeling. A central component of this elaborate inflammatory response is the activation and recruitment of T cells into the airways.[35] These cells are predominantly of the Th2 subclass, and it is thought that they orchestrate the inflammatory response to allergens in the lung. The asthmatic response can be divided into an early and a late phase.[36] The early phase (5–60 minutes) occurs following allergen exposure and leads to mast cell degranulation and release of lipid and protein chemoattractants. The late phase (4–24 hours) is characterized by the recruitment of lymphocytes and eosinophils into the airways. Murine models of asthma recapitulate some, but not all, of the features of human asthma.[37] However, many of the key features of human allergic asthma are preserved, including eosinophilic lung inflammation, mucus production, recruitment of Th2 lymphocytes, increased Th2 cytokines and allergen-specific IgE, airway hyperresponsiveness, and airway remodeling.

Role of Chemokines and Lipid Chemoattractants in Recruitment of T Lymphocytes in Asthma

Chemokines play an important role in the recruitment of T lymphocytes into the airway and lung during an asthmatic response. Several chemokines and lipid chemoattractants have been detected in the airways of atopic asthmatics and following allergen challenge in both mice and humans.[36] In a mouse model of asthma, ligands of the chemokine and lipid chemoattractant receptors—CCR1, CCR2, CCR3, CCR4, CCR5, CXCR1, CXCR3, and BLT1—were induced in the lung at an early time point after allergen challenge.[38,39] Similarly, in human segmental allergen challenge studies, the ligands for CCR3, CCR4, CCR5, CXCR1/2, CXCR3, and DP2, but not CCR8, were increased in bronchoalveolar lavage (BAL) samples following allergen challenge.[40–47] These data implicate a wide variety of both Th1- and Th2-inflammatory chemokines in recruitment of cells to the airways following allergen challenge and suggest that chemokines and lipid chemoattractants play an important role in the recruitment of T lymphocytes to the BAL and lung during an asthmatic response. Consistent with this supposition, studies on T cells isolated from the BAL of normal and atopic subjects demonstrated high-level expression of CXCR3 and CCR5 and intermediate-level expression of CCR4 and CCR6.[48] Also, CCR4 and CCR8 expression has been detected on T cells from endobrochial biopsies from asthmatic patients.[49] Although asthma has generally been described as a Th2-mediated disease, these data indicated that both Th1- and Th2-associated chemokines and chemokine receptors were expressed in the BAL after allergen challenge and that recruitment of lymphocytes was not dependent on a single chemokine–chemokine receptor pair.

Studies of chemokine receptor–knockout mice have also yielded information about the role of chemokine receptors in the development and pathogenesis of asthma. Although the Th2-associated chemokine receptors, CCR3, CCR4 and CCR8, have been associated with the asthmatic phenotype, only CCR3 and CCR4 have been shown to contribute to the allergic asthmatic response in studies that used genetically modified mice. CCR3 played a significant role in the recruitment of eosinophils and mast cells to the airway and lung in a mouse model of asthma but was not responsible for the recruitment of T lymphocytes.[50] A role for CCR4 in airway hyperresponsiveness, but not airway remodeling, was observed during chronic allergic responses to *Aspergillus funigatus*[51] In contrast, a role for CCR8 in the development of the allergic asthmatic response has been controversial, with one study suggesting it is important,[52] but two other similar studies demonstrating no role for this receptor.[53,54]

In addition to these Th2-associated receptors, other chemokines, chemokine receptors, and lipid chemoattractant receptors have been demonstrated to mediate allergic airway responses in mice. CXCL10 (CXCR3 ligand) contributed to airway hyperreactivity and inflammation in a murine model of asthma.[55] In the absence of CXCL10, mice demonstrated reduced allergic airway inflammation, whereas the converse was true in a mouse that overexpressed this chemokine ligand. The chemokine receptor–ligand pair, CCR6 and CCL20, has also been implicated in the allergic asthmatic response. In a mouse model of asthma, CCL20 was increased following allergen challenge, and the CCR6-knockout mouse displayed reduced airway resistance, eosinophilia, interleukin 5 (IL-5) production, and serum IgE level.[56] This defect appears to be due primarily to an alteration in T-cell activation.[57] Finally, studies of the BLT1-knockout mouse have indicated a critical role for BLT1 in early effector T-cell egress from the lungs to the airways following allergen challenge.[12] This finding suggests that CXCR3, CCR6, and BLT1 also play a role in promoting the inflammation observed in the allergic asthmatic response.

A recent study examined the chemokine receptor expression profile on BAL T cells from atopic asthmatics before and 42 hours after segmental allergen challenge.[58] Prior to antigen challenge, the authors found that BAL T cells from asthmatics expressed significantly more CCR2, CCR4, CCR5, CCR6, and CXCR3 than did peripheral blood T cells. Also, after dividing subjects into those with low and high recruitment of eosinophils, the investigators observed increased expression of CCR4 and CCR7 on BAL T cells but decreased expression of CXCR3 on these cells following allergen exposure. The authors concluded that although some of these receptors may play a role in baseline recruitment to the BAL, other receptors contribute to the recruitment of T cells to the airway during allergic inflammation.

We have recently performed similar studies examining the chemokine receptor expression on BAL and peripheral blood T cells before and 24 hours after segmental allergen challenge. Rather than group all $CD3^+$ T cells together as in the study by Kallinich *et al.*, we have examined the expression of chemokine receptors by flow cytometry on $CD4^+$ and $CD8^+$ T cells as two separate groups. At baseline, we observed statistically significant increases in the expression of CCR1, CCR5, CCR6, CCR9, CXCR1, CXCR2, CXCR3, CXCR4, CXCR6, and BLT1 on $CD4^+$ BAL T cells compared with $CD4^+$ peripheral blood T cells, as well as of CCR5, CCR6, and BLT1 on $CD8^+$ BAL T cells compared with $CD8^+$ peripheral blood T cells (manuscript in preparation). Because specific chemokine receptors are expressed differentially on $CD4^+$ and $CD8^+$ T cells, including but not limited to CCR4, CCR5, CCR6, and CXCR6, grouping all $CD3^+$ T cells together may mask (or amplify) alterations in the chemokine receptor profile due to differences in the CD4:CD8 ratio in the BAL and peripheral blood.

We initially hypothesized that following segmental allergen challenge the percentage of $CD4^+$ and $CD8^+$ BAL T cells that express the Th2-associated chemokine receptors, CCR3 and CCR4, would increase and that the percentage of cells that express the Th1-associated chemokine receptors CXCR3, CCR5, and CXCR6 would decrease. In our studies, we observed that the chemokine receptors CXCR3 and CCR6 were significantly decreased on both $CD4^+$ and $CD8^+$ T cells, and the chemokine receptor CXCR5 was significantly decreased on $CD4^+$ T cells (manuscript in preparation). Also, the chemokine receptors, CCR1, CCR7, CCR9, CXCR1, and CXCR6, increased on BAL T cells following segmental allergen challenge, whereas CCR2, CCR3, CCR4, CXCR2, CXCR4, CX_3CR1, and BLT1 remained relatively unchanged (manuscript in preparation). In comparison with the study by Kallinich *et al.*, we observed similar decreases in CXCR3 and increases in CCR7 expression on BAL T cells following segmental allergen challenge. However, we did not observe an increase in CCR4 expression on either $CD4^+$ or $CD8^+$ BAL T cells but did observe a statistically significant decrease in CCR6 expression on both $CD4^+$ and $CD8^+$ BAL T cells following segmental allergen challenge. We think that because CCR4 and CCR6 are differentially expressed on $CD4^+$ and $CD8^+$ T cells, our data provide a clearer analysis of the alterations in the expression of these receptors following segmental allergen challenge.

In addition to the expression of specific chemokine receptors on BAL T cells, chemokine ligands play a critical role in the recruitment of T cells to the airways. As previously discussed in this review, specific chemokine ligands have been measured in the BAL before and following segmental allergen challenge, including CCR3, CCR4, CCR5, CXCR1/2, and CXCR3 ligands.[40–47] To correlate with our studies of chemokine receptor expression on BAL T cells, we measured the production of the ligands for CXCR3 and CCR6, as well as other inflammatory chemokines for these subjects before and 24 hours after segmental allergen challenge by enzyme-linked immunosorbent assay (manuscript in preparation). CCL20 (CCR6 ligand) and CXCL8 (CXCR1 and CXCR2 ligand) were significantly increased in the BAL following segmental allergen challenge. Also, CXCL9, CXCL10, and CXCL11 (CXCR3 ligands) and CCL2 (CCR2 ligand) were increased in the BAL following segmental allergen challenge, whereas CCL5 (CCR1, CCR3, and CCR5 ligand) and CXCL16 (CXCR6 ligand) remained at similar levels before and after segmental allergen challenge. These data imply that ligands for CXCR1/2, CXCR3, CCR2, and CCR6 could play a role in recruitment of cells to the BAL following segmental allergen challenge.

Overall, the data from Kallinich *et al.* and our work in progress suggest that both Th1/Tc1- and Th2/Tc2-associated BAL T cells are recruited into the airways following segmental allergen challenge and that specific chemokine receptors play a role in this process. This hypothesis implies that both Th1- and Th2-associated processes mediate the development of allergic asthma. Also, the chemokine receptor profile before and following segmental allergen challenge in the BAL is unique to BAL T cells compared with peripheral blood T cells and argues that several chemokine receptors participate in the process of recruitment to this tissue-specific site.

Lung Transplantation

For patients with severe lung disease, lung transplantation offers the opportunity for a better quality of life and longer survival.[59–62] However, despite improvements in surgical techniques and immunosuppressive drugs, survival after lung transplantation is only 42.6% after 5 years. These are relatively poor outcomes when compared with those of heart or liver transplantation, which have a 5-year survival of 70%.[63] The relatively worse outcomes after lung transplantation compared with other solid-organ transplants relates predominantly to the development of obliterative scarring of the airways, so-called obliterative bronchiolitis (OB). OB is the major cause of morbidity and mortality after lung transplantation,[64] with more than 60% of lung transplant recipients developing this complication over time.[65,66]

OB is a fibroproliferative response in the small airways or bronchioles of the lung. It is characterized by increased collagen and increased numbers of myofibroblasts as well as infiltration of the lesions with lymphocytes. By narrowing the small airways and increasing resistance to airflow, OB can significantly reduce lung function in transplant recipients. OB can be difficult to diagnose by bronchoscopic biopsy, so patients are often diagnosed clinically when they demonstrate reduced lung function in the absence of infection. Unfortunately at this point the changes are often irreversible; thus, early diagnostic markers for OB would be extremely valuable in the management of these patients. It is hypothesized that OB results from repeated injuries to the airways, which directly damage the airway epithelium leading to the partial denudation of the airway surface. This is followed by inflammation and then luminal obliteration from an exuberant repair process marked by connective tissue synthesis and mesenchymal cell recruitment and/or proliferation.[67,68] Studies into the pathogenesis of OB in lung transplantation, have shown a strong correlation with previous episodes of acute rejection, suggesting that immune-mediated injury may be the predominant mechanism causing OB.[69] Since rejection is a specific injury to donor tissue orchestrated by reactive T lymphocytes,[70] it follows that T-cell recruitment into the transplanted lung is a critical component in the development of OB. Support for this hypothesis has come from experiments that have demonstrated donor-specific T lymphocytes in the BAL fluid and lung tissue taken from transplant recipients with OB.[71,72] These T-cell responses have selective clonal expansions presumably against alloantigens.[73] Also, other studies have shown that patients with persistent donor-specific lymphocytes in the BAL have a high incidence of OB, whereas patients with donor-specific alloantigen hyporeactivity in peripheral blood lymphocytes have a low incidence of OB.[69,74,75] Thus, a better understanding of the mechanisms that recruit T cells into lung allografts could provide important insight into the pathogenesis of OB.

Studies in humans and animals following transplantation have demonstrated expression of specific chemokines during rejection and the development of chronic allograft dysfunction.[76] In cardiac, liver, and lung allografts, the expression of the chemokine CXCL10 and its receptor CXCR3 have been shown to correlate with acute rejection.[77–79] In the study on lung transplant recipients, the intensity of CXCR3 staining and the level of CXCL10 expression correlated with the degree of rejection seen in transbronchial biopsy samples, suggesting that CXCR3 and its ligands are important for the rejection process.[78] Further conformation comes from a separate study, which demonstrated increased levels of the CXCR3 ligands CXCL9, CXCL10, and CXCL11 in the BAL from patients with acute rejection or OB.[80] Furthermore, in animal models, targeted inhibition of CXCL10 and CXCL9 can dramatically improve graft survival.[80] Although these data strongly implicate CXCR3 as an important mediator of lymphocyte trafficking in allograft rejection, a full analysis of the chemokines and chemokine receptors necessary for leukocyte recruitment in this process has not been done. Previous data in other diseases suggests that it is highly unlikely that a limited chemokine–chemokine receptor axis fully mediates leukocyte recruitment.[81]

Alloreactive T cells are thought to orchestrate rejection following transplantation and are numerous in lavage specimens. We hypothesized that these T cells traffic into the transplanted lung in response to the production of specific chemokines.

Thus, the T cells recruited into the airway should have a unique profile of chemokine receptors depending on the type of injury and the resulting chemokine production.

Chemokine Receptor Profile in BAL of Patients with OB

After obtaining human studies approval, we collected cells from BAL fluid taken from lung transplant patients undergoing surveillance bronchoscopy at the Massachusetts General Hospital. After lung transplantation, patients undergo bronchoscopic surveillance according to a predetermined protocol. Bronchoscopic surveillance includes collection of BAL fluid and transbronchial biopsies from the allograft. The BAL was performed by standard techniques.[82] The samples were coded and after analysis the diagnosis of the patient was revealed. Isolated cells were analyzed by flow cytometry and antibodies to 11 different chemokine–chemoattractant receptors (CXCR1, CXCR2, CCR3, CXCR3, CCR4, CXCR4, CCR5, CXCR5, CCR7, CCR9, BLT1) to determine the unique profile of chemokine receptors expressed on the T cells recruited into the transplanted lung. Using flow cytometric analysis and cell counts, we calculated the number of $CD4^+$ and $CD8^+$ T cells isolated and determined their chemokine receptor expression profile. Biopsy specimens were reviewed by a pathologist and graded according to the revised International Society for Heart and Lung Transplantation working formulation.[64]

The patients were at least 45 days out from their transplants and were not acutely ill. Twenty-two lung transplants were classified as clinically normal, 17 were diagnosed with OB, and the rest were diagnosed with either acute rejection ($n = 3$) or infection ($n = 9$) (excluded from analysis). The diagnosis of OB was based on specific criteria published by the International Society of Heart and Lung Transplantation[64,83] Characteristics of the lung transplants in the two groups were not different except for the lung function, which was significantly worse in the transplants with OB, as expected (data not shown). Also, there were no significant differences in the time since transplant, the amount of fluid recovered, the number of cells recovered, or total lymphocyte number recovered between patients with and without OB.

The chemokine receptor profile on T cells isolated from the BAL of lung transplants with OB demonstrated several differences with T cells isolated from the BAL of normal lung transplants (FIG. 1A and 1B). There were significantly more $CD4^+$ and $CD8^+$ T cells expressing the chemokine receptors CCR3, CCR4, and CXCR4. Also, CCR5 was expressed on more $CD4^+$ T cells in the transplants with OB. We also saw significantly more T cells expressing the LTB_4 receptor BLT1 in OB, as we have recently reported.[34] We saw similar levels of CXCR3 expression on T cells from patients with OB and normal lungs posttransplant. These results differ from those of Agostini *et al.*;[78] however, other groups have also reported that the percentage of $CXCR3^+$ T cells is high in the lung under normal conditions.[48,58]

These data suggest that there is a different subset of T cells recruited into the lung during the development of OB. Expression of the chemokine receptors CCR3 and CCR4 on activated effector T cells has been associated with Th2 polarization.[84] Th2-type inflammatory responses have been found to be important in the development of fibrosis in some lung diseases and in animal models of pulmonary fibrosis.[85–88] Specifically for sarcoidosis, some authors have suggested that a switch from Th1- to Th2-polarized inflammation accompanies the development of progressive lung dis-

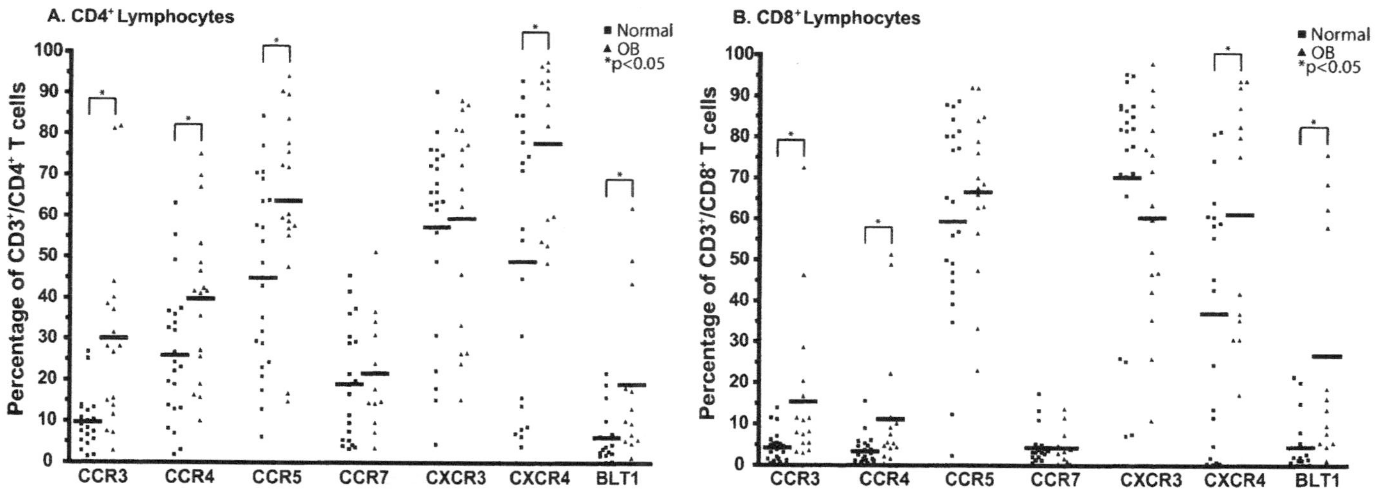

FIGURE 1. Chemokine receptor expression on $CD4^+$ T lymphocytes (**A**) and $CD8^+$ T lymphocytes (**B**) isolated from the BAL of patients post lung transplantation. $CD4^+$ T lymphocytes recovered from patients with OB had significantly higher expression of CCR3, CCR4, CCR5, CXCR4, and BLT1 than did lymphocytes from normal patients. Similarly, $CD8^+$ T lymphocytes recovered from patients with OB had significantly higher expression of CCR3, CCR4, CXCR4, and BLT1 than did lymphocytes from normal patients.

TABLE 1. Multvariate analysis of T-cell chemokine receptor profiles

	Odds ratio	95% CI	*P* value
CD4–CCR3	1.27	(1.05, 1.54)	.015
CD8–CXCR4	1.06	(1.00, 1.12)	.048

ease with fibrosis.[89] Our data are consistent with this concept in lung transplantation whereby the recruitment of Th2-polarized T cells into allografts correlates with the development of airway fibroproliferation in OB. Consistent with this finding, the cytokines IL-4 and IL-13, which are produced by Th2 cells, have been linked to the development of pulmonary fibrosis.[90–93] These data suggest that the recruitment of Th2-polarized T cells into the airways following lung transplantation could modulate airway fibrosis and lead to OB.

In addition to providing insight into the mechanisms of OB, the results of our investigation could be used for the diagnosis of OB post–lung transplant. Currently, lung biopsies have a sensitivity of only 20% for OB, so clinical criteria are used to make the diagnosis.[64] Unfortunately the clinical criteria for OB use a drop in lung function and thus identify patients late in the course of disease, when treatment is less effective. The identification of biomarkers for OB would potentially allow early intervention in the disease process, which could improve treatment outcomes. To test whether the chemokine receptor profile could be used as a diagnostic tool for OB, we performed multivariate analysis on the chemokine receptor profiles, using the logistic regression model with forward selection. The dependent variable was a diagnosis of OB, and the independent variables were chemokine receptors expressed on $CD4^+$ and $CD8^+$ T lymphocytes. The forward selection found that CCR3 expression on $CD4^+$ lymphocytes and CXCR4 expression on $CD8^+$ lymphocytes correlated best with OB (TABLE 1). A receiver operating characteristic (ROC) curve of CCR3 and CXCR4 expression indicate that BAL lymphocyte expression of CCR3 and CXCR4 could have utility as a diagnostic test with reasonable sensitivity and specificity (FIG. 2).

Future studies will try to link expression patterns of chemokines or their receptors to the future development of OB. Since a diagnosis of OB is usually made after the patient has already developed significant and often irreversible disease, early diagnostic markers of OB would be extremely valuable. Also, the information gathered may reveal novel therapeutic targets to treat this process.

Sarcoidosis

Sarcoidosis is an inflammatory disease of unknown cause that is characterized by granulomatous inflammation in several different organ systems. By far the most commonly affected organ is the lung, where the inflammatory response is characterized by infiltration by activated T lymphocytes (predominantly $CD4^+$) and macrophages. The clinical presentation of pulmonary sarcoidosis can be variable, with some patients presenting with acute disease that resolves whereas others progress to lung fibrosis and chronic respiratory failure. The underlying pathogenesis of this disorder remains unknown; however, T cells are thought to help mediate the inflammatory process, perhaps in response to an environmental antigen or occult infection.[94]

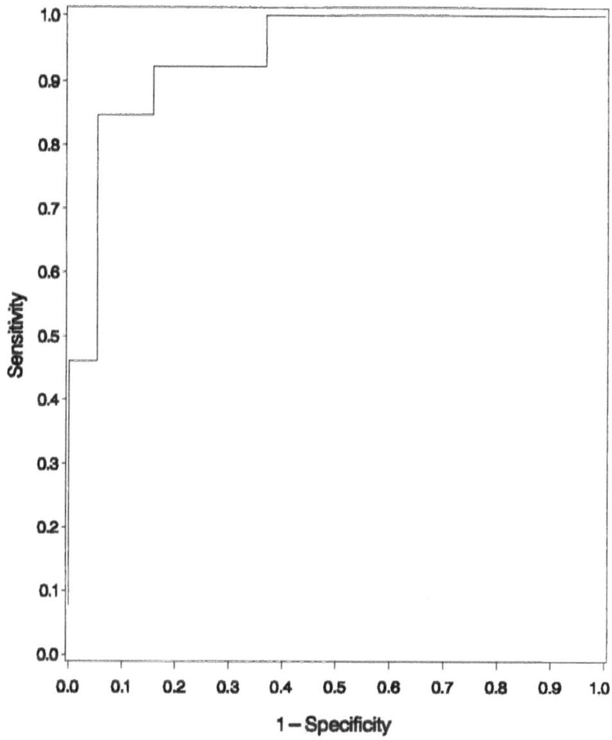

FIGURE 2. ROC curve of CCR3 and CXCR4 expression. The logistic regression model with forward selection was used. The dependent variable was a diagnosis of OB, and the independent variables were chemokine receptors expressed on $CD4^+$ and $CD8^+$ T lymphocytes. The forward selection found that CCR3 expression on $CD4^+$ lymphocytes and CXCR4 expression on $CD8^+$ lymphocytes correlated best with OB. These data indicate that BAL lymphocyte expression of CCR3 and CXCR4 could be useful as a diagnostic test with reasonable sensitivity and specificity.

Activated $CD4^+$ T cells preferentially accumulate in the airways of patients with sarcoidosis. Phenotypic analysis of these cells demonstrates that they are Th1 polarized with increased expression of interferon γ and IL-12.[95,96] It is thus not surprising that these cells express the chemokine receptor CXCR3, which is preferentially expressed on Th1-type T cells, and that there is upregulation of its ligand, CXCL10, predominantly in the macrophages found in granulomas.[97,98] Other studies have also shown that CCL5 (the ligand for CCR5), another receptor preferentially expressed by Th1 cells, is upregulated in the lungs of patients with sarcoid.[99] A more recent analysis of BAL samples from 18 patients with sarcoidosis confirmed that the chemokine receptors CXCR3 and CCR5 are expressed on many BAL lymphocytes and the levels were significantly increased when compared with expression on lymphocytes isolated from the blood. Another chemokine receptor associated with Th1-

polarized T cells, CXCR6, has also recently been reported to be enriched on T cells isolated from the lung in sarcoidosis.[100] In contrast, the receptors CCR4 and CXCR4 were expressed at similar levels compared with that in the blood.[101] In a study focusing on the role of CCR7 in sarcoidosis, the chemokine CCL19 was found to be upregulated in the BAL from patients with sarcoidosis compared with healthy subjects, as was the RNA copy level of its receptor, CCR7, in samples taken from total BAL cells.[102] Furthermore, the levels of CCL19 and CCR7 expression seemed to correlate with T-cell infiltration into the lung in these patients.[102]

We have also examined chemokine receptor expression on T cells isolated from the BAL on seven patients with biopsy-proven sarcoidosis. Our analysis confirms high-level expression of CCR5 and CXCR3, with low expression of CCR4 and CXCR4 on T cells in the BAL (FIG. 3A and 3B). We did not see high-level expression of CXCR6 or CCR7, however, as reported previously by others.[100,102] Our data, along with those from other groups, are consistent with the theory that sarcoidosis results from a Th1-type inflammatory response mediated by $CD4^+$ T lymphocytes. Furthermore, the data would suggest that therapies that target Th1-polarized T cells, CXCR3, and/or CCR5 may be of value in this disease.

Chronic Eosinophilic Pneumonia

Chronic eosinophilic pneumonia (CEP) is a rare idiopathic inflammatory lung disease characterized by eosinophilic infiltration of the pulmonary interstitium. Patients usually have a history of asthma and present with slowly progressive shortness of breath with peripheral pulmonary infiltrates on chest X-ray.[103] Little is known about its pathogenesis; however, studies have suggested that $CD4^+$ T cells in the lung modulate the pulmonary eosinophilia and contribute to the development of disease.[104–106] High levels of IL-5 have been documented in the BAL of CEP patients, consistent with this being a Th2-type inflammatory disease.[107] Studies in CEP have demonstrated increases in the Th2-associated CCR3 and CCR4 ligands, specifically CCL11, CCL17, and CCL22.[108–110] Further analysis has shown that $CCR4^+$ T lymphocytes were enriched in the BAL relative to blood in patients with CEP and the number of cells correlated with expression levels of CCL17 and CCL22. These data implicated CCR4 as a primary mediator of T-cell recruitment to the lung in this disease.[108] Our own data on three patients with biopsy-proven CEP confirmed high-level CCR4 expression on T lymphocytes isolated from the BAL in this disease (FIG. 4A and 4B). Based on these data, therapy targeting CCR4 or its ligands may be beneficial in CEP.

Potential Therapies

There are many antibodies and small-molecule inhibitors of chemokine and chemokine receptors that are currently being tested in pulmonary inflammatory disorders.[3] The chemokines and their receptors are attractive therapeutic targets in inflammatory diseases because they can specifically inhibit the accumulation of a subset of leukocytes, allowing one to interrupt the inflammatory cascade without the use of broadly immunosuppressive therapy. For example, in certain pulmonary disorders, such as sarcoidosis and asthma, where recruitment of T cells into the lung is thought to orchestrate the inflammatory response, inhibition of key T-cell–specific

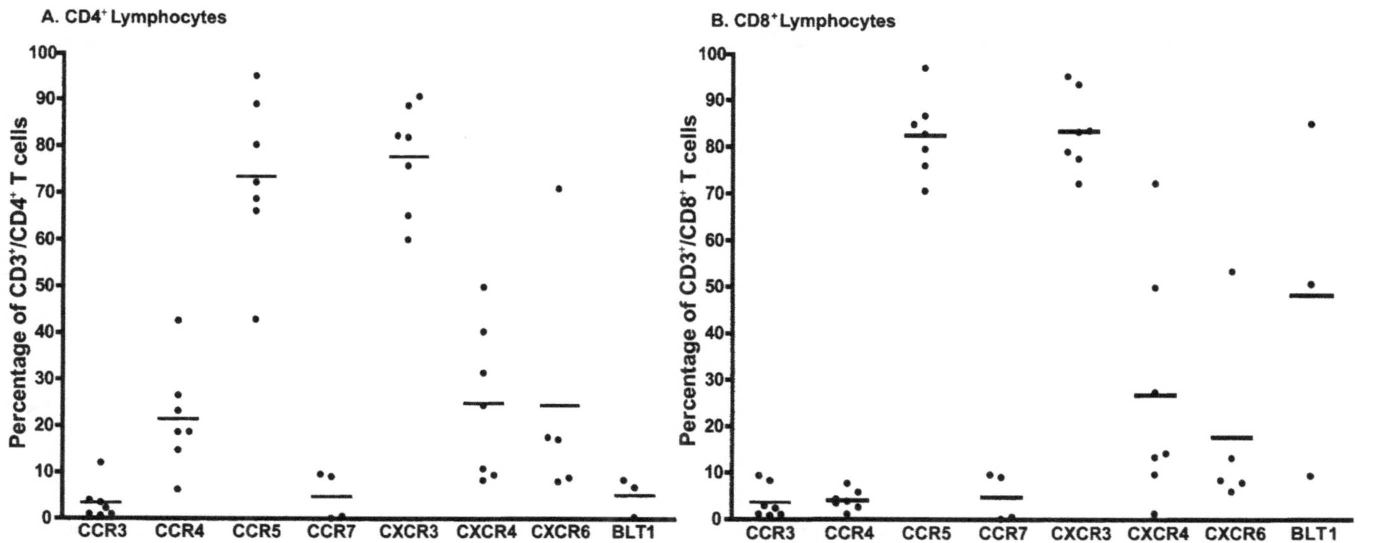

FIGURE 3. Chemokine receptor expression on CD4$^+$ T lymphocytes (**A**) and CD8$^+$ T lymphocytes (**B**) isolated from the BAL of patients with sarcoidosis. CD4$^+$ and CD8$^+$ T lymphocytes recovered from patients with sarcoidosis have high expression of CXCR3 and CCR5 and relatively low expression of CCR4 and CXCR4.

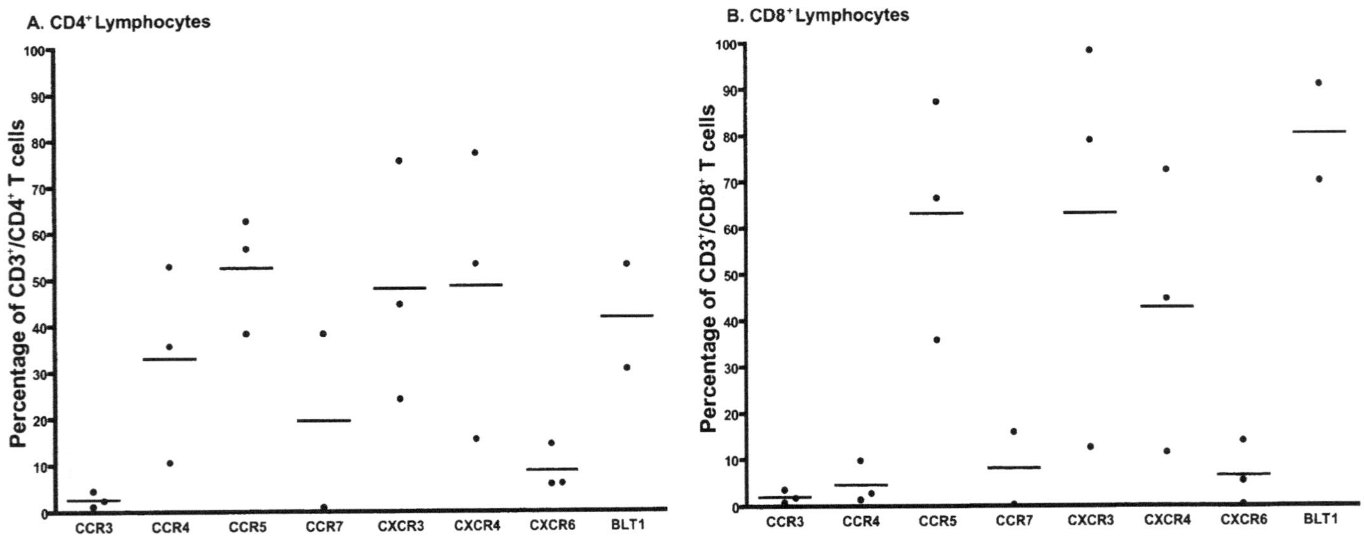

FIGURE 4. Chemokine receptor expression on CD4$^+$ T lymphocytes (**A**) and CD8$^+$ T lymphocytes (**B**) isolated from the BAL of patients with CEP. CD4$^+$ and CD8$^+$ T lymphocytes recovered from patients with CEP have relatively high expression of CCR4.

TABLE 2. Chemokine receptor profiles on BAL T cells in pulmonary disease

	CCR1	CCR2	CCR3	CCR4	CCR5	CCR6	CCR7	CCR9	CXCR1	CXCR2	CXCR3	CXCR4	CXCR5	CXCR6	BLT1	CX3CR1
Normal																
CD3	+	++++	+	++	+++++	++++	++	+	+	+	+++++	++++	+	—	—	+
Asthma: prechallenge[c]																
CD4	+	+	+	+++	++++	++++	++	+	+	+	+++++	++++	+	+	+	+
CD8	+	+	+	+	++++	++	++	+	+		+++++	++++	+	++	+	+
Asthma: postchallenge																
CD4	+	+	+	+++	+++	++[b]	+++	+	++	+	++[b]	++++	+[b]	+++	+	+
CD8	+	+	+	+	++++	+[b]	++	+	+	+	++[b]	++++	+[b]	+++	+	+
CEP																
CD4	—	—	+	++	++	—	+	—	—	—	++	+++	—	+	+++	—
CD8	—	—	+	+	+++	—	+	—	—	—	+++	+++	—	+	+++++	—
Sarcoidosis																
CD4	—	—	+	++	++++	—	+	—	—	—	++++	++	—	++	+	—
CD8	—	—	+	+	+++++	—	+	—	—	—	+++++	++	—	+	+++	—
Normal posttransplant																
CD4	—	—	+	++	+++	++	+	—	+	+	+++	+++	—	—	+	+
CD8	—	—	+	+	+++	+	+	—	+	+	++++	++	—	—	+	+
OB posttransplant																
CD4	—	—	++[a]	++[a]	++++[a]	+++	++	+	+	+	+++	++++[a]	+	—	+[a]	+
CD8	—	—	+[a]	+[a]	++++	+	+	+	+	+	++++	++++[a]	+	—	++[a]	+

NOTATION: +++++: >80%; ++++: 60–80%; +++: 40–60%; ++: 20–40%; +: <20%; —: not measured.
[a]Significant compared to normal posttransplant.
[b]Significant compared to asthma prechallenge.
[c]Unpublished observations.

chemokines or their receptors could reduce lung inflammation and thus reduce the need for corticosteroids. Although many therapies are in early clinical trials, there are no conclusive human studies demonstrating clinical benefit from an anti-inflammatory approach that targets chemokines or chemokine receptors. Also, inhibition of leukocyte accumulation in the lung could increase the sensitivity of the patient to certain infections. Although these agents have great promise for therapy in pulmonary inflammatory diseases, extensive testing is still necessary before they can be used clinically.

CONCLUSION

The recruitment of T cells into the lung in inflammatory pulmonary diseases is an active process under the control of chemokines and their receptors. We and others have defined disease-specific profiles of chemokine receptors expressed on T cells isolated from the lungs of patients with various pulmonary disorders (TABLE 2). These profiles provide important insights into the pathogenesis of these diseases as well as the mechanisms that recruit T cells into the lung. Also, the profiles could be used in diagnostic strategies and may suggest potential therapeutic targets for these disorders.

ACKNOWLEDGMENTS

Benjamin D. Medoff and Seddon Y. Thomas contributed equally to this report.

[*Competing interests*: The authors declare that they have no competing financial interests.]

REFERENCES

1. HOGAN, R.J., L.S. CAULEY, K.H. ELY, *et al.* 2002. Long-term maintenance of virus-specific effector memory CD8+ T cells in the lung airways depends on proliferation. J. Immunol. **169:** 4976–4981.
2. WOODLAND, D.L., K.H. ELY, S.R. CROWE, *et al.* 2002. Antiviral memory T-cell responses in the lung. Microbes Infect. **4:** 1091–1098.
3. D'AMBROSIO, D., M. MARIANI, P. PANINA-BORDINGNON & F. SINIGAGLIA. 2001. Chemokines and their receptors guiding T lymphocyte recruitment in lung inflammation. Am. J. Respir. Crit. Care Med. **164:** 1266–1275.
4. HERRICK, C.A. & K. BOTTOMLY. 2003. To respond or not to respond: T cells in allergic asthma. Nat. Rev. Immunol. **3:** 405–412.
5. BRIGHTLING, C.E., A.J. AMMIT, D. KAUR, *et al.* 2005. The CXCL10/CXCR3 axis mediates human lung mast cell migration to asthmatic airway smooth muscle. Am. J. Respir. Crit. Care Med. **171:** 1103–1108.
6. VON ANDRIAN, U.H. & C.R. MACKAY. 2000. T-cell function and migration. Two sides of the same coin. N. Engl. J. Med. **343:** 1020–1034.
7. WARDLAW, A.J., C. GUILLEN & A. MORGAN. 2005. Mechanisms of T cell migration to the lung. Clin. Exp. Allergy **35:** 4–7.
8. LUSTER, A.D., S. ABI-YOUNES & A. TAGER. 2000. Chemokines and disease. *In* Chemokines in Allergic Disease. M.E. Rothenberg, Ed.: 339–382. Marcel Dekker AG. New York.
9. ROLLINS, B.J. 1997. Chemokines. Blood **90:** 909–928.

10. BAGGIOLINI, M. 1998. Chemokines and leukocyte traffic. Nature **392:** 565–568.
11. COSMI, L., F. ANNUNZIATO, M.I. GALLI, *et al.* 2000. CRTH2 is the most reliable marker for the detection of circulating human type 2 Th and type 2 T cytotoxic cells in health and disease. Eur J. Immunol. **30:** 2972–2979.
12. TAGER, A.M., S.K. BROMLEY, B.D. MEDOFF, *et al.* 2003. Leukotriene B4 receptor BLT1 mediates early effector T cell recruitment. Nat. Immunol. **4:** 982–990.
13. SALLUSTO, F., C.R. MACKAY & A. LANZAVECCHIA. 2000. The role of chemokine receptors in primary, effector, and memory immune responses. Annu. Rev. Immunol. **18:** 593–620.
14. WELLS, T.N., C.A. POWER & A.E. PROUDFOOT. 1998. Definition, function and pathophysiological significance of chemokine receptors. Trends Pharmacol. Sci. **19:** 376–380.
15. CAMPBELL, J.J., K.E. MURPHY, E.J. KUNKEL, *et al.* 2001. CCR7 expression and memory T cell diversity in humans. J. Immunol. **166:** 877–884.
16. CAMPBELL, J.J., G. HARALDSEN, J. PAN, *et al.* 1999. The chemokine receptor CCR4 in vascular recognition by cutaneous but not intestinal memory T cells. Nature **400:** 776–780.
17. HUDAK, S., M. HAGEN, Y. LIU, *et al.* 2002. Immune surveillance and effector functions of CCR10(+) skin homing T cells. J. Immunol. **169:** 1189–1196.
18. HOMEY, B., H. ALENIUS, A. MULLER, *et al.* 2002. CCL27-CCR10 interactions regulate T cell-mediated skin inflammation. Nat. Med. **8:** 157–165.
19. KUNKEL, E.J., J.J. CAMPBELL, G. HARALDSEN, *et al.* 2000. Lymphocyte CC chemokine receptor 9 and epithelial thymus-expressed chemokine (TECK) expression distinguish the small intestinal immune compartment: epithelial expression of tissue-specific chemokines as an organizing principle in regional immunity. J. Exp. Med. **192:** 761–768.
20. PAPADAKIS, K.A., J. PREHN, V. NELSON, *et al.* 2000. The role of thymus-expressed chemokine and its receptor CCR9 on lymphocytes in the regional specialization of the mucosal immune system. J. Immunol. **165:** 5069–5076.
21. KIM, C.H., E.J. KUNKEL, J. BOISVERT, *et al.* 2001. Bonzo/CXCR6 expression defines type 1-polarized T-cell subsets with extralymphoid tissue homing potential. J. Clin. Invest. **107:** 595–601.
22. MATLOUBIAN, M., A. DAVID, S. ENGEL, *et al.* 2000. A transmembrane CXC chemokine is a ligand for HIV-coreceptor Bonzo. Nat. Immunol. **1:** 298–304.
23. QIN, S., J.B. ROTTMAN, P. MYERS, *et al.* 1998. The chemokine receptors CXCR3 and CCR5 mark subsets of T cells associated with certain inflammatory reactions. J. Clin. Invest. **101:** 746–754.
24. RE, F. & J.L. STROMINGER. 2001. Toll-like receptor 2 (TLR2) and TLR4 differentially activate human dendritic cells. J. Biol. Chem. **276:** 37692–37699.
25. INNGJERDINGEN, M., B. DAMAJ & A.A. MAGHAZACHI. 2001. Expression and regulation of chemokine receptors in human natural killer cells. Blood **97:** 367–375.
26. LOETSCHER, P., M. SEITZ, M. BAGGIOLINI & B. MOSER. 1996. Interleukin-2 regulates CC chemokine receptor expression and chemotactic responsiveness in T lymphocytes. J. Exp. Med. **184:** 569–577.
27. NISHIMURA, M., H. UMEHARA, T. NAKAYAMA, *et al.* 2002. Dual functions of fractalkine/CX3C ligand 1 in trafficking of perforin+/granzyme B+ cytotoxic effector lymphocytes that are defined by CX3CR1 expression. J. Immunol. **168:** 6173–6180.
28. QIN, S., G. LAROSA, J.J. CAMPBELL, *et al.* 1996. Expression of monocyte chemoattractant protein-1 and interleukin-8 receptors on subsets of T cells: correlation with transendothelial chemotactic potential. Eur J. Immunol. **26:** 640–647.
29. MATHEW, A., J.A. MACLEAN, E. DEHAAN, *et al.* 2001. Signal transducer and activator of transcription 6 controls chemokine production and T helper cell type 2 cell trafficking in allergic pulmonary inflammation. J. Exp. Med. **193:** 1087–1096.
30. LIAO, F., R.L. RABIN, C.S. SMITH, *et al.* 1999. CC-chemokine receptor 6 is expressed on diverse memory subsets of T cells and determines responsiveness to macrophage inflammatory protein 3 alpha. J. Immunol. **162:** 186–194.
31. CHARBONNIER, A.S., N. KOHRGRUBER, E. KRIEHUBER, *et al.* 1999. Macrophage inflammatory protein 3alpha is involved in the constitutive trafficking of epidermal langerhans cells. J. Exp. Med. **190:** 1755–1768.

32. DIEU, M.C., B. VANBERVLIET, A. VICARI, *et al.* 1998. Selective recruitment of immature and mature dendritic cells by distinct chemokines expressed in different anatomic sites. J. Exp. Med. **188:** 373–386.
33. LUSTER, A.D. & A.M. TAGER. 2004. T-cell trafficking in asthma: lipid mediators grease the way. Nat. Rev. Immunol. **4:** 711–724.
34. MEDOFF, B.D., E. SEUNG, J.C. WAIN, *et al.* 2005. BLT1-mediated T cell trafficking is critical for rejection and obliterative bronchiolitis following lung transplantation J. Exp. Med. **202:** 97–110.
35. BUSSE, W.W. & R.F. LEMANSKE, JR. 2001. Asthma. N. Engl. J. Med. **344:** 350–362.
36. LUKACS, N.W. 2001. Role of chemokines in the pathogenesis of asthma. Nat. Rev. Immunol. **1:** 108–116.
37. EPSTEIN, M.M. 2004. Do mouse models of allergic asthma mimic clinical disease? Int. Arch. Allergy Immunol. **133:** 84–100.
38. FULKERSON, P.C., N. ZIMMERMANN, L.M. HASSMAN, *et al.* 2004. Pulmonary chemokine expression is coordinately regulated by STAT1, STAT6, and IFN-gamma. J. Immunol. **173:** 7565–7574.
39. HENDERSON, W.R., JR., D.B. LEWIS, R.K. ALBERT, *et al.* 1996. The importance of leukotrienes in airway inflammation in a mouse model of asthma. J. Exp. Med. **184:** 1483–1494.
40. LILLY, C.M., H. NAKAMURA, O.I. BELOSTOTSKY, *et al.* 2001. Eotaxin expression after segmental allergen challenge in subjects with atopic asthma. Am. J. Respir. Crit. Care Med. **163:** 1669–1675.
41. BOCHNER, B.S., S.A. HUDSON, H.Q. XIAO & M.C. LIU. 2003. Release of both CCR4-active and CXCR3-active chemokines during human allergic pulmonary late-phase reactions. J. Allergy Clin. Immunol. **112:** 930–934.
42. SUR, S., H. KITA, G.J. GLEICH, *et al.* 1996. Eosinophil recruitment is associated with IL-5, but not with RANTES, twenty-four hours after allergen challenge. J. Allergy Clin. Immunol. **97:** 1272–1278.
43. PILETTE, C., J.N. FRANCIS, S.J. TILL & S.R. DURHAM. 2004. CCR4 ligands are up-regulated in the airways of atopic asthmatics after segmental allergen challenge. Eur. Respir. J. **23:** 876–884.
44. NOCKER, R.E., T.A. OUT, F.R. WELLER, *et al.* 1999. Influx of neutrophils into the airway lumen at 4 h after segmental allergen challenge in asthma. Int. Arch. Allergy Immunol. **119:** 45–53.
45. VIRCHOW, J.C., JR., C. WALKER, D. HAFNER, *et al.* 1995. T cells and cytokines in bronchoalveolar lavage fluid after segmental allergen provocation in atopic asthma. Am. J. Respir. Crit. Care Med. **151:** 960–968.
46. MURRAY, J.J., A.B. TONNEL, A.R. BRASH, *et al.* 1986. Release of prostaglandin D2 into human airways during acute antigen challenge. N. Engl. J. Med. **315:** 800–804.
47. WENZEL, S.E., J.Y. WESTCOTT, H.R. SMITH & G.L. LARSEN. 1989. Spectrum of prostanoid release after bronchoalveolar allergen challenge in atopic asthmatics and in control groups. An alteration in the ratio of bronchoconstrictive to bronchoprotective mediators. Am. Rev. Respir. Dis. **139:** 450–457.
48. CAMPBELL, J.J., C.E. BRIGHTLING, F.A. SYMON, *et al.* 2001. Expression of chemokine receptors by lung T cells from normal and asthmatic subjects. J. Immunol. **166:** 2842–2848.
49. PANINA-BORDIGNON, P., A. PAPI, M. MARIANI, *et al.* 2001. The C-C chemokine receptors CCR4 and CCR8 identify airway T cells of allergen-challenged atopic asthmatics. J. Clin. Invest. **107:** 1357–1364.
50. HUMBLES, A.A., C.M. LLOYD, S.J. MCMILLAN, *et al.* 2004. A critical role for eosinophils in allergic airways remodeling. Science **305:** 1776–1779.
51. SCHUH, J.M., C.A. POWER, A.E. PROUDFOOT, *et al.* 2002. Airway hyperresponsiveness, but not airway remodeling, is attenuated during chronic pulmonary allergic responses to *Aspergillus* in CCR4–/– mice. FASEB J. **16:** 1313–1315.
52. CHENSUE, S.W., N.W. LUKACS, T.Y. YANG, *et al.* 2001. Aberrant in vivo T helper type 2 cell response and impaired eosinophil recruitment in CC chemokine receptor 8 knockout mice. J. Exp. Med. **193:** 573–584.

53. ARAI, T. K. ABE, H. MATSUOKA, *et al.* 2000. Introduction of the interleukin-10 gene into mice inhibited bleomycin-induced lung injury in vivo. Am. J. Physiol. Lung Cell Mol. Physiol. **278:** L914–L922.
54. KIPS, J.C., G.P. ANDERSON, J.J. FREDBERG, *et al.* 2003. Murine models of asthma. Eur. Respir. J. **22:** 374–382.
55. MEDOFF, B.D., A. SAUTY, A.M. TAGER, *et al.* 2002. IFN-gamma-Inducible protein 10 (CXCL10) contributes to airway hyperreactivity and airway inflammation in a mouse model of asthma. J. Immunol. **168:** 5278–5286.
56. LUKACS, N.W., D.M. PROSSER, M. WIEKOWSKI, *et al.* 2001. Requirement for the chemokine receptor CCR6 in allergic pulmonary inflammation. J. Exp. Med. **194:** 551–555.
57. LUNDY, S.K., S.A. LIRA, J.J. SMIT, *et al.* 2005. Attenuation of allergen-induced responses in CCR6–/– mice is dependent upon altered pulmonary T lymphocyte activation. J. Immunol. **174:** 2054–2060.
58. KALLINICH, T., S. SCHMIDT, E. HAMELMANN, *et al.* 2005. Chemokine-receptor expression on T cells in lung compartments of challenged asthmatic patients. Clin. Exp. Allergy **35:** 26–33.
59. TENVERGERT, E.M., M.L. ESSINK-BOT, A. GEERTSMA, *et al.* 1998. The effect of lung transplantation on health-related quality of life. Chest **113:** 358–364.
60. AURORA, P., B. WHITEHEAD, A. WADE, *et al.* 1999. Lung transplantation and life extension in children with cystic fibrosis. Lancet **354:** 1591–1593.
61. LANUZA, D.M., C. LEFAIVER, M. MC CABE, *et al.* 2000. Prospective study of functional status and quality of life before and after lung transplantation. Chest **118:** 115–122.
62. TRULOCK, E. 2001. Lung and heart-lung transplantation: overview of results. Semin. Respir. Crit. Care Med. **22:** 479–488.
63. ARCASOY, S.M. & R.M. KOTLOFF. 1999. Medical progress: lung transplantation. N. Engl. J. Med. **340:** 1081–1091.
64. ESTENNE, M., J.R. MAURER, A. BOEHLER, *et al.* 2002. Bronchiolitis obliterans syndrome 2001: an update of the diagnostic criteria. J. Heart Lung Transplant **21:** 297–310.
65. SUNDARESAN, S., E.P. TRULOCK, T. MOHANAKUMAR, *et al.* 1995. Prevalence and outcome of bronchiolitis obliterans syndrome after lung transplantation. Ann. Thorac. Surg. **60:** 1341–1346.
66. REICHENSPURNER, H., R.E. GIRGIS, R.C. ROBBINS, *et al.* 1996. Stanford experience with obliterative bronchiolitis after lung and heart-lung transplantation. Ann. Thorac. Surg. **62:** 1467–1472; discussion 1472–1473.
67. TULLIUS, S.G. & N.L. TILNEY. 1995. Both alloantigen-dependent and -independent factors influence chronic allograft rejection. Transplantation **59:** 313–318.
68. WAAGA, A.M., M. GASSER, I. LASKOWSKI & N.L. TILNEY. 2000. Mechanisms of chronic rejection. Curr. Opin. Immunol. **12:** 517–521.
69. TRULOCK, E.P. 1997. Lung transplantation. Am. J. Respir. Crit. Care Med. **155:** 789–818.
70. BRADLEY, J.A. & E.M. BOLTON. 1992. The T-cell requirements for allograft rejection. Transplant. Rev. **6:** 115–129.
71. RABINOWICH, H., A. ZEEVI, I.L. PARADIS, *et al.* 1990. Proliferative responses of bronchoalveolar lavage lymphocytes from heart-lung transplant patients. Transplantation **49:** 115–121.
72. DUQUESNOY, R.J., J.D. TRAGER & A. ZEEVI. 1991. Propagation and characterization of lymphocytes from transplant biopsies. Crit. Rev. Immunol. **10:** 455–480.
73. DUNCAN, S.R., V. VALENTINE, M. ROGLIC, *et al.* 1996. T cell receptor biases and clonal proliferations among lung transplant recipients with obliterative bronchiolitis. J. Clin. Invest. **97:** 2642–2650.
74. DUQUESNOY, R. & A. ZEEVI. 1992. Immunological monitoring of lung transplant patients by bronchoalveolar lavage analysis. Transplant. Rev. **6:** 218–230.
75. REINSMOEN, N.L., R.M. BOLMAN, K. SAVIK, *et al.* 1994. Improved long-term graft outcome in lung transplant recipients who have donor antigen-specific hyporeactivity. J. Heart Lung Transplant **13:** 30–36; discussion 36–37.

76. El-Sawy, T., N.M. Fahmy & R.L. Fairchild. 2002. Chemokines: directing leukocyte infiltration into allografts. Curr. Opin. Immunol. **14:** 562–568.
77. Goddard, S., A. Williams, C. Morland, *et al.* 2001. Differential expression of chemokines and chemokine receptors shapes the inflammatory response in rejecting human liver transplants. Transplantation **72:** 1957–1967.
78. Agostini, C., F. Calabrese, F. Rea, *et al.* 2001. CXCR3 and its ligand CXCL10 are expressed by inflammatory cells infiltrating lung allografts and mediate chemotaxis of T cells at sites of rejection. Am. J. Pathol. **158:** 1703–1711.
79. Zhao, D.X., Y. Hu, G.G. Miller, *et al.* 2002. Differential expression of the IFN-gamma-inducible CXCR3-binding chemokines, IFN-inducible protein 10, monokine induced by IFN, and IFN-inducible T cell alpha chemoattractant in human cardiac allografts: association with cardiac allograft vasculopathy and acute rejection. J. Immunol. **169:** 1556–1560.
80. Belperio, J.A., M.P. Keane, M.D. Burdick, *et al.* 2002. Critical role for CXCR3 chemokine biology in the pathogenesis of bronchiolitis obliterans syndrome. J. Immunol. **169:** 1037–1049.
81. Gerard, C. & B.J. Rollins. 2001. Chemokines and disease. Nat. Immunol. **2:** 108–115.
82. Ward, C. & E.H. Walters. 2001. Bronchoalveolar lavage: critical evaluation of techniques. *In* Human Airway Inflammation. D.F. Rogers & L.E. Donnelly, Eds.: 31–60. Humana Press. Totowa, NJ.
83. Estenne, M. & M.I. Hertz. 2002. Bronchiolitis obliterans after human lung transplantation. Am. J. Respir. Crit. Care Med. **166:** 440–444.
84. Sallusto, F., A. Lanzavecchia & C.R. Mackay. 1998. Chemokines and chemokine receptors in T-cell priming and Th1/Th2-mediated responses. Immunol. Today **19:** 568–574.
85. Agostini, C., U. Basso & G. Semenzato. 1998. Cells and molecules involved in the development of sarcoid granuloma. J. Clin. Immunol. **18:** 184–192.
86. Kunkel, S.L., N.W. Lukacs, R.M. Strieter & S.W. Chensue. 1996. Th1 and Th2 responses regulate experimental lung granuloma development. Sarcoidosis Vasc. Diffuse Lung Dis. **13:** 120–128.
87. Wallace, W.A. & S.E. Howie. 1999. Immunoreactive interleukin 4 and interferon-gamma expression by type II alveolar epithelial cells in interstitial lung disease. J. Pathol. **187:** 475–480.
88. Wallace, W.A., E.A. Ramage, D. Lamb & S.E. Howie. 1995. A type 2 (Th2-like) pattern of immune response predominates in the pulmonary interstitium of patients with cryptogenic fibrosing alveolitis (CFA). Clin. Exp. Immunol. **101:** 436–441.
89. Agostini, C., F. Adami & G. Semenzato. 2000. New pathogenetic insights into the sarcoid granuloma. Curr. Opin. Rheumatol. **12:** 71–76.
90. Huaux, F., T. Liu, B. McGarry, *et al.* 2003. Dual roles of IL-4 in lung injury and fibrosis. J. Immunol. **170:** 2083–2092.
91. Jakubzick, C., E.S. Choi, B.H. Joshi, *et al.* 2003. Therapeutic attenuation of pulmonary fibrosis via targeting of IL-4- and IL-13-responsive cells. J. Immunol. **171:** 2684–2693.
92. Kolodsick, J.E., G.B. Toews, C. Jakubzick, *et al.* 2004. Protection from fluorescein isothiocyanate-induced fibrosis in IL-13-deficient, but not IL-4-deficient, mice results from impaired collagen synthesis by fibroblasts. J. Immunol. **172:** 4068–4076.
93. Sandler, N.G., M.M. Mentink-Kane, A.W. Cheever, *et al.* 2003. Global gene expression profiles during acute pathogen-induced pulmonary inflammation reveal divergent roles for Th1 and Th2 responses in tissue repair. J. Immunol. **171:** 3655–3667.
94. Fanburg, B.L. & O. Villa. 2000. Sarcoidosis. *In* Textbook of Respiratory Medicine, Vol. 2. J.F. Murray & J. A. Nadel, Eds.: 1717–1732. W.B. Saunders. Philadelphia.
95. Moller, D.R., J.D. Forman, M.C. Liu, *et al.* 1996. Enhanced expression of IL-12 associated with Th1 cytokine profiles in active pulmonary sarcoidosis. J. Immunol. **156:** 4952–4960.
96. Robinson, B.W., T.L. McLemore & R.G. Crystal. 1985. Gamma interferon is spontaneously released by alveolar macrophages and lung T lymphocytes in patients with pulmonary sarcoidosis. J. Clin. Invest. **75:** 1488–1495.

97. AGOSTINI, C., M. CASSATELLA, R. ZAMBELLO, *et al.* 1998. Involvement of the IP-10 chemokine in sarcoid granulomatous reactions. J. Immunol. **161:** 6413–6420.
98. MIOTTO, D., P. CHRISTODOULOPOULOS, R. OLIVENSTEIN, *et al.* 2001. Expression of IFN-gamma-inducible protein; monocyte chemotactic proteins 1, 3, and 4; and eotaxin in TH1- and TH2-mediated lung diseases. J. Allergy Clin. Immunol. **107:** 664–670.
99. IIDA, K., J. KADOTA, K. KAWAKAMI, *et al.* 1997. Analysis of T cell subsets and beta chemokines in patients with pulmonary sarcoidosis. Thorax **52:** 431–437.
100. AGOSTINI, C., A. CABRELLE, F. CALABRESE, *et al.* 2005. Role for CXCR6 and its ligand CXCL16 in the pathogenesis of T cell alveolitis in sarcoidosis. Am. J. Respir. Crit. Care Med. **172:** 1290–1298.
101. KATCHAR, K., A. EKLUND & J. GRUNEWALD. 2003. Expression of Th1 markers by lung accumulated T cells in pulmonary sarcoidosis. J. Intern. Med. **254:** 564–571.
102. GIBEJOVA, A., F. MRAZEK, D. SUBRTOVA, *et al.* 2003. Expression of macrophage inflammatory protein-3 beta/CCL19 in pulmonary sarcoidosis. Am. J. Respir. Crit. Care Med. **167:** 1695–1703.
103. GOETZL, E.J. & J.M. LUCE. 2000. Eosinophilic lung diseases. *In* Textbook of Respiratory Medicine, Vol. 2. J.F. Murray & J.A. Nadel, Eds.: 1757–1773. W.B. Saunders. Philadelphia.
104. FUJIMURA, M., M. YASUI, S. SHINAGAWA, *et al.* 1998. Bronchoalveolar lavage cell findings in three types of eosinophilic pneumonia: acute, chronic and drug-induced eosinophilic pneumonia. Respir. Med. **92:** 743–749.
105. HAYAKAWA, H., A. SATO, M. TOYOSHIMA, *et al.* 1994. A clinical study of idiopathic eosinophilic pneumonia. Chest **105:** 1462–1466.
106. WALKER, C., W. BAUER, R.K. BRAUN, *et al.* 1994. Activated T cells and cytokines in bronchoalveolar lavages from patients with various lung diseases associated with eosinophilia. Am. J. Respir. Crit. Care Med. **150:** 1038–1048.
107. TANIGUCHI, H., S. KATOH, J. KADOTA, *et al.* 2000. Interleukin 5 and granulocyte-macrophage colony-stimulating factor levels in bronchoalveolar lavage fluid in interstitial lung disease. Eur. Respir. J. **16:** 959–964.
108. KATOH, S., K. FUKUSHIMA, N. MATSUMOTO, *et al.* 2003. Accumulation of CCR4-expressing CD4+ T cells and high concentration of its ligands (TARC and MDC) in bronchoalveolar lavage fluid of patients with eosinophilic pneumonia. Allergy **58:** 518–523.
109. KATOH, S., N. MATSUMOTO, K. FUKUSHIMA, *et al.* 2000. Elevated chemokine levels in bronchoalveolar lavage fluid of patients with eosinophilic pneumonia. J. Allergy Clin. Immunol. **106:** 730–736.
110. MIYAZAKI, E., S. NUREKI, T. FUKAMI, *et al.* 2002. Elevated levels of thymus- and activation-regulated chemokine in bronchoalveolar lavage fluid from patients with eosinophilic pneumonia. Am. J. Respir. Crit. Care Med. **165:** 1125–1131.
111. BROMLEY, S.K., S.Y. THOMAS & A.D. LUSTER. 2005. Chemokine receptor CCR7 guides T cell exit from peripheral tissues and entry into afferent lymphatics. Nat. Immunol. **6:** 895–901.

Toll-Like Receptor Activation in the Pathogenesis of Systemic Lupus Erythematosus

TERRY K. MEANS AND ANDREW D. LUSTER

Center for Immunology and Inflammatory Diseases, and Division of Rheumatology, Allergy and Immunology, Massachusetts General Hospital and Harvard Medical School, Boston, Massachusetts 02129, USA

ABSTRACT: Systemic lupus erythematosus (SLE) is characterized by the production of pathogenic autoantibodies to nucleoproteins and DNA. The level of anti-DNA antibodies correlates with disease severity, and the deposition of these immune complexes (ICs) in the kidneys is thought to contribute to disease pathogenesis. Recent evidence suggests that the DNA component of ICs purified from SLE patients (SLE DNA-ICs) contributes to the development of SLE pathology. SLE DNA-ICs induce proliferation of self-reactive B cells and cytokine production by plasmacytoid dendritic cells (PDCs) in a TLR9-dependent manner. One of the cytokines induced by DNA-containing ICs is interferon α (IFN-α). Elevated serum levels of IFN-α and overexpression of interferon-induced genes have been observed in SLE patient blood and shown to correlate with disease severity. We have recently found that the mechanism of IFN-α production by PDCs depends on TLR9 and FcγRIIa (CD32), and CD32 delivers SLE DNA-ICs to intracellular lysosomes containing TLR9. This CD32–TLR9 pathway, which is operative in PDCs, is distinct from the BCR/TLR9 pathway in B cells and may prove to be a novel target for future SLE therapies. In this article, the role of toll-like receptors, cytokines, and Fc receptors expressed by PDCs in the pathogenesis of SLE is summarized.

KEYWORDS: toll-like receptors; plasmacytoid dendritic cells; systemic lupus erythematosus; autoimmune disease; chemokines; cytokines; immune complexes; autoantibodies

INTRODUCTION

Systemic lupus erythematosus (SLE) is a systemic autoimmune disease characterized by autoantibodies to nuclear DNA and/or nuclear proteins.[1] The serological hallmark of the disease is the high level of antinuclear antibodies present in 99% of individuals with SLE. With a prevalence of 40–50 cases per 100,000, SLE is the second most common autoimmune disease behind rheumatoid arthritis.[2] Sixty-five percent of patients with SLE have disease onset between the ages of 16 and 55 years. In adults there is a 10–15 times higher frequency of SLE in women, typically during

Address for correspondence: Terry K. Means, Ph.D., Massachusetts General Hospital, 149 13th St., Charlestown, MA 02129. Voice: 617-726-6497; fax: 617-726-5651. tmeans@partners.org

Ann. N.Y. Acad. Sci. 1062: 242–251 (2005). © 2005 New York Academy of Sciences. doi: 10.1196/annals.1358.027

the childbearing years, which is thought to be due to an estrogen hormonal effect. Clinical manifestations of SLE include skin rash, joint inflammation, and organ injury (e.g., kidney). SLE is characterized by chronic inflammation initiated by the deposition of immune complexes (ICs) in the target organs. This deposition of ICs induces a local inflammatory response by activating resident tissue cells that secrete cytokines and chemokines. These secreted chemokines recruit dendritic cells, neutrophils, and monocytes to the sites of IC deposition, amplifying the inflammatory response. These observations suggest that cellular activation by ICs plays an important role in the pathogenesis of SLE. Sadly, during the last 40 years no new FDA-approved drugs for SLE have come to market. In this review we will discuss the mechanism for cell activation by SLE DNA-ICs, the understanding of which may provide clues for potential new therapies for SLE.

AUTOANTIBODIES AND IMMUNE COMPLEXES IN SLE

Immunoglobulins play an important role in host defense; however, they are also involved in autoimmune diseases, in which antibodies recognize the host's own tissue, triggering unwanted inflammatory responses that result in organ damage. In SLE, several types of autoantibodies have been shown to be associated with disease. These include anti-dsDNA, anti–Smith antigen, antihistones, anti-ssDNA, anti-RNP, anti-Ro, anti-La, anti–proliferating cell nuclear antigen, anti-Ku, and anti–Laminin B.[3] Although some of these autoantibodies are found in other rheumatic diseases, anti-dsDNA antibodies are uniquely present in SLE.[4] Furthermore, the anti-dsDNA antibody is regarded as a marker for SLE, and the American College of Rheumatology classification criteria for the disease include antibody binding to DNA.[5]

BIOLOGY OF TOLL-LIKE RECEPTORS

Toll-like receptors (TLRs) are an evolutionarily conserved family of type I transmembrane receptors that play an important role in innate immunity.[6,7] These germ line–encoded receptors share extended homology in their intracellular tail with receptors for the cytokines interleukin 1 (IL-1) and IL-18.[8,9] A variety of viral, bacterial, and fungal products that serve as TLR ligands have been identified. To date, 10 human TLRs have been identified, and conserved pathogen-associated molecular patterns (PAMPs) found on microbes leads to a signal-transduction cascade that results in cellular activation, thereby stimulating innate immune defenses. TLR1, -2, -4, -5, and -6 are expressed on the cell surface, where they serve to recognize bacterial products such as triacylated lipopeptides (TLR1/2 heterodimer), diacylated lipopeptides (TLR2/6 heterodimer), lipopolysaccharide (TLR4), and flagellin (TLR5).[10–13] TLR3, -7, -8, and -9 are localized to intracellular compartments and serve to recognize viral products such as dsRNA (TLR3), ssRNA (TLR7/8), and unmethylated CpG DNA from bacteria and viruses (TLR9).[14–21] Upon ligand binding, TLRs trigger a signal transduction cascade beginning with the recruitment of MyD88, IRAK, and TRAF6, which activate downstream mediators such as mitogen-activated protein kinase and NF-κB. Finally, the activation of transcription factors leads to the production of chemokines and cytokines that amplify the immune response. Recent studies suggest that TLR signaling is protective in acute infections and for maintenance of homeostasis of the gut; however, chronic or dysregulated TLR signaling can be destructive to the host and may exacerbate disease.[22]

ROLE OF IFN-α IN SLE

The interferons (IFNs) were the first cytokine family discovered and include type I IFNs (IFN-α and IFN-β) and type II IFN (IFN-γ). The type I IFNs are produced primarily by myeloid cells in response to viruses and endotoxin, whereas type II IFN is secreted by lymphocytes in response to a variety of specific antigens. Both types of IFN have antiviral activity and immunoregulatory functions that affect the development of cell-mediated immunity and self-tolerance. A role for type I IFN in SLE was first reported in 1979.[23] In this study, the sera of patients with SLE were found to contain high levels of type I IFN, which correlated with disease activity, disease severity, and the presence of anti-DNA antibodies.[23] These data provided the first clue that this cytokine might play a central role in this autoimmune disease. Interestingly, these findings were nearly forgotten until a decade later, when the Ronnblom and Alm groups noticed that patients receiving recombinant IFN-α as treatment for cancer and hepatitis C infections began developing autoantibodies and symptoms that mimic those of SLE.[24] In hindsight, the toxicity of IFN-α is probably not surprising considering its many immunoregulatory effects, including differentiation of T and B cells, cell survival, and maturation of monocytes and dendritic cells.[25] Finally, work by the Banchereau and Pascual groups has found that peripheral blood mononuclear cells (PBMCs) isolated from patients with active SLE have a signature gene expression pattern with overexpression of 12 IFN-induced genes.[26] Together, these data support the hypothesis that overproduction of IFN-α plays a critical role in SLE.

IFN-INDUCING FACTOR IN LUPUS SERUM

Since patients with active SLE often have persistent production of circulating type I IFNs, in the late 1990s Ronnblom, Alm, and colleagues began searching for an endogenous IFN inducer in SLE patients.[27] SLE serum was found to induce IFN production in cultures of PBMCs isolated from normal donors, and fractionation of SLE serum revealed that the molecular mass of the IFN-inducing factor was between 300 and 1000 kDa.[28] These data indicate that the IFN-inducing factor may be an antigen–antibody IC.[29] This hypothesis is supported by the fact that passage of SLE serum over a protein G column removed the IFN-inducing activity from the serum. Also, DNase, but not RNase, abolished the IFN-inducing activity of the SLE serum. Together these data suggest that DNA–anti-DNA ICs could be part of the IFN-inducing activity in SLE serum. Interestingly, a possible role for the DNA component of ICs in cell activation was suggested after the DNA contained in these complexes was characterized. The DNA in DNA–anti-DNA ICs purified from SLE patient serum was sequenced and found to contain CpG dinucleotides at a five times higher frequency than that expected in the genome.[30,31] In vertebrates, CpG dinucleotides are suppressed; however, they are found in clusters near the 5′ coding region of genes and are called CpG islands. Interestingly, the CpG frequency in these islands is one in every 12 bp, similar to the average CpG frequency found in the cloned lupus IC DNA. Later, synthetic oligonucleotides based on the sequences of the lupus IC DNA were found to be immunostimulatory and induced cytokine production from primary human monocytes.[31] Finally, unmethylated but not methylated CpG DNA mixed with anti-DNA antibodies induced IFN-α production from normal PBMCs. Together, these data suggest that ICs composed of hypomethylated CpG-containing DNA with anti-DNA antibodies are at least one of the IFN-α–inducing factors in SLE serum.

PLASMACYTOID DENDRITIC CELLS IN SLE

In 1999 the elusive cell type responsible for producing large amounts of IFN-α in response to viral stimulation was isolated from white blood cells.[32] This IFN-producing cell (IPC) was shown to be an immature form of a specialized dendritic cell. This rare population of IPCs, now called plasmacytoid dendritic cells (PDCs), represents only 0.1% of PBMCs but produces 1000 times more IFN-α than other blood cells following microbial stimulation.[32] PDCs are $CD123^+$, $CD4^+$, $CD11c^-$, and blood dendritic cell antigen (BDCA) 2^+ and 4^+.[33] This rare population of cells is now routinely separated from whole blood through the use of anti-BDCA4 magnetic beads, and further characterization has demonstrated that these cells selectively express TLR7 and TLR9, which is consistent with their specialized function as viral sensors.[34] PDCs were also found to be the major cell type responsible for IFN-α production following *in vitro* stimulation with lupus serum or purified SLE DNA-ICs.[35,36] Interestingly, SLE patients were found to have reduced numbers of circulating PDCs, but increased numbers of PDCs in skin lesions.[37] These findings are consistent with recent studies showing that upon activation, PDCs upregulate expression of the chemokine receptors CXCR3 and CCR7, which direct trafficking of cells to peripheral sites of inflammation and the lymph nodes, respectively.[38] Because PDCs are the major IFN-producing cell type activated by SLE DNA-ICs, they may play an important role in the pathogenesis of SLE.

CELL ACTIVATION BY SLE DNA-ICs

In agreement with others, we found that sera isolated from lupus patients induces cellular activation. Specifically, we found that normal human PDCs could be stimulated by SLE serum, but not by serum isolated from Sjogrens syndrome or rheumatoid arthritis patients.[39] Moreover, the activity of SLE serum correlated with the presence and levels of anti-DNA antibodies present in the SLE serum. Also, we confirmed that purified DNA-containing ICs from SLE serum were responsible for the stimulatory activity of SLE serum and that these SLE DNA-ICs could stimulate cytokine production from PDCs, monocytes, and B cells, but not T cells or monocyte-derived DCs. Since other cytokines besides IFN-α have been implicated in the pathogenesis of SLE, we examined the full profile of cytokines and chemokines induced by SLE DNA-ICs in PDCs. We found that SLE DNA-ICs induced the expression of 16 chemokines and nine cytokines by PDCs (FIG. 1). SLE DNA-ICs induced

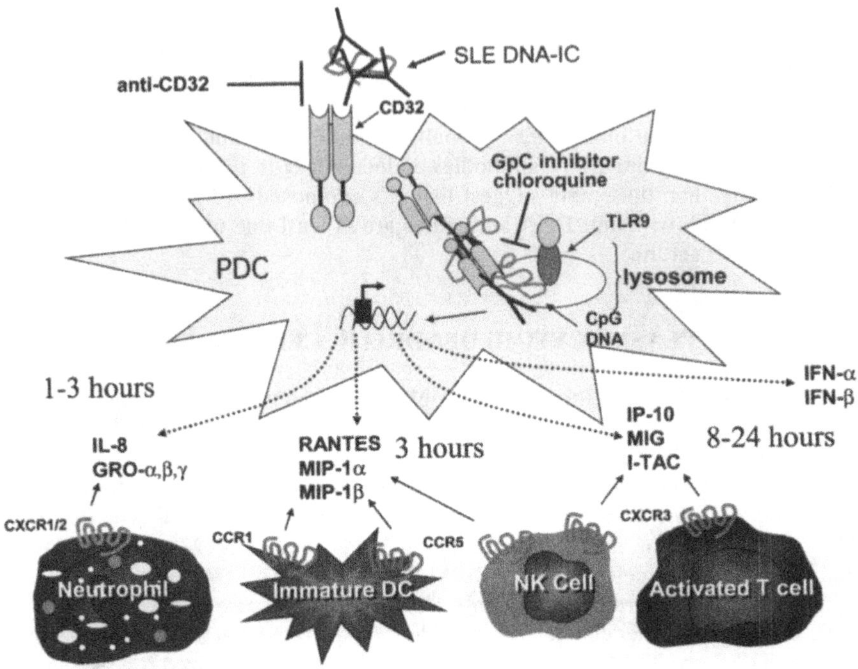

FIGURE 1. SLE DNA-ICs activate PDCs through cooperation of CD32 and TLR9. CD32 sequentially binds, internalizes, and delivers SLE DNA-ICs to intracellular lysosomes containing TLR9, triggering a signaling cascade that leads to the production of cytokines and chemokines that exacerbate disease.

chemokines active on neutrophils (CXCL8\IL-8/, CXCL1\GRO-α, CXCL2\GRO-β, CXCL3\GRO-γ), NK cells (CCL5\RANTES), immature DCs (CCL3\MIP-1α, CCL4\MIP-1β), and effector T cells (CXCL9\MIG, CXCL10\IP-10, CXCL11\I-TAC, CCL22\MDC, CCL1\I-309). We found no induction of chemokines active on B cells (CXCL13\BCA-1) or eosinophils (CCL11\Eotaxin1). SLE DNA-ICs also induced the expression of the proinflammatory cytokines IL-1β, IL-6, TNF-α, IL-18, IFN-α, IFN-β, iNOS, and Th1 cytokines (IFN-γ, IL-12), but not Th2 cytokines (IL-4, IL-5, IL-10, IL-13). These data demonstrate that SLE DNA-ICs have robust stimulatory activity, being capable of inducing cytokines and chemokines, many of which have been previously implicated in autoimmunity.[40]

TLR9 RECOGNITION OF DNA-CONTAINING ICs

Since the DNA contained in SLE DNA-ICs is enriched for CpG dinucleotide sequences, we hypothesized that SLE serum containing anti-DNA antibodies activates cells through TLR9. Furthermore, we hypothesized that chronic stimulation of TLR9 by SLE DNA-ICs leads to the overproduction of IFN-α, which may not be the cause of disease, but at the very least exacerbates SLE pathogenesis. To test this hypothesis, we stably transfected human embryonic kidney (HEK) cells, which are normally unresponsive to SLE serum and SLE DNA-ICs, with TLR9, TLR2, TLR3, or TLR4/MD2. We found that only HEK cells expressing TLR9 were activated by lupus serum and SLE DNA-ICs. Furthermore, the TLR9-dependent activity in these experiments was shown to be specific for the DNA component of SLE ICs, as DNase treatment of SLE serum or SLE DNA ICs greatly reduced its activity. We also found that TLR9 is involved in PDC activation by SLE DNA ICs. Both chloroquine and GpC oligonucleotides, known inhibitors of TLR9 signaling, blocked SLE DNA-IC–induced IFN-α production in PDCs (FIG. 1). Chloroquine inhibition is interesting because hydroxychloroquine is one of the few FDA-approved drugs used as a treatment for SLE.[41] These data suggest that inhibitors of TLR signaling, which block SLE DNA-IC–induced IFN-α production (and other cytokines and chemokines), would be promising candidates for clinical trials.

Fc RECEPTORS IN SLE

Recently, SLE pathogenesis has been linked to several genetic factors, including polymorphisms in FcγRs.[42] Of particular interest are studies of FcγRIIa (CD32), as polymorphisms in this receptor have been shown to have a strong correlation with the pathogenesis and susceptibility to SLE.[43–47] CD32 is a membrane-bound 40-kDa glycoprotein, with two extracellular immunoglobulin (Ig)-like domains and a cytoplasmic domain.[48] This receptor is unique to humans and higher primates and is the most widely expressed FcγR. Human CD32 is a low-affinity receptor for monomeric IgG, but binds avidly to complexed IgG. CD32 binds preferentially to IgG1, IgG3, and IgG2a, which are the most common isotypes for autoantibodies in SLE. CD32 forms a dimer with itself and has an immunoreceptor tyrosine–based activation motif (ITAM) located in its cytoplasmic tail. In humans, antigen–antibody interactions form ICs, which induce FcγR-mediated cell activation. The activation induced by binding of immune complexes to CD32 is usually curtailed by antibody binding to FcγRIIb, which contains an ITIM located in its cytoplasmic tail.

Mice deficient for FcγRI or FcγRIII have impaired inflammatory responses to immune complexes, whereas mice deficient in the inhibitory FcγRIIb have enhanced responses.[49–51] Recently, it was shown that increasing the expression of FcγRIIb on B cells in lupus-prone strains of mice reduced mortality, autoantibody production, and kidney pathology.[52] These data suggest that FcγRIIb plays a pivotal role in B-cell tolerance and that FcγRs may be a useful target in therapeutic approaches for SLE. The role of CD32 in IC-mediated inflammation has been difficult to study because mice do not express this receptor. Recently, transgenic mice expressing human CD32 were made using the human promoter for its expression.[53] These mice spontaneously developed autoimmunity with symptoms similar to those of SLE (i.e., antinuclear antibodies, IC deposition). These findings clearly indicate that CD32 plays an important role in mediating IC-induced inflammation. Human CD32 is expressed on neutrophils, eosinophils, B lymphocytes, platelets, mast cells, Langerhans cells, and dendritic cells. Recently, CD32 expression was found on a subset of BDCA4$^+$/BDCA2$^+$ PDCs by FACS.[54] Also, an anti-CD32 antibody, but not antibodies to FCγRI or FcγRIII, blocked IFN-α production by PDCs stimulated with ICs isolated from lupus patients (FIG. 1).[39,54,55] Moreover, treatment of SLE ICs with papain or pepsin, enzymes that cleave IgG into Fc/Fab and $F(ab)_2$ fragments, inhibited IFN-α production by PDCs.[39,54] These data suggest that both the DNA and antibody components of SLE ICs are necessary for inducing maximal IFN-α production and that the Fc portion of the antibody is required. Together these data suggest that CD32 is expressed on some PDCs and is necessary for mediating IC-induced IFN-α production.

CD32 INTERNALIZATION OF SLE DNA-ICs

Since TLR9 signaling takes place in intracellular lysosomes, we hypothesized that CD32 expressed on PDCs is involved in the uptake of SLE DNA-ICs.[56] To test this hypothesis, we incubated PDCs with fluorescently labeled SLE DNA-ICs. We found that the $CD32^+$, but not the $CD32^-$, subset of PDCs efficiently internalized SLE DNA-ICs.[39] Moreover, SLE DNA-ICs induced robust IFN-α production from $CD32^+$ PDCs, but not $CD32^-$ PDCs. To determine whether CD32 cross-linking signals contribute to SLE DNA-IC–induced IFN-α production, we stimulated PDC with papain/pepsin-treated SLE DNA-ICs in the presence of FuGENE6. FuGENE6 is a liposomal carrier used to transfect DNA and proteins into cells. Papain/pepsin-treated SLE DNA-ICs in the presence, but not absence, of FuGENE6 were internalized and induced IFN-α production by PDCs to a similar level as untreated SLE DNA-ICs. These data demonstrate that CD32 cross-linking alone does not induce IFN-α production by PDCs and support a mechanism whereby CD32 facilitates cellular uptake of SLE DNA-ICs and delivers it to intracellular lysosomes containing TLR9, where signaling is initiated (FIG. 1).

INTRACELLULAR LOCALIZATION OF TLR9, CD32, AND DNA–ANTI-DNA ICs

To determine whether trafficking of SLE DNA-ICs into cells was related to TLR9 signaling, we performed confocal microscopy studies on U373 cells stably transfected with yellow fluorescent protein (YFP)–tagged TLR9 and cyan fluorescent protein (CFP)–tagged CD32. In the quiescent state, these transfected cells expressed CD32–CFP on the plasma membrane and TLR9–YFP in the endoplasmic reticulum. Following stimulation with Alexa Fluor–tagged SLE DNA-ICs, CD32 colocalized with SLE DNA-ICs into intracellular vesicles containing TLR9. Concurrent with movement of SLE DNA-IC/CD32 into the cells, TLR9 redistributed from the endoplasmic reticulum to CD32/SLE DNA-IC–containing vesicles. The intracellular structures where CD32/SLE DNA-ICs/TLR9 colocalized were identified as acidic lysosomes. The interaction of TLR9 with SLE DNA-ICs in the lysosomes was rapid, but transient, occurring as quickly as 5 minutes with no interactions after 30 minutes. Also, ICs from other rheumatic diseases failed to colocalize with TLR9. Thus CD32 sequentially binds, internalizes, and delivers SLE DNA-ICs to lysosomes, where they interact with TLR9, triggering a signaling cascade that induces IFN-α production (FIG. 1).

CONCLUSIONS

Recent studies have demonstrated that ICs purified from the serum of patients with active SLE stimulate PDCs; however, the mechanism of activation was poorly understood. Our recent studies show that PDCs express CD32, which facilitates the internalization of SLE DNA-ICs into subcellular lysosomes containing TLR9, where binding and signaling are initiated. These data suggest a functional interaction between TLRs and Fc receptors and raise the possibility that ICs containing ligands for other TLRs, such as RNA, activate cells through similar pathways (i.e., FcR/TLR7). There appear to be species-specific differences in TLR9 expression. TLR9 is functionally expressed on mouse but not human DCs. Also, human PDCs express BDCA2, BDCA4, and CD123, whereas mouse PDCs express B220, Ly6C, and CD11c. These differences might render mouse models of SLE less directly relevant to human SLE and suggest the need for further study in humans.

[*Competing interests*: The authors declare that they have no competing financial interests.]

REFERENCES

1. Mok, C.C. & C.S. Lau. 2003. Pathogenesis of systemic lupus erythematosus. J. Clin. Pathol. **56:** 481–490.
2. Lawrence, R.C., C.G. Helmick, F.C. Arnett, *et al.* 1998. Estimates of the prevalence of arthritis and selected musculoskeletal disorders in the United States. Arthritis Rheum. **41:** 778–799.
3. Tan, E.M. 1989. Antinuclear antibodies: diagnostic markers for autoimmune diseases and probes for cell biology. Adv. Immunol. **44:** 93–151.
4. Hahn, B.H. 1998. Antibodies to DNA. N. Engl. J. Med. **338:** 1359–1368.
5. Tan, E.M., A.S. Cohen, J.F. Fries, *et al.* 1982. The 1982 revised criteria for the classification of systemic lupus erythematosus. Arthritis Rheum. **25:** 1271–1277.
6. Takeda, K., T. Kaisho & S. Akira. 2003. Toll-like receptors. Annu. Rev. Immunol. **21:** 335–376.
7. Means, T.K., D.T. Golenbock & M.J. Fenton. 2000. Structure and function of toll-like receptor proteins. Life Sci. **68:** 241–258.
8. Bell, J.K., G.E. Mullen, C.A. Leifer, *et al.* 2003. Leucine-rich repeats and pathogen recognition in toll-like receptors. Trends Immunol. **24:** 528–533.
9. O'Neill, L.A. & C. Greene. 1998. Signal transduction pathways activated by the IL-1 receptor family: ancient signaling machinery in mammals, insects, and plants. J. Leukoc. Biol. **63:** 650–657.
10. Hayashi, F., K.D. Smith, A. Ozinsky, *et al.* 2001. The innate immune response to bacterial flagellin is mediated by toll-like receptor 5. Nature **410:** 1099–1103.
11. Poltorak, A., X. He, I. Smirnova, *et al.* 1998. Defective LPS signaling in C3H/HeJ and C57BL/10ScCr mice: mutations in the *tlr4* gene. Science **282:** 2085–2088.
12. Takeuchi, O., A. Kaufmann, K. Grote, *et al.* 2000. Preferentially the R-stereoisomer of the mycoplasmal lipopeptide macrophage-activating lipopeptide-2 activates immune cells through a toll-like receptor 2- and myd88-dependent signaling pathway. J. Immunol. **164:** 554–557.
13. Ozinsky, A., D.M. Underhill, J.D. Fontenot, *et al.* 2000. The repertoire for pattern recognition of pathogens by the innate immune system is defined by cooperation between toll-like receptors. Proc. Natl. Acad. Sci. USA **97:** 13766–13771.
14. Hemmi, H., O. Takeuchi, T. Kawai, *et al.* 2000. A toll-like receptor recognizes bacterial DNA. Nature **408:** 740–745.
15. Hemmi, H., T. Kaisho, O. Takeuchi, *et al.* 2002. Small anti-viral compounds activate immune cells via the TLR7 MyD88-dependent signaling pathway. Nat. Immunol. **3:** 196–200.

16. JURK, M., F. HEIL, J. VOLLMER, *et al.* 2002. Human TLR7 or TLR8 independently confer responsiveness to the antiviral compound R-848. Nat. Immunol. **3:** 499.
17. HEIL, F., H. HEMMI, H. HOCHREIN, *et al.* 2004. Species-specific recognition of single-stranded RNA via toll-like receptor 7 and 8. Science **303:** 1526–1529.
18. DIEBOLD, S.S., T. KAISHO, H. HEMMI, *et al.* 2004. Innate antiviral responses by means of TLR7-mediated recognition of single-stranded RNA. Science **303:** 1529–1531.
19. ALEXOPOULOU, L., A.C. HOLT, R. MEDZHITOV & R.A. FLAVELL. 2001. Recognition of double-stranded RNA and activation of NF-kappaB by toll-like receptor 3. Nature **413:** 732–738.
20. TABETA, K., P. GEORGEL, E. JANSSEN, *et al.* 2004. Toll-like receptors 9 and 3 as essential components of innate immune defense against mouse cytomegalovirus infection. Proc. Natl. Acad. Sci. USA **101:** 3516–3521.
21. WANG, T., T. TOWN, L. ALEXOPOULOU, *et al.* 2004. Toll-like receptor 3 mediates West Nile virus entry into the brain causing lethal encephalitis. Nat. Med. **10:** 1366–1373.
22. RAKOFF-NAHOUM, S., J. PAGLINO, F. ESLAMI-VARZANEH, *et al.* 2004. Recognition of commensal microflora by toll-like receptors is required for intestinal homeostasis. Cell **118:** 229–241.
23. HOOKS, J.J., H.M. MOUTSOPOULOS, S.A. GEIS, *et al.* 1979. Immune interferon in the circulation of patients with autoimmune disease. N. Engl. J. Med. **301:** 5–8.
24. RONNBLOM, L.E., G.V. ALM & K.E. OBERG. 1990. Possible induction of systemic lupus erythematosus by interferon-alpha treatment in a patient with a malignant carcinoid tumour. J. Intern. Med. **227:** 207–210.
25. BLANCO, P., A.K. PALUCKA, M. GILL, *et al.* 2001. Induction of dendritic cell differentiation by IFN-alpha in systemic lupus erythematosus. Science **294:** 1540–1543.
26. BENNETT, L., A.K. PALUCKA, E. ARCE, *et al.* 2003. Interferon and granulopoiesis signatures in systemic lupus erythematosus blood. J. Exp. Med. **197:** 711–723.
27. VALLIN, H., S. BLOMBERG, G.V. ALM, *et al.* 1999. Patients with systemic lupus erythematosus (SLE) have a circulating inducer of interferon-alpha (IFN-alpha) production acting on leucocytes resembling immature dendritic cells. Clin. Exp. Immunol. **115:** 196–202.
28. VALLIN, H., A. PERERS, G.V. ALM & L. RONNBLOM. 1999. Anti-double-stranded DNA antibodies and immunostimulatory plasmid DNA in combination mimic the endogenous IFN-alpha inducer in systemic lupus erythematosus. J. Immunol. **163:** 6306–6313.
29. LOVGREN, T., M.L. ELORANTA, U. BAVE, *et al.* 2004. Induction of interferon-alpha production in plasmacytoid dendritic cells by immune complexes containing nucleic acid released by necrotic or late apoptotic cells and lupus IgG. Arthritis Rheum. **50:** 1861–1872.
30. SANO, H., O. TAKAI, N. HARATA, *et al.* 1989. Binding properties of human anti-DNA antibodies to cloned human DNA fragments. Scand. J. Immunol. **30:** 51–63.
31. SATO, Y., M. MIYATA, Y. SATO, *et al.* 1999. CpG motif-containing DNA fragments from sera of patients with systemic lupus erythematosus proliferate mononuclear cells *in vitro*. J. Rheumatol. **26:** 294–301.
32. SIEGAL, F.P., N. KADOWAKI, M. SHODELL, *et al.* 1999. The nature of the principal type 1 interferon-producing cells in human blood. Science **284:** 1835–1837.
33. BLOMBERG, S., M.L. ELORANTA, M. MAGNUSSON, *et al.* 2003. Expression of the markers BDCA-2 and BDCA-4 and production of interferon-alpha by plasmacytoid dendritic cells in systemic lupus erythematosus. Arthritis Rheum. **48:** 2524–2532.
34. HORNUNG, V., S. ROTHENFUSSER, S. BRITSCH, *et al.* 2002. Quantitative expression of toll-like receptor 1-10 mRNA in cellular subsets of human peripheral blood mononuclear cells and sensitivity to CpG oligodeoxynucleotides. J. Immunol. **168:** 4531–4537.
35. BAVE, U., G.V. ALM & L. RONNBLOM. 2000. The combination of apoptotic U937 cells and lupus IgG is a potent IFN-alpha inducer. J. Immunol. **165:** 3519–3526.
36. BAVE, U., H. VALLIN, G.V. ALM & L. RONNBLOM. 2001. Activation of natural interferon-alpha producing cells by apoptotic U937 cells combined with lupus IgG and its regulation by cytokines. J. Autoimmun. **17:** 71–80.
37. CEDERBLAD, B., S. BLOMBERG, H. VALLIN, *et al.* 1998. Patients with systemic lupus erythematosus have reduced numbers of circulating natural interferon-alpha-producing cells. J. Autoimmun. **11:** 465–470.

38. Asselin-Paturel, C., G. Brizard, K. Chemin, *et al.* 2005. Type I interferon dependence of plasmacytoid dendritic cell activation and migration. J. Exp. Med. **201:** 1157–1167.
39. Means, T.K., E. Latz, F. Hayashi, *et al.* 2005. Human lupus autoantibody-DNA complexes activate DCs through cooperation of CD32 and TLR9. J. Clin. Invest. **115:** 407–417.
40. Qing, X. & C. Putterman. 2004. Gene expression profiling in the study of the pathogenesis of systemic lupus erythematosus. Autoimmun. Rev. **3:** 505–509.
41. The Canadian Hydroxychloroquine Study Group. 1991. A randomized study of the effect of withdrawing hydroxychloroquine sulfate in systemic lupus erythematosus. N. Engl. J. Med. **324:** 150–154.
42. Risch, N. 2000. Searching for genes in complex diseases: lessons from systemic lupus erythematosus. J. Clin. Invest. **105:** 1503–1506.
43. Salmon, J.E., S. Millard, L.A. Schachter, *et al.* 1996. Fc gamma RIIA alleles are heritable risk factors for lupus nephritis in African Americans. J. Clin. Invest. **97:** 1348–1354.
44. Schur, P.H. 1995. Genetics of systemic lupus erythematosus. Lupus **4:** 425–437.
45. Sullivan, K.E. 2000. Genetics of systemic lupus erythematosus. Clinical implications. Rheum. Dis. Clin. North Am. **26:** 229–256, v–vi.
46. Sullivan, K.E., A.F. Jawad, L.J. Piliero, *et al.* 2003. Analysis of polymorphisms affecting immune complex handling in systemic lupus erythematosus. Rheumatology (Oxford). **42:** 446–452.
47. Davies, K.A., M.G. Robson, A.M. Peters, *et al.* 2002. Defective Fc-dependent processing of immune complexes in patients with systemic lupus erythematosus. Arthritis Rheum. **46:** 1028–1038.
48. Ravetch, J.V. & S. Bolland. 2001. IgG Fc receptors. Annu. Rev. Immunol. **19:** 275–290.
49. Bolland, S. & J.V. Ravetch. 2000. Spontaneous autoimmune disease in Fc(gamma)RIIB-deficient mice results from strain-specific epistasis. Immunity **13:** 277–285.
50. Clynes, R., J.S. Maizes, R. Guinamard, *et al.* 1999. Modulation of immune complex-induced inflammation *in vivo* by the coordinate expression of activation and inhibitory Fc receptors. J. Exp. Med. **189:** 179–185.
51. Clynes, R., C. Dumitru & J.V. Ravetch. 1998. Uncoupling of immune complex formation and kidney damage in autoimmune glomerulonephritis. Science **279:** 1052–1054.
52. McGaha, T.L., B. Sorrentino & J.V. Ravetch. 2005. Restoration of tolerance in lupus by targeted inhibitory receptor expression. Science **307:** 590–593.
53. McKenzie, S.E., S.M. Taylor, P. Malladi, *et al.* 1999. The role of the human Fc receptor Fc gamma RIIA in the immune clearance of platelets: a transgenic mouse model. J. Immunol. **162:** 4311–4318.
54. Bave, U., M. Magnusson, M.L. Eloranta, *et al.* 2003. FcgammaRIIa is expressed on natural IFN-alpha-producing cells (plasmacytoid dendritic cells) and is required for the IFN-alpha production induced by apoptotic cells combined with lupus IgG. J. Immunol. **171:** 3296–3302.
55. Batteux, F., P. Palmer, M. Daeron, *et al.* 1999. FCgammaRII (CD32)-dependent induction of interferon-alpha by serum from patients with lupus erythematosus. Eur. Cytokine Netw. **10:** 509–514.
56. Latz, E., A. Schoenemeyer, A. Visintin, *et al.* 2004. TLR9 signals after translocating from the ER to CpG DNA in the lysosome. Nat. Immunol. **5:** 190–298.

Index of Contributors

Printed and bound by CPI Group (UK) Ltd, Croydon, CR0 4YY

15/09/2026

14962391-0002